From Birth until Sunset:
POISONED *to* DEATH

Marie DiMercurio RT(R)MHSc

PAGE PUBLISHING, INC.
New York, NY

First originally published by Page Publishing, Inc. 2016

ISBN 978-1-68289-153-7 (pbk)
ISBN 978-1-68289-154-4 (digital)

Printed in the United States of America

Acknowledgments

First, I want to thank God for my amazing journey into the field of health and natural hygiene. It was He who gave me a passion and inspiration for learning about the human body along with the fields of nutrition and pathology and how they all connect. He allowed me to look into the human body as He does. He also led me to a book written by Harvey Diamond, *Living without Pain.* This book was the opening to a beautiful adventure of a new life, health, healing and restoration of my own body. It led me back to school to get my master's degree in natural hygiene.

I offer a sincere thanks to all the people at the Fit for Life Sciences Institute for their help with my journey in discovering the treasures of knowledge and wisdom.

I appreciate the phone conversations of these helpful and compassionate doctors, especially in my times of need: the late Dr. John Lee, Dr. Dan Chesnut and Dr. Stanley Bass. They are special people with big hearts. I send out a great big hallelujah and a round of applause to all the folks at Hallelujah Acres for their selfless efforts as well as their God-given wisdom and knowledge through their ministry, e-mail health tips, and books, especially to George Malkmus, Olin Idol, Michael Donaldson, and Paul and Ann Malkmus. There is a living God who works through others.

I also want to thank Mark Heuslin and Mike Covher for all their energy, time, and efforts. Whenever I called and needed "Book stuff done again."

My editor, Jeff Archer is a gem who has worked overtime for me. A huge thank you is not enough for all he has done.

Also a special thank you for the man who chooses to remain anonymous for the beautiful cover photograph. You are a blessing.

I offer a special appreciation for all the folks who contributed to the processing of this book.

I always save the best until last to savor. I am most appreciative of my husband, John, for all his love, patience, and support throughout this journey. He became a big part of this entire process because of his health challenge of CLL since 1998. It's a joy working side by side with your life partner. We just want to continue to follow the diet and lifestyle that God designed for our bodies. Thank you for being my husband and for the encouragement through the journey of life and health.

Contents

Foreword

This wonderful book, *From Birth to Sunset* is a detailed and resourceful introduction to the field of natural hygiene, interlaced with the powerful experiences of Marie's personal journey toward a healthier and more abundant life. Marie explores many aspects of health and well-being and questions the long-lived "standards" regarding diet, nutrition, and exercise in the US. It will stimulate you to query things that you may have taken for granted in our healthcare system as well as challenge you to evaluate *your* personal lifestyle choices and truly *listen* to the dialogue between you and your body. It is a very personal choice.

In my more than thirty years in the field of chiropractic, I have yet to see a book that ties in so beautifully with the concepts of my daily practice, removing interference from the body's natural, God-given wisdom, and amazing ability to heal itself. If you take a moment and look around, you will see a world of wonder many hesitate to explore. The physiological systems that are in play on a second-by-second basis in our bodies are truly remarkable. They must be properly acknowledged and maintained for achieving optimal health and restoration.

Many people suffer needlessly from debilitating disease and dysfunction, desperate for answers. Marie provides invaluable information on how to gain/regain control of your body. Her research and knowledge of food combining, its effect on digestion, and other physiologic responses of our bodies provides very useful tools in getting back on track to experience unparalleled vitality.

I have been inspired by witnessing Marie's amazing journey, and this book will serve a wonderful purpose for many readers as they embark on their own individual voyage. You will learn about the laws of nature, the cycles of the body, ways to improve your health, and vitality through healthy techniques for combining and preparing food, how to maximize the nutrients from the foods you already eat, and which foods to eliminate or avoid altogether. It will change your thinking on how you view your diet and your environment and the effects the many poisonous toxins have on your body.

With chronic disease on the rise in the US, it is necessary to evaluate these principles and incorporate them into our lives to achieve the necessary changes for the abundant and healthy life we all desire. Don't wait for desperation. Read and listen.

Cathryn H. Dilliard
Doctor of Chiropractic
El Cajon, CA

Introduction

This book is a lifelong journey given to me by God. It is based on life experiences, lessons, and teachings of my own life as well as those of other people given to me as we passed through the pathways of life together. I had a very immature interest in the health of the body. Then about a year into my sobriety, I started to exercise and take supplementation, but I was still ignorant of what a good, healthy diet consisted of beyond the food pyramid. When I moved to San Diego, I was recovering from a back surgery, but I started having pain in my neck, shoulders, arms, wrists, and feet; in fact, much of my body had varying degrees of pain. I suffered from severe pain and fibromyalgia and took massive doses of MSM (methylsulfonyl-methane), which was the only way to gain relief. When I didn't take it, the joints and muscles of my whole body became inflamed. I definitely didn't want to go on pain pills because of my past addictions.

I was working in a small hospital, doing bone density/radiology exams and began to study about osteoporosis and nutrition from the medical and supplementation view. In 1999, my husband was diagnosed with CLL (chronic lymphacytic leukemia), and I became aware of the supplementation/natural cures for cancer. The only good thing that came from this was that we shipped out all chemicals from our house and started reading labels with a little more discernment. Still, the supplements increased along with the many vitamin/herb distributorships I had become a part of, but looking back, our diet was still horrendously unhealthy.

My journey started when I reached the crossroads of life, and I felt like I wanted to jump off the face of the Earth. It began when I realized that I could not do a single thing to change myself, my life, my body or the situations of my existence. My weight was the highest it ever was, at 165 pounds, and I weighed more than my husband. A woman is supposed to weigh less than her man. The criterion was that one would continue to gain five pounds a year as they age. (I found out later it was by eating the standard American diet.) I thought that I was doomed to be obese for the remainder of my days. I continued to struggle with that issue. I had spent the better part of my life dieting, yo-yo dieting, then finally realized that I would not be fat if I had never dieted in the first place. I suffered with bulimia and anorexia in my youth just trying to attain a perfect image, and now I face regrets. When I thought of the word diet, I just ate into oblivion and gained more weight. I was at my turning point.

I have gone through too many addictions and withdrawals, such as alcohol, drug abuse, caffeine, nicotine, and refined sugars, all painful journeys of recovery, and I could not go there again. When one goes through a time of trauma, and it has been implanted in the memory as a bad experience, it will never be repeated ever again, and these addictions finally cease. I have no desire to ever return to past issues.

Slowly, throughout the years, I dealt with my food addictions and the scale quit ruling my life, but one doesn't stop eating and the cravings continued to plague me. I love to eat, and I live to eat. What can I say? I'll admit to being a food addict, especially for all the wrong kinds of foods. I didn't know how to stop the horrible food cravings that made me want to continue to eat even though I'd be stuffed. I felt like I was caught in a web of despair with no way out. I tried different supplements and herbs that were marketed for relief but to no avail.

Based on what I consumed, my body became depleted, fatter, and sicker while more chronic, "unknown" diseases were developing. For years, I went to the gym several days a week, ate healthy—at least I thought so—took loads of supplements and herbs to stay healthy, but I wasn't healthy. I was a distributor of most supplement companies to be able to buy everything at wholesale prices, and some of them helped for a time, but nothing really *kept* me *well*. I was tired all of the time, just physically exhausted and could never get enough sleep I continued to get colds several times a year. Flu season came and went, and of course, even though I received the yearly vaccinations, I continued to get sick again. I felt that I had lost control of my body.

I had unknown, but persistent, allergies and carried Kleenex wherever I went because I always had a runny nose and was constantly clearing my throat. I suffered from skin rashes; dry, cracked hands and feet; and constant bouts of skin cancer. I only had one surgically removed. For the rest, I rubbed on my progesterone cream, and that seemed to cure them at least for a time, but they always seemed to come back. If I got too much sun, I'd end up with sun poisoning because of past overexposure to sun tanning lamps. My bone density was low, and I didn't realize that it was the result of my earlier destructive years of addictive behavior. My digestive system had so many upsets that no matter what I ate, I would get gassiness, indigestion, and hypoglycemic reactions. My food allergies created hives, bronchial spasms, and an occasional anaphylactic reaction, projectile vomiting, and diarrhea. I thought I was dying. I remember asking my allergist to test me for food preservatives and additives. He said it was impossible because there were thousands of them and people just couldn't eliminate all of them. The standard American diet consists of bottled, frozen, canned, and packaged foods. I thought, "What will I eat? What can I snack on?" I was clueless. I was killing myself, and I didn't even know it. I was living a so-called healthy life, including lots of herbs and vitamins, and yet my body was out of control, and I couldn't stop it. I could give up the alcohol, cigarettes, and caffeine, but I couldn't stop eating. There was some insanity occurring, but what? I had a history of deep depression, which was alleviated without drugs when I became a serious advocate of working out at the gym, but I now sensed with despair it was trying to creep back into my life.

I was desperate. I was sick and tired of being sick and tired. One day, I learned from an herbal distributor about the power of fruit smoothies in the morning with herbal products to promote health. Well, the demonstrated product didn't taste very good, so eliminating most of the herbs, I continued that regimen of just the fruit. Our mornings included fruit smoothies and herbal tea only. I started losing weight in significant amounts. I didn't tell anyone of the sometimes large amounts, sometimes two–three pounds in a day. I lost forty pounds in five months, and I thought it was the tea that did it, but years later, after I received my degree in natural hygiene, I realized that it was the fruit only in the morning that allowed my body to cleanse itself of toxins and lose the excess baggage that I had been carrying for years. But that still didn't bring complete health to me, not until I started following the principles of the natural hygienic lifestyle and eating raw fruits, vegetables, nuts, seeds and drinking distilled water. I did not only keep the sixty-pound weight loss off, but I finally gained my coveted health and wellness. My true journey really began with the study of natural hygiene and living it, not as a diet, but as a lifestyle.

When I eat processed foods, even if they are organic, I consistently gain weight, so these are also eliminated. All of my health challenges have now disappeared, and my body remains free of disease and sickness. I have a focused clarity of mind that I never had before, which feels great, and I have finally gained control over my own body. If I do get sick, it is because I was disobedient to the laws of nature and the principles of natural hygiene. My life has been filtered throughout the pages of this book.

The experiences that we have in our lives are supposed to help us to learn, but unfortunately, many don't step up to the challenge whether out of ignorance, denial, stubbornness, or sheer rebellion. How we look at our experiences and deal with them are parts of learning. But other factors include how we overcome them, and how we deal with each one of our struggles, that is, through acceptance, adaptation, change or battling. What I am speaking of is the total combination of all of life's experiences and challenges. We must exit from the victim role and take responsibility for all of the consequences of our actions, thereby learning, growing, and changing from each. We are not an aloof entity; our lives and experiences do affect all of those around us, in our examples, as well as our speech. We can create a nightmare in our examples as well as our speech for others close to us by our wrong choices that create disastrous consequences.

Disclaimer

The nutritional and health information in this book is for reference purposes only and is no way intended as medical counseling or medical advice. Nutritionists and other experts in the field of health and nutrition will embrace many extensively changeable views. The information and sole purpose of this book is to give information and education about health. It should not be used to treat, diagnose, or prevent any disease or medical condition without the advice of a competent medical professional, especially one trained in the science of nutrition and wellness.

Because there is always some risk involved when changing a diet and lifestyle, the author and publisher are not responsible for any adverse effects or consequences that might result. Please do not adhere to the teachings of this book if you are not willing to assume the risk.

If you do use the information contained in this book without the approval of a healthcare professional, you are prescribing for yourself, which is your constitutional right, but the author and publisher assume no responsibility with respect to loss, damage, or injury or alleged to be caused directly or indirectly by the information contained in this book.

PART I

The Problem

C H A P T E R   1

Fearfully and Wonderfully Made

The human body is fearfully and wonderfully made. According to God's word, Psalm 139:14–16a: "I will praise You, for I am fearfully and wonderfully made; Marvelous are Your works, and that my soul knows You very well. My frame was not hidden from You, when I was made in secret, and skillfully wrought in the lowest parts of the earth. Your eyes saw my substance, being yet unformed."[1]

We begin life from one tiny cell. Incorporated (impacted) into this cell is the imprint of all the characteristics of each person—gender, eye color, shoe size, hand and foot size and shape, intelligence, hair color and texture, skin color, etc. This is all determined at fertilization by the baby's genetic code that comes from the DNA of both the parents, which resides in the human chromosomes in that one tiny cell.

Life itself is a miracle! It begins at conception with one cell; it begins with a fertilized egg, and that one cell continues to divide into many cells, organs, and systems. Then at birth, a miniature human being is born into this world. The events of the fetal development are just remarkable, even the birthing process happens with the body knowing and following its Creator's plan. It is an amazing process, the human body. We are fearfully and wonderfully made.

19

The human body consists of more than two hundred trillion different cells of different shapes, sizes, and function; each cell having its own powerhouse and function. These cells are designed to communicate within each organ and system, thereby helping the body to function together as a whole. All the cells have their own lifespan, and the body compensates, taking charge of replacing the old and worn-out ones. The body is fearfully and wonderfully made.

Our skin is our protective covering and weighs about six pounds (Anatomy & Pathology 4th Edition. Page 29. The World's Best Anatomical Charts Lippincott, Williams, and Wilkins. Stokie, Illinois). There are miles of capillaries, and whatever we put onto our skin will penetrate into our bodies throughout this vascular system. In fact, millions of our skin cells fluff off every day and we get a whole "new look" every month; all new skin. Amazing, we are fearfully and wonderfully made.

The bones of the body are considered to be an organ. Did you know that a baby has 305 bones and an adult has 206? The child's bones on a radiograph have many extra spaces (cartilage) that need to grow together. This keeps a child a lot more pliable and flexible. The child falls down the stairs and is generally not harmed. An adult will break bones doing the same thing. It is so awesome how bones grow from the cartilage. The bone cells are fully replaced in about one year. We are fearfully and wonderfully made.

Our hearts will continue to beat throughout our lives. They beat ten thousand times per day and pump five quarts of blood per minute. The cardiac cells of the heart are not dependent on the nervous system to work. In fact, if all nerves were cut off to the heart it would continue to beat rhythmically for some time on its own. The body is fearfully and wonderfully made.

The blood vessels carry the blood on a sixty-thousand-mile journey throughout the body. This is an amazing journey too. The blood and the lymphatic system along with its organs of the kidneys and liver, clean and filter the blood of the entire body; getting rid of the toxins in the cells, tissues, and body without our ever thinking or doing anything about it. Ask a dialysis patient. The body is fearfully and wonderfully made.

If a person were to experience smoke inhalation from a fire scene, his/her red blood cells will be carrying carbon monoxide instead of oxygen. The good news is the body will replace all of those red blood cells in two–three months with new ones to carry oxygen. Platelets are replaced every two weeks. The body is equipped to heal and restore the nerve cells, muscle cells, bone cells, or any other cells if the body is nourished and cleansed properly and continually. The body is fearfully and wonderfully made.

Capillaries are the most ignored part of the circulatory system. They should be given more credit for what they do than people realize. Michael Dye quotes Dr. Richard Passwater, PhD, who emphasizes "that in our circulatory system, the capillaries are where the action takes place." He explains, "The sole function of the circulatory system is to exchange nutrients for waste products…the capillaries *allow* the cells to live by exchanging nutrients for wastes."[2] The heart just pumps the blood, and the arteries and veins transport the blood. The capillaries are the main provider. The body is fearfully and wonderfully made.

The brain and the nervous systems, central and peripheral, send signals and messages to the entire body, helping the body to communicate as a whole. The myelin sheath covers and protects the nerve cells. The nerve signals with this myelin sheath can travel at thirty-two feet per second, but without it, the response travel time is three–six feet per second, such as what occurs with the disease of multiple sclerosis. Those with this disease have encountered a self-destructing myelin sheath.

The pancreas creates its own anti-acid (sodium bicarbonate) to settle an upset stomach. The liver, which is the heaviest and largest organ of the body, handles more than five hundred functions for the body. The liver has the most amazing powers of regeneration. If a person were to cut off more than half of the organ, it would grow back into a whole organ again. When a person contracts liver cancer, all functions cease, and it's usually terminal because there isn't any liver dialysis. The body is fearfully and wonderfully made.

The quality of the cells that are replacing the old ones depends on what we are feeding our bodies. If we eat *dead,* non-garden foods, i.e., cooked, fragmented, processed foods, our bodies will reap diseased, poor quality cells that will not aid in the proper functioning of the body. God created the human body to receive proper nourishment from garden-fresh produce to produce and maintain health, thus obtaining freedom from disease.

Some may say, "I wished that I would have taken better care of my health," but I hear quite often, "The golden years are not so golden. Just don't get old. It's horrible." They didn't realize that their health problems were their own responsibility. They go through their lives with a sense of despair and hopelessness, seeing numerous doctors who conduct many series of tests and procedures, also prescribing many different medications, only to have their health deteriorate more intensely. It's a sad, sad state. The quality of their lives is whittled away because of this practice. We need to take responsibility for our own health, not giving that responsibility to the medical profession. As a friend so truthfully stated, "They are just practicing at medicine. They don't really know what they are doing."

Endnotes

1. The New King James Version the Holy Bible, copy. 1994, Thomas Nelson Inc. Publisher. Psalm 139:14-16a
2. Michael Dye, *God's Way to Ultimate Health* (Hallelujah Acres, 1995), 139.

CHAPTER 2

The Owner's Manual to the Body

When we were born into this world, we did not receive an owner's manual on the functioning and repair of our body. If we had, we would all turn out different and better for it. The body, in its incredible wisdom, is an amazing and awesome being. We should all take an anatomy and physiology lesson on how the body is made and how it all works together. In the owner's manual, each human body was created in its own unique way, different yet with many similarities. The differences are in our own manual, but the similarities are in everyone's manual. Those are the ones to be focused on, especially on how we can avoid diseases. God, our Creator, wrote many of them into His word, the Bible. He gave commands to observe, follow, and live each day. When we are obedient, we will thrive in health. When we disobey, we wallow in sickness.

Our genes have been designated in a unique code for self-protecting and self-healing. God designed our human body, how it is to function, and how the body responds to food and drink. In the health of this body, homeostasis is the normal natural state, and disease is abnormal and unnatural. We've been given a gift, and we are expected to respect it, the gift of life. We cannot put all types of chemicals in the perfect human specimen and expect it to thrive and function optimally, just as you would never put anything but the correct form of gasoline in your car engine or it would cease to run. Your body is the same way; it needs pure fuel (food) to run, or rather, function optimally and stay well-tuned. When a person will clean out a car (body) and add the correct fuel (food), it's insane to go back to the old ways. Insanity is doing the same thing over and over and expecting different results. It's abusive to do anything else, and we are told to love ourselves. And if our bodies are not the temple of the Holy Spirit, we should treat them like a temple, not a cesspool or garbage dump.

We will live out a certain number of days, but if we fail to observe the laws of nature, the days will be marked with suffering and made significantly shorter. The observance of the laws will bring us good health, freedom from pain and disease, properly functioning organs, perfect and optimal weight without the dieting and counting calories. We will feel good, vibrant, and energetic. The laws of nature have to do with what we feed our bodies and what we must neglect to put in.

The laws of nature are coherent to the owner's manual from our Creator. Throughout the Bible, God told his people what to eat and what not to eat. God differentiated between clean and unclean foods. These are for the protection of His people. After these continued readings in the Bible, I finally discovered why. For example, no Jewish person eats pork. For God said, "Do not eat swine, it is unclean" (Leviticus 11:7 KJV).[1] God in His wisdom knows what's best for humans, even if people don't. A pig is a diseased animal; its body has no way of eliminating the bacteria and diseases. Even after it's cooked, humans, in their consumption of pork, absorb all of the poisons into their own body. Bacon, in fact, is totally indigestible in the human body especially with all of its chemicals. God said fish is okay, but nothing else. No shrimp or other shellfish. Why? Toxins and protection from them. The Israelites, as well as the people of today, think that these are just religious rite. Wrong. They are for our protection, so we should heed these commands. God knows that our human bodies cannot handle many of the foods that man chooses to consume. Man will eat just about anything, but then, man destroys and God delivers. We need to be protected from our perverse ways and ourselves.

He commanded these things to protect and preserve His people. Many times, people were, and still are, disobedient to these commands and suffer tremendously. At the beginning of creation, God said in Genesis 1:29, "Behold I have given you every herb (vegetable), bearing seed, which is upon the face of all the earth for food."[1] In fact, before Noah's Ark and the flood of the world came about, according to the Bible, the beasts of the earth and the birds of the air, all of these creatures were herbivores (Genesis 1:30, 6:21, 9:3–4).[1] There were not any carnivores, including man, until after the flood, because the green plants and fruits weren't available. The waters covering the earth destroyed all of them.

God gave perfect bodies to all living creatures that would live hundreds of years with instructions on how man was to take care of himself. We are not to conform to the standard American diet. The Bible states, "Be not conformed to this world, but be transformed by the renewing of your mind, that you may prove what is that good and acceptable and perfect will of God" [1]

Therefore, when we look at the wisdom of the body, we come to know that it was created in the wisdom of an Intelligent Creator and Spiritual Being. The normal functioning of the human body is beyond the scope of what we see. It is a marvelous and awesome creation in how it all works together. When we do our bodies right in all its needs, it will continue to perform with perfection as it was meant to be. So each body does come with an owner's manual if we are wise enough to 'read' it: it is the body itself.

Endnote

1. Romans 12:2 (New King James Version).

CHAPTER 3

What Is Health and Natural Hygiene?

Health is a state of optimal wellness, wholeness, and homeostasis. A healthy person is a perfectly-functioning organism. Optimal health is within reach. It cannot just be desired, as it must be lived each day of life. It is also actively seeking and living the truth of the laws of nature, of the human body.

The health of the human body is normal and natural; therefore, sickness and disease is unnatural and abnormal. One can look at another person and *see* if there is health or not based first of all on outer looks and appearance. Thus, the body's anatomy and function is in a perfect state. Therefore, health must be maintained for disease to be prevented.

Healthy people have a joyous attitude and a peaceful spirit. They have a delight and passion for living, loving, and giving. They look radiant and feel well and refreshed. True health involves a pain-free, sound body with fluid movements, vital organs that work optimally, and mental functions that are at their peak of alertness and attunement. They look forward to waking up each morning, are energetic, look forward to each day with joy, and anticipate each new learning experience. They enjoy doing for others and seem to be on a mission; one that promotes health. It emits from their spirit with a passion.

They are a joy to be around. A healthy person is a beautiful person who shines from the inside out. His/her body is one of health. It functions perfectly as the Creator of the universe created the human body to be, to perform with magnificence.

Optimal and perfect health is attainable if the healthy conditions are observed and lived. It does take a disciplined spirit and a determined attitude—determined enough to march to a different beat—one that doesn't follow the crowd or at least the pattern of this world, of which the standard American diet is an example of.

A healthy body is a well-rested and refreshed one. This is very important because to rest properly and sleep well, one must be free of stress and toxins. It is important to keep one's priorities straight. Many will go through their day rushed, trying to make up all the things that they failed to get done yesterday. People never seem to get a moment's peace to just to sit down and refresh themselves. The saying, "Take time to smell the roses," is a powerful statement that is quite misunderstood and ignored. People are geared to get to their destinations but never enjoyed life's journey along the way. Slowing down and relaxing are so important. If everything does not get done, oh well. I am not promoting procrastination by any means; I am just saying prioritize. Take the important things first. Most of the things that we stress about are not important, but people just don't know how to say no. As human beings, we do have our limits, and they must be learned. Being patient with ourselves and with others is one of the most important priorities.

No one who lives in this world, except those who study natural hygiene and live by its principles, can understand what health really is. Those who have health are the envy of those who do not have health. Beauty fades with loss of health. Those who do not have health are set in their ways, and those who do have health have been set apart in this world as special. They have been presented a gift by their Creator, a gift of life and freedom from disease. It is conditional; there must be obedience to the laws of nature and the laws of life. These laws will sustain the conditions of health. In obedience, we will maintain a healthy body, and it will maintain us with a wonderful existence of joy. The healthy body will just turn and laugh at all of the diseases of mankind, for they will not apply at all. There aren't the germs, viruses, bacteria, and fears that plague others. Herbert Shelton states the truth of health in his review: "Genuine health is an active vigorous state of the body in which all the structures are sound and unimpaired, all its functions efficient and in which, by reason of its own vigor and energy, the body can wade through all the common emergencies of life with flags flying and banners streaming."[1]

Let us celebrate life.

The practice of natural hygiene is parallel to what our Creator designed for the human body. Dr. Herbert Shelton defines natural hygiene as "the branch of biology that relates to the preservation and restoration of health"[2] using the laws of nature. I personally call natural hygiene a science that correlates with the wisdom of God. It is a system of mind and body care. This includes caring for what is in the environment externally as well as the inward one because this is vital to life. It *is* life itself. It is based on the principles and laws of nature.

Natural hygiene teaches the way to optimal health and to live an abundant life by eating fresh whole foods produced by nature itself, exercising, and getting sufficient rest and sleep. It is also important to get a daily allotment of fresh air and sunshine. An internal and external cleanliness must be achieved along with learning to manage stress and maintaining a positive perspective toward others and life in general. It is imperative to avoid negative influences and continue to maintain a great and loving attitude. Loving and long lasting friendships are encouraging and supportive, for they can be the anchors during the storms of life.

People need to be social and use their network of people that is placed in the pathways of life. It is important to practice what we preach, to live a life based on example.

According to Dr. Paul Goldberg, natural hygiene teaches that one cannot disobey nature's laws without suffering the consequences.[3] Some people depending on their genetic structure may get away with the abuse longer, but in the end, it will still bite good and hard. There is a price tag to everything in life. It may or may not be monetary, but it's still there. If one violates through excesses, abuses, bad habits, poor choices, and unwise decisions, there will be a paid consequence. It may be right away or into the near or distant future, but we do reap what we sow. We can no longer plead ignorance; there aren't any victims. So just as sickness is a choice, wellness is a choice. Choose well; choose wisely.

One must begin to look at life as well as live life in all of its aspects, not just as diet, exercise, or pure water. One must come to appreciate and respect the natural laws and what they mean to life itself. These were created in conjunction with life with our Creator, for preservation, protection, endurance, vitality, vital power, inertia, and limitations.

People cannot function on diets, for these are only a temporary facade. Natural hygiene is a living program designed for the whole completeness of the body. It can now be called a "live it" program, not a "die it."

Each and every cell cleans and drains its waste products into the blood and lymph systems to be excreted and eliminated. This drainage process depends on the purity of the body and its tissues.[4]

If there is a slowdown of the elimination, the wastes will accumulate and the body becomes slowly poisoned. It is important to remove these wastes quickly from the blood, lymph, and body's tissues, for only then can the body get back to normal and its functions maintained.

A way of helping the body in this process of the backup of toxins is fasting.[5] In this case, a distilled water and vegetable juice fast may be recommended. Food hinders the process because the body has to work at digestion and elimination, and the fasting body needs to just eliminate and cleanse. The digestive system gets put to a rest as well as the remainder of the body. It is important to rest during a fast because the body will detoxify and cleanse much more effectively. As the body rests, fewer toxins are generated, and more energy is produced. Therefore, the body will begin the detoxification process to improve and once again function optimally.

Often, as the body is fasting, many may experience uncomfortable symptoms as the body is doing its housecleaning. In the body's cleansing, these symptoms must not be masked over or encouraged to cease. The cleansing must continue until the body becomes well.

Good new habits must be allowed for maintaining optimal health. Health comes from correct living. Unless one does change to a correct living standard after a fast, there will never be any permanent health.[6] Bad practices produce human wreckage. Natural hygiene is a way of *life*, and it is to be lived daily.

Exercise helps people in so many ways because being functional helps our bodies to stay in a healthy mode. Exercise, such as daily walks and stretching help us to relieve stress, relax, and sleep well at night. Activities for the body are essential for all the muscle groups to have strength and function. Atrophy is a weakening and eventual deadening from none use of muscles or organs. Exercise adds to the proper functioning of the mechanical aspects of muscle, nerve, and hormone function and also helps the body to stay alert and focused. It really eases the depressive spirits and gives a joyous and peaceful attitude. Exercise helps the circulation of our blood and lymph in proper flow and especially keeps the immune system strong so the body can continue the elimination of toxins and wastes.

Daily sunbaths and fresh air expedite the healing process and health of the body. The days of "baking out in the sun" are over for me after a few bouts of sun poisoning. Everything done in moderation is beneficial, but extremes must be avoided. They destroy the organism and put a tension on our wellbeing.

Sunshine for a small period daily warms our bones and allows the skin to formulate vitamin D, which helps the calcium to absorb and keep our bones dense. Daily park walks in the sunshine to me are heaven. I've got my exercise, vitamin D bath, and fresh air in one hour of my day. That's living. Instead of all of the dangerous suntan lotions which block vitamin D from entering the body, I have found that powdered vitamin C mixed with a good organic (less harmful ingredients to the skin and body itself) body lotion works as a wonderful sunscreen, applied through the time in the sun and a great skin healer (see resources for powdered vitamin C and organic body lotion). A natural, hygienic diet allows the body not only internal health and healing, but the skin no longer burns when going out in the sun. My skin used to burn, blister, and get sun poisoning if I was out too long. I can walk, work in the garden, and still not burn. It's wonderful. I have heard this of others who had the same experience.

Fresh, clean air keeps the lungs, blood, and body clean, oxygenated, and free of carbon dioxide. When people walk in parks, mountainous areas, and reserves, the trees filter and keep the air clean of pollutants. Trees not only are beautiful to look at but also are our friends. While sleeping, fresh air is very beneficial for the body because during resting time, the body is refreshed, cleansed, and healed; and at the same time, the fresh air cleans out the lungs, blood and cells.

To maintain a clean body, it must have pure clean water. The body consists of mostly water, and to flush out the toxins, the water one drinks must be free of chemical pollutants and toxins. Tap water is full of these poisons, making it dangerous to drink it. Only distilled water is pure enough and free of all harmful contaminants to be consumed by the human body.

People need to drink only when the body demands it, when thirsty. It is important not to drink water with one's meals for it dilutes and interferes with the digestive process. Many people have a need to drink water or other beverages with their spiced, cooked, and processed foods. But whole raw foods, which are full of water and nutrients, will digest properly without added water. Even if nuts are consumed as part of the vegetable meal, it isn't necessary to consume any water because the raw vegetables *are* the water. These foods contain the water that the body needs.

Speaking of foods, the most important part of the healthy lifestyle is to eat wholesome raw foods properly combined to meet the standards of optimal health. Proper food combining allows optimal digestion for the absorption and assimilation of vitamins, minerals, and nutrients. Raw, fresh, organically-grown fruits, vegetables, seeds, and nuts are types of foods that supply all the vitamins, minerals, and other nutrients the body demands. The human body does not have the physical capability to digest meats, dairy products, grains, refined sugars and flours, starches, processed foods with all of their chemicals, colorings, and additives, and other such SAD (standard American diet) items. The body is very sluggish as it attempts to rid the meats and other toxic foods; it requires much nerve energy that sleep is supposed to generate. People get up each morning and are so tired from lack of sleep, also from the unreleased toxins that they must start their day with stimulants to get going. A natural, hygienic body is cleansed throughout the morning, refreshed because of a clean, relaxed body that feels rejuvenated and ready to go and face the world.

If the body is impaired in any way, its digestive functioning processes slow down and the foods that are eaten are not able to be processed. Even overeating of good whole foods adds a burden to the body because it creates toxins due to the undigested and fragmented foods. The body, therefore, cannot assimilate and metabolize; it just becomes filled with waste products and buildup of the already toxic overload, creating a burden on the elimination process. The body needs complete rest, through fasting, to allow these toxins to be eliminated.

The human body, in its optimal state of health, will digest, assimilate, metabolize, and eliminate waste products without any problem. From mouth to anus, a fruitarian and all-raw vegetable diet will eliminate waste products within twenty-four hours, whereas, the standard American diet takes longer, from forty-eight–seventy-two hours, sometimes up to one hundred hours because of the processing of the additives and chemicals in these foods. The body is unable to digest these things; therefore, poisonous substances just keep building up within the body and saturate the body with a chemical overload that does not add to good health but takes from it.

Comfort for the human body is important. The temperature in the environment needs to be neither too hot nor too cold. If it is too cold, the body shivers trying to stay warm and if it is too hot, the body is sluggish and sweats trying to cool down. The variation of temperature creates stress in the body. If, for example, we eat a meal while the body is cold, whether in the air or food temperature, the digestion will slow down because of all the energy going elsewhere trying to warm up. The homeostasis of the body's temperature is 98.7°F, and everything in the body's internal environment works optimally at that temperature.

Proper-fitting clothes comfort the body. Tight clothes add stress and strain on the body, creating an unhealthy tension. Some synthetic combinations of clothing materials can cause toxic reactions to the skin, such as rashes, hives, etc. Therefore, cotton or other porous clothing may be more beneficial to wear.

Human emotions, especially intense and lengthy, can have a devastating effect on the body because of the stressful nature of these emotions. One can have a great diet and life, but when stress arises, it can still take the body into the pits of despair. The effects of the digestive system during these times can bring terrific demands that inhibit the digestive process. It is best not to eat when one is highly emotional. Wait until the next meal, if possible, when one is calmer. In the Bible, one can read, "A merry heart does good like medicine."[7] Laughter and humor stimulate the endorphins of the body, adding a feeling of health through the body processes, relieving nervous tension. When one is happy, life is joyful. Someone once said to me, "Happiness is peacefulness and contentedness, you can be content at times and not peaceful, and the other way around, at other times though you will have both and enjoy those moments of happiness, but you will never have it all of the time." People are always looking for happiness from outside of themselves. Removing this burden produces freedom. Positive emotions are life-giving experiences.

Sleep is the state of rest in which the eyes are closed, the muscles are relaxed, the mind is unconscious, and the nervous system is inactive. During restful and uninterrupted sleep, the body can generate and restore its nerve energy and assimilation process. Daily, adequate sleep is essential for the body's recovery process and to maintain optimal function. The healthier a person is, the less sleep the body requires, but a minimum of six to ten hours is needed.

Rest and relaxation are important for quick short periods to give the body a needed break during the day. Just sitting down can help the body recoup. It has been told that a ten-minute rest or nap can be equal to an hour's sleep at night in regard to the resulting recovery of the body's capacity and function. A moment of revitalization is a quick recovery for the busy person to recover one's strength and vigor.

Concerning recreation and play, the old saying goes, "All work and no play make Jack a dull boy." There is a pearl of wisdom to this. Everything in life needs to be in balance and moderation and recreation are parts of that balance. People need constructive and pleasurable playtime, games, and hobbies. It helps to make people more rounded, joyful, and also able to forget about the burdens of life for a short while. Moments of disconnect are necessary to keep a balance within life and to maintain a joyful spirit. People must have some leisure and fun time. Playtime helps to reduce stress. Life needs to be enjoyable and can be fun. In this leisure time, people need to share pleasant moments with friends and family. Many of these activities are also social events. The conversations and times must be kept in proper prospective, not a negative cycle, but to encourage one another.

Humans are social beings. "No man is an island" is an old saying, but that statement concludes, "And when he does, he becomes a volcano." People do not like loneliness. Many, out of fear and insecurity, do tend to isolate themselves even though it does not serve any useful purpose. It will only tend to harm the one who isolates.[8] "People who need other people are the luckiest people in the world," states an old song with much truth to it. It may take much practice to come out of one's shell, but it is well worth it the self-esteem and self-confidence. People grow and blossom when in social relationships. They are our mirrors, and we learn from others about ourselves.

Socializing can bring encouragement and support from others who share similarities to us. Relationships are the important part of life, and people will wither and die without them. It has been said, "If you have at least one best friend, you are a success, and if you have two best friends, you are truly blessed."

Touch is important. Every human being craves loving touch, hugs, kisses, and tender strokes. If babies aren't touched, hugged, and cuddled, they will emotionally and physically die. Adults can emotionally die as well. There are a lot of withered adults walking around in this world who are emotionally needy. Human bodies are engrained for touch; all the hormones in the body will thrive because of the touch of another human being. Trust for another human is developed by touch. Relationships develop, becoming deeper, more meaningful and genuine through loving and hugging. To gain friendships, one must reach out and be a friend and give love to be loved. Relationships and touch are give and take, mutual sharing for intimacy to be developed. Intimacy is not always sexual; it's just human to need others.

Cleanliness isn't just the cleaning and bathing of the outer body. Cleanliness also includes the inner body and all of the cellular structures. Internal filth builds up with a polluted diet and lifestyle, and the cells also become constipated. The accumulations need to be eliminated daily for the health of the organism thorough the elimination of waste products, the purer and cleaner the body will be.

Our Creator created the body, with its own daily physiological cycles, without any help or assistance from any outside source. Without these cycles, there isn't any health. One must respect this and be accountable to receive health and healing of the body to eliminate disease.

These cycles are:

4:00 a.m. to 12:00 noon – Elimination
12:00 noon to 8:00 p.m. – Appropriation
8:00 p.m. to 4:00 a.m. – Assimilation [9]

They are followed one-after-another in complete perfection. The eating process is followed by assimilation, which is the process of converting these nutrients into usable products for the body to use for function and repair, to maintain optimal wellness. The body then will continue into the next following process; to eliminate all of the waste products, and to purge toxins from the body. These processes are consistent with those persons who are diligent in following the laws of nature and live a healthy lifestyle.

Disease is considered to be a cleansing process as it helps the body to slow down and rid itself of built-up toxic overload. Human beings, in their perverted lifestyles and diets, go beyond the body's capabilities of the elimination process. Therefore, the body says it's had enough; now it needs a rest and thorough cleansing.

Other cleansing processes that are important but are often left unheeded are ones of the mind, emotions, bad habits, and spirituality. There needs to be a daily inventory to make the wrongs right and to have an emotionally healthy balance. In the Alcoholics Anonymous program, the twelve-step recovery is an excellent program for all to live an emotionally, spiritually balanced life. The tenth step of recovery, "Continued to take a personal inventory and when we were wrong promptly admitted it"[10] needs to be lived continually on a daily basis throughout one's life to bring about a change of behavior. This in turn will rid us of bad habits, and exercise a positive loving attitude to each and every person in the pathways of life. The burdens of emotional baggage are lifted off and now a sense of freedom from hopelessness and despair can be enjoyed. There comes peacefulness and security with oneself and God our Creator. I personally have a motto, "Learn from the mistakes of others because we will never live long enough to make them all by ourselves." This is all a part of the growing experience and continued life's learning processes.

Endnotes

1. Herbert M Shelton, "The Healthy Body Laughs at Viruses," *INHS Hygienic Review,* February 2004.

2. Herbert M Shelton, "Natural Hygiene-What Is It?" *INHS Hygienic Review*, February 2010.

3. Dr. Paul Goldberg, "Theme-What is Natural Hygiene?" *INHS Hygienic Review*, January 2004.

4. Herbert M Shelton, "Living vs Dieting," bk. 3, in *Fit for Life – Basic Health Library*, Winnepeg, Canada, 1999, 7.

5. Marti Wheeler, "The Enormous Value of Resting and Fasting in Disease," in book 3, *Fit for Life – Basic Health Library*, 7.

6. Hannah Allen, "Fasting Does Not Make the Body Disease-Proof," Fasting, 1070.

7. Proverb 17: 22 (NKJV).

8. Robert and Elizabeth McCarter, "Belonging to A Group or Social Circle," bk. 3, in *Fit for Life – Basic Health Library*, 24.

9.   Harvey Diamond, "Living Without Pain," Osprey FL, VP Nutrition LLC 2007, p194–197.
10. Alcoholics Anonymous, *World Service, Inc.*, Grand Central Station, NY, NY. 3rd ed. (1978), 9.

CHAPTER 4

What Is Disease?

What *is* disease? According to *Webster's Dictionary*, disease is an illness; disorder of health, discomfort.[1] *The Oxford Dictionary of Current English* says disease is a disorder in a human, animal, or plant caused by an infection, diet or by faulty functioning of a process.[2] *The Home Medical Dictionary* states simply that disease is a sickness[3] and *Mosby's Medical Nursing and Allied Health Dictionary* says that disease is "(1) a condition of abnormal vital function involving any structure, part, or system of an organism" and "(2) a specific illness or disorder characterized by a recognizable set of signs and symptoms, attributable to heredity, infection, diet, or environment."[4]

Disease is an *emergency crisis* of the body.

The roots of all disease are toxicity and deficiency. Toxicity is caused by the consumption and over-accumulation of chemicals and pollutants from the foods, environment, lifestyle, and stress. Toxicity is of the accumulation of poisons in the body. Deficiency consists of a lack or a shortage of what the body needs, necessities that is insufficient and fails to be contained within the body. Examples include nutrients, enzymes, and dietary components.

There are so many different definitions of disease, most have common themes, but many blame outside sources instead of what disease is really meant to do. Disease is the process of healing.

Everyone believes they have caught something, or they are fighting a cold or flu, a virus, or germs have overtaken them. They take pills, drugs, herbal supplements or other concoctions to get rid of the horrible symptoms. Supposedly, the drugs, etc. are going to cure them. Diseases are not cured, but alleviating the causes of the disease allows the body to heal itself. Trying to stop the disease will only stop the body's clean-up methods and allow the disease to linger longer.

Epidemics of mass hysteria are created by a world in which people follow each other in their destructive lifestyles. Each person eats the same types of food although there may be differences in the preparation of these foods. Many live somewhat the same life practices and get the same diseases. People believe that their disease was a result of receiving it from another person. Everyone is paranoid of germs, and they will receive vaccines to prevent disease. The big problem is that people fail to see that the vaccine only brings on the disease that they dread because the body needs to get rid of the additional toxins of these drugs. It is just a vicious cycle. The causes haven't been taken away, so the person becomes ill again as the body is still attempting to cleanse and purify itself. The body is trying to accomplish and stay in homeostasis.

The body that cleanses itself of toxins through illness has less of a chance of developing damaging chronic diseases. Some people will claim that they can do and eat anything they want but never seem to suffer any illnesses. They are just continuing to overload their body throughout the years, and then as the internal damage unknowingly continues to develop, the body has had enough and will cease to function, thereby losing momentum. Finally, full-force disease is impacted, sometimes to the point of tragic suffering that leads to the death of the organism.

The body is like a fine piece of well-tuned machinery. If it is well-oiled (fed), it will run with absolute precision and clarity. But if one does not keep it clean and starts adding inferior and improper oils (foods), it will break down and cease to run. When people insist that they cannot give up their foods of choice, they are just adding nails to their coffins.

People are responsible for the health they have or don't have, and for the diseases that wreak havoc in their bodies. God created individuals with a free will and told them all to choose life, not destruction. When people choose processed foods over fresh whole foods that are grown, not manufactured, they are making the choice to have sickness plague their bodies. People cannot really complain about all of their health challenges; these exist because people continue to give in to the lusts of the flesh. People are very stubborn and continue to deny optimal health with their unhealthy actions.

When one gets a cold, flu, or injuries of some kind, the body immediately goes into action. It starts the cleaning and healing process. The body recognizes anything that enters it, and if the body knows that it doesn't belong there, it seeks to get rid of the invader, attempting to destroy it and maintain the homeostasis of the organism.

Diseases of any kind trigger the housecleaning processes of the body. Disease affects the entire body, not just one or two areas, although these one or two areas may be the only ones seemingly affected. People believe disease represents something outside of the themselves. Disease begins and is transported throughout the body. It is a course of accumulated and not eliminated toxins. The levels become unbearable for the body and under the burden, the body starts breaking down the systems of the body. Those people who use drugs to try and abolish the symptoms of disease harm themselves even more. The disease process lasts longer because the body's purging process has ceased because of drug ingestion and continued eating. The body must be allowed to go through the whole cleansing process directly and unhurriedly, or it will continue to degenerate even further, spiraling downward from bad to worse. Take away the cause of disease, and the body may rebound, regenerating and trying to heal itself. The well body seeks balance and homeostasis. Disease and health fall into the same equation. Disease is produced by the body to keep us healthy. It is the body's housecleaning or body cleaning.

In the beginning of creation, there weren't any of this world's diseases. It was survival of the fittest, but other than that, people just died of old age. The average age is stated at 912 years, and then he died. At that time, a year still consisted of 365 days. People didn't die of strokes, cancers, heart attacks, diabetes, and the like, maladies that exist now. These people just simply lay down and went to sleep and died, painless and free. People do not want to have a painful death. They fear that more than anything, but what are they doing to themselves? Because of their diet and lifestyles, they are creating the most painful way to die: lethal poisoning through horrible and painful diseases. Many of these diseases lead to a painful, "existing only" life that is a slow suicide.

Then people will pay millions of dollars during their painful existence to pharmaceutical companies and doctors to fix them and make them better, looking for a cure. Everyone has this freedom and gift at their disposal, at their beck and call. All that is required is to accept the gift of life through a change in diet and lifestyle. The problem is that most don't believe the concept; it's too simple to comprehend. Many will even, on their last breath, continue to do what they are doing even though it is killing them.

If drugs were to really cure people then it would have been announced on every radio and television station, every news broadcast, and newspaper worldwide. Well, there hasn't been any news as such because it's not true. Drugs don't heal and neither does food heal. Given the right circumstances and environment, the human body heals itself.

This self-healing is built right into the body. It is God's amazing gift to all of us. We can watch and experience this wonderful healing. If we receive a cut, we can watch as the blood cleanses the wound, then it clots and scabs without any interference from our part. It will start its healing process from the inside out. The deepened inner layer starts healing first as the healing continues, going upward toward the scabbed area, which then pushes off the scab. In less than a week, in a healthy body, we see that the skin is back to normal. People must realize that this same healing occurs within the body if it is fed and nourished properly, if people feed their bodies and treat and maintain them properly as God designed them. The body was not designed to be a dump for processed foods, additives, drugs, or anything made by humans. Only what God created for the body to feed on should enter the body. People need to be obedient to the laws of nature and God. People do not need to cook their foods, so that eliminates a lot of things, especially animal products.

Cooked foods harm the body because they create acid waste products within the body. Animal proteins when cooked, in fact all cooked proteins, putrefy within the intestinal tract, and because these foods do not contain fiber, they move very sluggishly through the intestines, coating the walls. In many cases, this coating starts to harden and impact itself and does not get eliminated.

Raw vegetable proteins, seeds, and nuts along with raw fruits that are all properly combined, contain all the fiber-rich protein that the body needs and uses for proper functioning of the digestive intestinal system. Thereby, the entire body will utilize and benefit from these real foods.

There are seven stages of disease, and the common ground of all these stages is toxemia. It has many sources: insufficient rest, stress, improper food choices, and improper food combinations. Stress may be one of the main contributors to disease. The body loses nerve energy and becomes exhausted, overburdened, and unable to remove and eliminate poisons from the cells, tissues, and organs. These poisons have a degenerating effect on the entire organism; thus, this process burdens the body even more.

The first stage is enervation, the state in which the body doesn't have enough nerve energy to cleanse itself; thereby, it slowly loses its stamina. People will get insufficient sleep, work too hard and too long, burning the candle at both ends. They will then stress out because they cannot meet the high demands of the life they've placed upon themselves. When morning comes, they are a wreck trying to wake up, throwing in the coffee, sugary foods to stimulate their systems to attention. Therefore, they become wired up, but are still sleepy. The body and the brain function on empty—empty nutrition, empty nerve energy, and empty brainpower.

The second stage is toxemia. The toxins build up and the poisons accumulate and saturate to the point of overflow. If changes aren't made to their lifestyle and people continue with this degrading pathway, their organs and systems begin to slow down. The dead materials that need to be eliminated will not be evacuated. Dead decomposing cells and waste products continue to back up and accumulate even further which depletes the body and its functioning even more. The body lacks strength, it then "chokes, sputters, and coughs" like a car that's been deprived of good fuel and oil. It will eventually die, not peacefully but painfully.

The third stage is irritation. Irritation is just annoying and sometimes bothersome, many times just ignored or just overlooked, and usually it's not painful. The human cells and organ systems sense the body's overload of poisons not eliminated and try to release the toxic wastes. It then signals the nervous system, hormones, digestive system, and other parts of the body to react in such a way to discard the mess of wastes. Constipation is a problem of the digestive system as well as the entire body. The cells of the body in a diseased state become constipated as well. Constipation is just inability to eliminate. The sphincter muscles, colon muscles, and nerves along the rectum and colon become irritated at trying to move a cement block of compacted stool along for elimination, but it just won't empty. The buildup continues and gassiness gets worse. The colon starts to become inflamed, leading to the next stage that causes a variety of diseases, one called diverticulitis, an out pouching of the colon that creates serious problems that could be corrected by a diet and lifestyle change.

The next stage of disease is inflammation. This is the point when the body starts screaming to stop all of the abuse. The pain starts and spreads; swelling may also occur as the buildup of poisons continues to increase and the vital energy decreases. Pain/inflammation often occurs in the areas of past injuries and weakened locations. Toxins may accumulate in these areas; they are persistent areas of inflammation. When one eats foods not proper for the body's health, the toxins may direct first to these areas, for example, locations of recent surgery, past fractured bones, arthritis, etc. As the pain builds, the digestion ceases. Eaten foods sit in the stomach and add to the toxins as they ferment and putrefy. People will begin to take pain pills to alleviate the symptoms, slowing down the systems even more. Every person who continues to take pain pills generally does not have any bowel movements on their own accord. These toxic wastes build up and accumulate in the digestive tract and colon, creating a serious dilemma. At that point, they will take laxatives, suppositories, and enemas to seek relief when all that was necessary to prevent their health challenges is to cease taking the drugs and change their diet and lifestyle. Their burdens will cease. Pain pills can be continuously prescribed. People will live on these drugs even though they are destructive to the health of the body. The body can develop a resistance to the drug; therefore, the person requires more of the drug to get the same effect, creating an addiction to the pain drug. This continued effort will only set the stage for the next stage of disease.

Ulceration, the fifth stage of disease, is the destruction of cells and tissues. A fine example of ulceration is in the intestinal tract where ulcers form, creating large internal sores in the esophagus, the stomach, duodenum, small bowel, and colon, even on the skin. The toxic poisons eat away at the body, creating severe pathology. People will be treated for these conditions, which only worsen because the causes are not addressed; no changes have been made. Such diseases with ulcers in the digestive tract are stomach ulcers, Crohn's disease, and ulcerative colitis. Surgeries, drugs, and the like are attempted, but these only create horrifying effects on the already depleted and challenged body. They will go through life as the walking dead, only existing in a state of grief and despair. It will only get worse.

The sixth stage of disease is induration, a hardening of the tissue. This is the stage when tumors start to form. This process is the body's protective mechanism to provide protection for the rest of the body. It tries to keep all the toxins confined to one area. The accumulated poisons are altering the DNA at this point, and each cell begins to become mutated, and the destruction of the body continues to come to the last stage of disease.

Cancer is the last stage of disease. It is the body in a mass-destruction mode due to an improper lifestyle. If the body has gone over the threshold of irreversible disrepair, no matter what kind of healthy lifestyle may occur in revelation, it may be too late. It's a sorry mess of regrets. "I wish I took better care of myself," many will say. Cancer cells are mutated and uncontrollable. The hostile environment that protected them keeps going strong. No one can violate the laws of the Creator and His creation and not suffer the consequences.

Most people are cemented in the belief that their diseases are caused by germs, viruses, bacteria, genes, and other people. They are just the victims of all the unhealthy stuff that's going around in the world. People don't want to realize that by their unhealthy living practices, which everyone else is also doing. They have created their own sickness and disease. Each individual is responsible for his/her own health, whatever it is, good or bad. Our bodies are full of bacteria, but these little guys are not to blame for all of our problems that plague human beings. God created bacteria to clean up the pollutants that overwhelm our bodies. They are there to protect us. Unfortunately, if the bacteria are destroyed, as with the overuse of antibiotics, yeast infections can develop as well as other related diseases. The body does need a certain amount of bacteria to keep clean. These are the body's line of defense and should not be killed off as the medical doctors do with the ordering of and the use of drugs. Disease is simply the breakdown of the body and its systems due to the buildup of toxins without any way of eliminating them. The things that contribute to disease are the chemicals in our foods and environment, wrong food choices, improperly combined foods, and incorrect lifestyles. The person must be determined to take responsibility for his or her own health/sickness and begin to choose and practice wiser lifestyles—eating a healthier diet, giving up smoking, exercising, and becoming physically fit.

Health can only be achieved by healthful living practices. If these laws are violated, then the body will suffer the consequences of destruction. People must eliminate toxic, unproductive diets and lifestyles, which consist of the improperly combined foods, sugars, meats, sodas and herbs, drugs, vaccines, etc. These only destroy the body even further.

Endnotes

1. *Webster's Dictionary* (Larchment, NY: Webster's Book Essentials, 1990), s.v. "disease."

2.	*Oxford Dictionary of Current English* 4th ed., s.v. "disease."
3.	*Home Medical Dictionary* (Ottenheimer, 1998), s.v. "disease."
4.	*Mosby's Medical, Nursing, & Allied Health Dictionary* (C.V. Mosby, 1990), s.v., "disease."

CHAPTER 5

The Immune System

The immune system is the body's defense against all outside, foreign predators. The body is not on the lookout for germs; it is attempting to prevent diseases. The medical and science professions are geared into believing that germs, viruses, and bacteria are the main causes of all that goes wrong with the body; however, the chemicals and pollutants in our environment and foods, along with the destructive lifestyles create our health challenges.

The more sensitive a person is, the better chance he/she has of continually getting rid of toxins and disease within the body. Itching, sneezing, coughing, vomiting, and diarrhea are the body's ways of expelling these improper substances that have been put voluntarily or involuntarily into our bodies. Small particles will get caught into the lungs and airways; the body in all of its wisdom will try and expel these to keep the airway clean for fresh air.

The lymph system helps to circulate and clean the body of dead cells, poisons, and fluids from around the body's cells and soft tissue areas. The lymphatic system not only includes its lymphatic channels and lymph nodes but the spleen, thymus, tonsils, and adenoids. There are other areas, the importance of which people are unaware of. They also help clean and filter the body's debris. People may continue to get sore throats and ear infections from improper lifestyle and accumulations of toxins. In particular, an increasing number of small children get those so-called childhood diseases. The parents take the child to the doctor, who continues to administer drugs, which only add to the mess. The toxins are continuingly building up in the tonsils and adenoids, therefore, becoming very inflamed and swollen. At this point, doctors surgically remove these organs, telling the parents that these are useless anyway and "Everyone can live without them without any problems." The tonsils and adenoids are there for an important reason: they help the body rid itself of infectious toxins.

Doctors just go in and start cutting out things of less importance. Another one is the appendix at the base of the cecum. God created this to filter infections and toxins of the colon and digestive system. The improper foods that people consume add to the overload and buildup of poisons. The appendix then becomes severely inflamed, so much so that the doctors will require major surgery to remove it before it bursts its accumulated poisonous contents throughout the abdominal area. When it does burst, it can be life threatening. Doctors then scurry through the surgical process, trying to remove what they can and then administer a series of antibiotics and other drugs to clean up the mess and bring the patient back to health. The problem is that the patient does not gain their health back unless they take away the cause of the disease that created that disaster.

My sister is one of these medical disasters. I can't call her a victim because she believes that all of the medical profession is correct in its so-called cures. She claims that her burst appendix with the poisons that were dumped throughout her abdomen, and the drugs that were administered were the start of all her health challenges. These poisons created a condition that resulted in her hysterectomy and many other surgical procedures. The woman is partially right; the poisons did their damage, so did the drugs that were administered, but the lifestyle that she lives is far more severe. She takes so many different drugs, all self-diagnosed because of her nursing experience and drug knowledge. Now, her body is overwhelmed to the point of physical disrepair and breakdown. She has created a scientific experiment out of her own body. It is very sad because she has severe gastric reflux disease to the point of vomiting stomach acids because of what all the drugs have done to her stomach. She has severe osteoporosis because of the years of consuming colas, alcohol, Tums, and smoking coupled with improper diet and lack of exercise. Now because of her excessive use of drugs, she has developed peripheral neuropathy in both her feet, which is now spreading up her legs to the groin area. She has had two spinal surgeries due to tumors in her vertebra and still administers her own IG IV through intravenous ports. These drugs are costing the insurance companies $11,000 a month. She has gotten off the cigarettes and is supposedly juicing with some fresh raw juices but claims that people must have raw and cooked vegetables to get correct nutritional intake. Her body may have already passed the threshold of destruction. There may not be any way to rejuvenate this horrible mess of humanity. The body that was created in perfection, but because of free will, wrong choices, and ignorance has been severely abused to the point of no return. She is living a miserable, self-induced existence.

CHAPTER 6

Unhealthy Bodies
and Addictions

Why are many foods not suitable for maintaining a healthy human condition? A person can go through a grocery store and marvel at all of the aisles of foodstuffs, mostly packages, boxes, bottles, and canned goods up the main aisles. Produce may be a large section of the store, but most shoppers seemingly pass up these items. Processed foods, food additives, refined ingredients make up the foods that people crave. These foods are very addicting, and people keep going back repeatedly for these items. These chemicals that are ingested on a daily basis poison the body.

People who are seeking better health can and are continuously deceived into buying those so-called health foods. Instead of sugar, they will use honey, molasses, or pure maple syrup. All of these sugars are just another form and still do the body harm by affecting the body's chemistry the same way that sugar affects it possibly worse.

Honey is good for the bees and not meant for human consumption. Molasses is the waste product of the manufacturing of sugar; it is a totally harmful product. Maple syrup is the sap from the maple trees that is boiled in large vats, and it is still a refined sweetener that has no place in the human diet.

Other waste products bought by the deceived health seeker are brewer's yeast, a waste from the beer industry. Whey is a protein product bought by people who feel they need extra protein, especially body builders. Liver is another product that is supported by the medical profession to cure a body of anemia, lack of iron. Liver is one of the organs of detoxification and elimination. Therefore, a person will get all of the waste products and toxins by eating this portion of the animal flesh. Gelatin is supposed to be consumed for strong nails and hair. This product, by adding considerable amounts of sugar, coloring, artificial flavorings will compound these into a dessert, Jell-O. The deceived public eats this stuff, which is made a few steps different from glue, which is both made from horse's hoofs. This is all worthless garbage and not suitable for the human body.

Babies are fed chemically-induced powdered baby formulas and jars of baby food. The body in its pure state cannot take too much of this abusive treatment.

Babies are started on their perverted lifestyles by parents who feed them on the run. A mother who breast feeds her child calmly and at the same time has a healthy raw produce diet will have a baby who is calm and healthy, not colicky and sick. These processed-food-fed babies tend to be chubby and fat because of their diet. I have seen overweight babies, and it is very sad because these babies grow into childhood and adulthood plagued with obesity and a lifestyle that shackles them to it. It is abusive for the child to be living in this prison of despair and sickness. It is a vicious merry-go-round, a merry-go-round of ignorance that will be passed down to the next generation. This world is a victim of this ignorance, rebellion, and laziness.

Education is the clear factor, but when it is brought to the forefront, most often it is balked at because of the food cravings involved and the profits of the food manufacturing companies. A perverted palate and the comfort foods that feed it are hard to let go and surrender. This also feeds and continues an addictive cycle. When people were young and ill, they were given comfort foods to help cure the body, but mostly just for comfort. There are many memories attached to these foods, which is another reason they are so irresistible. People need to comfort themselves in more healthy ways. There will have to be some changes in thinking, behavior, and developing new habits and lifestyles. That is a tough one for most people, especially in the physical aspect. The addictions of these chemicals have a mild to severe withdrawal process.

Withdrawals can and do include the physical aspect. The withdrawals are the cleansing part of the elimination of the chemicals. A fast expedites the recovery process and speeds up the healing. Some foodstuff chemical withdrawals can be just as excruciating as illegal street drugs. My own experiences can tell their own story.

I started off through the doors of Alcoholics Anonymous on September 12, 1979. I went cold turkey on alcohol and prescription drugs, pain pills/codeine. The physical aspect was bad, but the mental and emotional part was an absolute nightmare. Now, looking back, I would have fared better throughout the healing process if I had better dietary habits. When I help those going through physical withdrawals, I get people to fast on raw juice and distilled water to help the body clean properly.

The hardest part of the addictive process is the mental attitudes. It is the attachments to the past that seem the hardest to surrender. That is the soul-wrenching part that takes the most effort. In fact, the founders of Alcoholics Anonymous spoke to my uncle and aunt (beginning members of this once fine organization), telling them that they wanted to somehow help the recovering alcoholic to learn to live sober. They wanted to incorporate into the program something to help the recovering alcoholic to live *and* to stay sober, but they died before that could be accomplished. Too many of the recovering alcoholics are too attached to their past crutches and have continued to be weakened by them. Many have atrophic spirits and souls, which in a spiritual sense haven't been used. Therefore, many remain as babies, resorting back to their drug of choice when life got in their face.

Coming off the hard drugs, one would think that it would be easier to deal with the world's drugs. Caffeine was a very difficult drug for me to escape from. I used caffeine to sustain me throughout the day while attending school, just to keep me awake through the horrendous schedule. I was a first-time student in my late thirties and caring for a home and family. I kept getting migraines on the weekends when I didn't need to use caffeine. A friend told me to just have a cup of coffee and the headache would go away. "You are just addicted to the caffeine." I was furious. I didn't need any more addictions in my life, so I used that anger to go through the most horrible physical withdrawals imaginable. I went off all caffeine on a Friday and continued to spend the next three days with the most head-crushing migraine I had ever had in my life. When I go through an extremely bad experience, it always remains forever engraved into my memory bank, which keeps me diligent and determined in my path. It is a blessing.

By far, the smoking withdrawal was my worst addiction to conquer. It took years to realize that no matter what or how I went about it. I was severely hooked on nicotine. My body would not allow me to be without a cigarette for long of a length of time. I started my mornings as my head lifted off the pillow, reaching for the first cigarette of the day until the time I lay down in the darkness to rest for the night, smoking the last one of the day, watching the glow of the cigarette. I did not want to be consumed by my addiction but felt trapped because I was unable to stop.

There were many mornings toward the end of my smoking career that I could not stop coughing. I just knew that I was going to die, but I hoped not that way. I would cut back but still couldn't stop, eventually smoking more again. It was such an endless cycle. I began to take an exercise class, which, looking back, was helpful to curb my nicotine cravings.

It was by divine intervention though that I quit. I knew that I didn't want to quit and accepted that downheartedly. So I just prayed for the desire to quit. Well, my prayer was answered the next day. (Be careful what you pray for, it may happen sooner that you think.) So I went for twelve hours without a cigarette, and then I went for another twelve hours again. I decided that I would just see how long I could go without smoking. When two days had passed, I wanted to smoke, but a well-intentioned friend pointed out the accomplishments of the past four days and said she wished that she could have that determination in her life, stating kindly that now I could just quit. She was still addicted and in admiration of what I was doing. People really do watch us; we just have to continue to struggle and be good examples.

I did try eating better at that point, and the daily exercise continued to help my body to release the cravings and cleanout the chemicals. People need to stay away from these addictive foods and drugs of all kinds. Yes, caffeine, alcohol and nicotine are drugs as well as all types of processed foods. We need to be free of these substances forever one day at a time. If we start on some of these substances, the cravings are awakened. Lay's Potato Chips have advertised, "Betcha can't eat just one!" They know better. That's why they created these addictive products to get people to continuously buy and eat more.

It is important to remember, it's like the alcoholic needs to stay out of the bar and away from the first drink. Well, people need to accept their addictions and stay out of the junk food areas of the grocery stores. Don't buy them, and they are not going to be eaten if they aren't brought into the home.

In fact, the health food stores carry so much junk foods—canned, processed, and packaged so-called foodstuffs. They are enough to stuff your face but do nothing to nourish the body. Health is a business, but the uninformed consumer isn't getting anything out of it except get sicker instead of becoming healthier. When we are sick and tired of being sick and tired, we will be more determined to do something differently.

Through our sufferings, we will remember that most can be, and are, blessings if they help us to change our lives and attitudes. They help us to remain on the pathways marked out for a healthy and fruitful life.

CHAPTER 7

Chronic, Debilitating Diseases

It seems to be the time and season for painful diseases. Everyone seems to be experiencing pain, especially in the joints and muscles. It seems that "everyone" has one or both of these debilitating diseases: fibromyalgia and arthritis. Well, at least everyone who is eating and living the standard American diet and lifestyle.

"Fibromyalgia is a condition affecting the muscles and the connective tissue associated with the muscles." *Living Without Pain*, Harvey Diamond page 48. Fibromyalgia symptoms include pain, tenderness, and aches in specific areas of the body. These are called tender points because they are extremely sensitive to touch. The pain disturbs sleep, making a person become stressed, irritable, and chronically tired.

Its cause, at least according to medical professionals, is unknown. They claim it is an autoimmune disease in which the body is attacking and destroying itself. Many doctors say, "It's all in your head," and prescribe tranquilizers or an antidepressant. The many drugs that a person will take to relieve the pain and sleeplessness only challenge the body and compound the symptoms. So a person has more side effects, therefore creating more health challenges and diseases than before originally seen. Do these drugs cure the person? Absolutely not. It is a guessing game with the patient as the victim.

Arthritis, at this time, is the most disabling disease of our nation. The joints are stiff and immobile; they have lost their flexibility. Pain with each movement is normal. There are other forms of arthritis—rheumatoid arthritis and osteoarthritis—and all of these, people are suffering tremendous pain in their bodies. Arthritis is joint inflammation and a disorder of the connective tissue. The cartilage is connective tissue that supports the joints, so there is a cushion between the moveable bones. Osteoarthritis is a degenerative joint disease. The cartilage is wearing away to the point that there is bone-on-bone contact. Most occurrences are in the back, knees, hips, shoulders, hands, and feet. As the spine develops degenerative disk disease, bone spurs form at the ends of the vertebral bodies, and these cause pain on the muscles that attach to the spine. The spine, at the loss of the disk, will begin to fuse together, sometimes crushing the nerve between the bones. This is extremely disabling and painful as the person loses all function and may become confined to a wheelchair or opts for surgery, which may or may not correct this condition. Most of this occurs because the standard American diet significantly ages the human body. Harvey Diamond states that osteoarthritis may be the result of rheumatoid arthritis. In fact, he claims that if it would be accurate to say that in most cases, osteoarthritis is the end result of rheumatoid arthritis gone to the extreme.[2]

Rheumatoid arthritis is the inflammation of the synovium of the joints. It becomes lost altogether; the joint and the cartilage are left unprotected. Pain, swelling and disfiguring become normal. If the cartilage deteriorates too much, this disease cannot be reversed, even if the underlying causes are taken away.

The body can't take any more when it is wracked with pain and over-accumulated amounts of toxins from improper diet and lifestyle become saturated beyond the overload. The body rebels and just wants to correct itself. This overload of chemicals wears on the delicate, but intricate systems of the body that begin to wear down. How does the body hold up to this abuse? Pain takes away the quality of life.

Drugs become habitual. These medicines are taken but the control of the body now turns over to the chemicals/drugs, not the person. In the standard American diet, chemicals equate disease. So these drugs only create even more problems, more pain, more toxins, and more problematic diseases. It's like getting caught up in a squirrel cage. The nerve energy of the body is drained; there is overwhelming fatigue, and they cannot go one step further. The whole body is screaming in despair. Unfortunately, the person isn't paying attention, and nothing is changed. Everyone, including the doctors, seems so clueless about what is going on.

People need to eliminate the chemicals/drugs, sugars, packaged processed foods, additives, sodas, alcohol, animal proteins, dairy products, refined flours, and most improper food combinations from their diets or the body will never rebound. Keep them away, and the body will do an amazing thing; it will heal itself, and may even become livable again as the pain diminishes and the body's energy is restored.

Depression is another debilitating disease that is rampantly plaguing the world's population and is due to too many hormonal changes within the brain and the body. The disease of depression may not be as physically challenging as arthritis or osteoporosis, but emotionally, it is devastating to those who are captured in its grip. These changes have been caused by the excess amounts of accumulated chemicals and toxins that have not and cannot be eliminated. The World Health Organization cites that depression currently affects 350 million people around the world. It affects 20 million Americans alone.[3] It silently attacks with many people suffering from it. The money lost because of depression is astounding because of the treatments, lost productivity, and disability every year. Unfortunately, this number continues to rise.

There are various mental illnesses that are parallel to each other with depression ranging from mild to severe: bipolar, manic depressive, schizophrenia, paranoia, and psychosis to name a few. Many of these people can suffer silently for years, and may go through the medical route as a tragic victim pumped full of drugs as everyone is looking for a so-called cure, which turns out to be a useless venture.

Countless people cannot continue this pathway of hell, but in many cases, they will try and commit suicide, just to end their misery, with some succeeding.

Numerous cases, if not all of them, could have been prevented. The fortunate ones have found the way out through a change of diet and lifestyle. Discontinuing the use of drugs is an important key to getting the body free of all the poisons that are contributing to the imbalanced emotional state.

The standard American diet and lifestyle contribute most to this sad state of mental anguish. Many people will say that it can be genetic. It may come from learned lifestyles and behavior rather than genes. A depressed pregnant mom can have a depressed child because of what she is doing throughout her pregnancy. The emotional state of the mother does affect the baby utero as well as her diet, even if she is not on medication during her pregnancy. It can be a squirrel-cage situation.

Depression is a rapidly growing problem in our society today with refined grains and refined sugars the major contributing factors. Hypoglycemic reactions also correlate with depression. These reactions include hypersensitivity, irrationality, emotional instability and sometimes aggressiveness. According to George Malkmus, the sugars that come from both the refined grains as well as the refined sugars may be involved in "mental illness, divorce, and crime as alcohol has been found to be." [4]

Children can suffer from depression, and if they eat a poor diet determined by their parents, the bad behavioral characteristic of ADD or ADHD resembles moods and acts of depression. These are contributed to refined sugars and refined grains in the diet. George Malkmus also claims, "Since 1965, scientists have repeatedly linked high gluten consumption coming from refined grains to learning disorders and schizophrenia."[5]

I suffered silent depression for years as I was growing up and was into my twenties. I had an existence but didn't have a life. I did not realize that it was depression, and the only medication consumed was occasional alcoholic binges and eating binges coupled with a very poor diet, lack of exercise, and continuous smoking of cigarettes. I tried to just quit drinking, but as an alcoholic who was dry and had no other change to heal the malnourishment of my body, my suffering only became worse. The lifestyle and diet I lived was passed on through learned experience.

After I entered Alcoholics Anonymous, I began to realize that I was suffering from depression and just stuck it out, sober at least. Eventually, through the years, I learned more about diet, nutrition, and most of all, the blessed daily exercise program that literally saved my life. When I started exercising every day, the depression, states of despair, and sadness became history. The fears passed as I stayed with this and sought recovery in other areas to help my mental state, as well as my emotional and physical state. The years of continued exercise kept me free from all the prescription drugs. Diet and exercise are so important to me because I do not want to live in that hell ever again.

A raw produce diet with fresh fruits and vegetables, nuts and seed with fresh pure water is the only way to keep the body healthy, emotionally stable, in continued recovery, and free from diseases. It is a whole lifestyle change that can be a godsend to those trapped in hell with the light at the end of their tunnel.

Processed foods, additives, drugs, and other chemicals paralyze a person to an existence instead of living a life. Food sensitivities and improper food combinations can cause depression because it upsets the delicate emotional and physical balances of the body. A person must be continually diligent; otherwise, they can lose more than they sought to gain. Prayer and a connection to God our Creator make the journey to health and healing a whole lot easier. Obedience to the laws of nature needs to be the ultimate life goal.

Osteoporosis is a silent killer. The disease weakens and destroys the bones. The person isn't even aware of it until it's too late. By that time, the bones are too brittle and too weak to handle the stresses of everyday life, including carrying the frame of the body, for the weight of it may be great, and there may come a time when the hip or vertebrae may fracture. Osteoporosis is now in epidemic proportions in our nation.

Osteoporosis is a disease of excessive bone loss and decreased bone density.[6] Overtime, there is less bone, and what is left is lighter and more porous. There is an increased risk of bone fractures due to brittleness. Fosomax, a drug given to osteoporotic women and men, makes the bones even more brittle.

The common factors that presupposes osteoporosis are smoking, sedentary lifestyle, deficiency of vitamin D, calcium or magnesium, a meat-based rather than a raw plant food diet, and too many grains and dairy products. Alcoholism is also a major risk.

According to the late John Lee, MD, who conducted extensive research on osteoporosis said there are two types of bone cells that are important to the osteoporosis process: osteoclasts and osteoblasts. Osteoclasts are the cells that dissolve or reabsorb old bone, leaving behind tiny, unfilled spaces. The osteoblasts move into these spaces and rebuild new bone. This process is called remodeling; it is the mechanism for the remarkable repair abilities and the continuing strength of our bones.[7] If these two processes remain in balance, bone mass and bone strength will continue to be constant. Osteoporosis is bone loss that occurs because of osteoclast dominance. More is being reabsorbed than is newly created.

The strongest the bones are is at the age of twenty-five–twenty-six, and according to medical sources, there is a decline after that. When a woman reaches menopause, supposedly, it declines faster after that. This is all because of a perverted diet and lifestyle.

The long bones of the body remain stronger than the rest of the skeletal bones. When they become weak enough to fracture, there is a very great problem indeed. People have been deceived in the prevention and treatment of osteoporosis. The medical profession will claim that it is a hormone change due to the loss of estrogen. I will totally disagree with them. What then can they say about osteoporosis in men? I operated a bone density machine in a small hospital and interviewed my patients. I had many young people with severe osteoporosis. As we talked, many indicated that they had diets consisting of hamburgers, fries, sodas, very little vegetables if any. They would be cooked. Their diets and lifestyles weren't healthy at all. I did get to do a lot of research in this field because of my job.

Many claim that drinking milk, eating Tums, and taking their calcium supplements were ways to beat osteoporosis. People have heard through the years of growing up, "Drink your milk; it will make your bones strong." Well this is faulty thinking and does greater damage to the body.

There aren't any substitutes for the faulty and perverse diet. The Tums, and anti-acid medication now have become pseudo substitutes for calcium. It is completely indigestible by the human body; it tends to create more acid in the stomach as the body in its wonderfulness desires to maintain its balance. The Tums, along with the added calcium supplements, are totally unabsorbable calcium, which settles in the joints, organs, and blood, creating arthritis, gallstones, kidney stones, and other hosts of problems.

Women are many times given HRT (hormone replacement therapy), Fosomax, and other drugs by the medical profession to treat osteoporosis. These drugs endanger the body, which will accumulate more toxins to an already acidic body. The cause has still not been addressed.

Milk, because it is an animal-based protein/calcium, creates acidity in the body also. The body in its created wisdom tries to maintain balance by making itself more alkaline, draws calcium from the bones to do this. In this way, the kidneys can excrete these wastes and excess calcium from the body via the urinary tract. Adding meats to this already acid equation only accentuates and compounds the burden on the body. People who eat a raw plant-based diet do not have this problem. That's where cows get their calcium from the plants they eat!

It is quite ironic because the medical profession is quite adamant about a lot of milk-drinking for good bone density. In fact, Leon Root, MD, in his book, *Beautiful Bones without Hormones*, contradicts himself by saying to take 1,500 mg. of calcium per day, and "how do you do that? We'll start out with dairy products, the foods with the highest calcium content of all. These foods can be high in fat, so try to use a low-fat variety whenever possible. Low-fat dairy products actually contain more calcium than those who still have their fat." He then promotes a lot of raw fruits and vegetables, contesting that dried figs contain 269 mg. of calcium.[8] That's about nine figs per day. Here's the contradictory part, the not-so-good food groups, the ones to avoid: meats. Meats are still animal protein the same as dairy products. They both deplete calcium from the bones. No wonder people are confused; they listen to too many contradictory things stated as facts by the so-called experts. People will believe these facts because, after all, he/she is the doctor and should know what they are talking about.

Successful prevention and treating of this disease will require proper diet, weight-bearing exercise, removal of all processed foods from the diet, eating instead properly combined raw fruits and vegetables, sunshine daily for vitamin D, and avoidance of all drugs and supplements. In fact, it has been noted that drinking a pint of freshly extracted organic carrot juice daily allows the body to assimilate more calcium than many bottles of calcium supplements, and these calcium pills are an inorganic, useless, and a toxic form of calcium for the body. They will tend to create kidney stones, gall stones, bursitis, and other joint problems, and the bones will still be deficient of calcium because they are unabsorbable.

Gastroesophageal reflux disease (GERD) is a disease of the abused body that hasn't been listened to. The body can only take so much abuse. In all of its intelligence the body speaks in its own language, but no one seems to or wants to listen to it. When the body suffers, it lets the recipient know. Americans have a love affair with food. They will continue to eat anything their hearts desire no matter what effect it has on their bodies. They will also continue to suffer the consequences of this affair: disease. They lust over these foods so much that they will resort to taking drugs, do tests and procedures, cut body parts out, *anything*. But don't let anyone take away their favorite, special, comfort foods. They have become their gods; their idols. As the Bible says, "You reap what you sow."[9] The American public hasn't figured it out yet or are they just that rebellious? People are killing themselves with their forks.

GERD or gastroesophageal reflux disease is a disease that is created by improper diet and lifestyle. The food will reflux back up into the esophagus from the stomach. God created the body's digestive tract to have one-way valves. The foods are eaten first by mouth, which in turn after it is chewed and swallowed is then propelled down the esophagus into the stomach.

After eating a meal of improperly combined foods, the stomach is unable to digest these foods, and continues to churn, dumping in more acids, placing a severe burden on the digestive system. The partially undigested matter will ferment as in the case of undigested fruits and starches and the proteins will putrefy. As the foods continue to stay in the stomach instead of exiting, as they should, this mess will create indigestion, heartburn, burping, bloating, and bad breath. This is the evidence of poor digestion. The foods need to exit the stomach quickly for proper assimilation and nutrition; and if it is held up in any way, it will reflux back up through the one-way sphincter. If this process continues too often, it weakens the sphincter muscle, and erodes the esophagus with the stomach acids, thus creating GERD. If this is left untreated, other types of esophageal problems can and will occur, including the risk of esophageal ulcers and cancers. Over-the-counter drugs are consumed by the truckloads with an attempt to "cure" these symptoms—Tums, Rolaids, and other anti-acid remedies. Also used are baking soda and poisonous aluminum products. All of these products decrease the stomach acid, but the body needs acid for digestion; thus, it secretes more. A change of diet and lifestyle should be attempted instead because it is wiser, healthier, and what the body was created to do. The cause needs to be addressed and accomplished.

This is a type of disease that people do not take any responsibility for as being caused by their own actions. It's far easier just to blame someone or something else. At this time, more than sixty million American people[10] suffer from heartburn at least once a month.

The biggest problem is that there are now more and more infants and children who are becoming diagnosed with GERD. These are children who are developing the adult diseases. Most are put on a regimen of drugs to cure instead of addressing their diets. The processed foods that are fed to them are destroying their little digestive systems and bodies. Many are to the point where they are vomiting these acids from their stomachs, and the drugs obviously are of no value. This society has become a drugged society.

Ms. Kristina Anderson states that the cost of GERD diagnosis and treatment in the United States estimates at $14,000,000 with 60 percent spent on drug treatment.[11] All for the sake of just feeding their taste buds and faces but not their body's health. This is the case of living to eat, not eating to live, and the parents aren't properly training their children in the way of health but in the way of sickness.

The proper combination of foods is important for optimal digestion. When people continually feed the body in times of distress, even eating good foods, the body cannot digest and assimilate these foods. In emotional upheaval, the digestion will cease, so it's best to wait until the next meal and eat with a calm attitude.

GERD is becoming more prevalent worldwide. Ms. Anderson's states that "7 percent of adult Americans claim to have GERD on a daily basis, whereas 20 percent report heartburn on a weekly basis and 44 percent on a monthly basis."[12] White men tend to have more severe forms of this disease, including Barrett's esophagus, which is a cancerous condition that develops when the cells of the esophageal lining are continually exposed to the back-up of stomach acids, and Zanker's diverticulitis, a large diverticuli of the esophagus where foods gets stuck and backs up; thus, nothing is going down in the proper direction and digestion is hindered.

I know of a gentleman who has gone through four or five (possibly more) esophagus surgeries for repairs because of hiatus hernias, esophagitis, and other problems. Many of these cannot continue to be treated without doing more damage. It becomes an endless cycle of destruction.

Most of the disease that Americans are plagued with is due to their diets and improper lifestyle choices. God created all things in His creation for a purpose, so each of His creations would be fed. Man is the only species that eats the foods of other species.

People have to learn to love and take care of their own bodies. If they really loved themselves as God loves them, they would not eat these so-called foods. They would obey the laws of nature and God. People need to eat foods that are designed to digest and assimilate, not foods that stay in the stomach, foods that stick to the ribs. Fresh, raw, and whole fruits and vegetable are what the body craves, uses, and needs to live, and they are optimally healthy. Fruits, vegetables, some seeds and nuts and pure water are all the human body desires. No more disease with obedience.

Cancer is a disease that plagues the body, which is depleted, exhausted, unable to optimally function—one that will wither up and die a slow, painful suicide of each cell and tissue of the body that had been fed the poisons of drugs of any kind. Chemicals, especially chemotherapy during the illness, will kill more people from the treatments than from the disease itself. The way it is now, the standard of care and today's protocol for cancer is chemotherapy and radiation therapy. According to David and Anne Frahm, "People don't get cancer unless their metabolism is severely damaged, their system becomes highly toxic, and their immune system does not work properly."[13] And Rev. George Malkmus adds, "Normal cells divide 50–60 times and then die. Cancer cells *divide* forever."[14]

People just want to continue what they are doing—how they are living and eating the foods they love and not wanting to change anything even if it means getting cancer. People are terrified of getting cancer and of dying but just refuse to see that what they are doing is leading them right through that door. People refuse to believe that food and their lifestyle is the issue, so they just want to be left alone.

No one can see how all the chemicals are destroying human bodies and the human race, especially the doctors, food companies, etc. Food, they say, can't be the problem; that's too simple. After all, everyone eats these foods, and why would poisons be sold in the stores? The government wouldn't allow it. They are all deceived and believe the lie. If anyone gets sick, he/she just takes drugs, and if a person isn't cured, oh well. There will be a series of tests and procedures to be run, and if all else fails then *you* die.

People who are dying of this exhaustive state are dying of cancer, and when they are administered chemotherapy drugs as well as other poisons in enormous amounts, they always expect a cure. The desperate ones are looking for hope, but they are looking in the wrong direction. The oncology doctors are pushing these treatments for these desperate patients who are pushed to the brink of an agonizing death a lot quicker. The success rate of these doctors is at zero. None will survive; all die from some form of cancer. Insanity is doing the same thing over and over while expecting different results. It's just normal; it's just what happens in this day and age, they all say, and everyone will get cancer at one point in his/her life. It's to be expected. The only ones who can heal from cancer are those who will change their entire life to an extremely healthy approach.

Of those oncology doctors surveyed and asked what they would do if they got cancer, most said would not take these drugs or go through what their patients are going through, nor could they do this to their family members. They know it's a horrible, ugly fate. They do know how devastating it all is.

What other options does the public have? The doctors do not give them any other choice, and people need to become responsible for the lifestyle they lead, the foods they consumed, the environment they live and work in. Let us *not vacate* our senses. People need to be educated.

I do know of one oncologist/hematologist who, in her medical practice, takes on ten new patients each week, 520 new cases each year. That's sad. What's wrong with this picture? She also states that there isn't any way that foods or diet can make any difference with the prevention or healing of the body of cancer.

Many people may be at the point where the years of abuse, damage, and destruction have been too great to reverse and regenerate to optimal health. Most of these regrets came too late. For example, according to Mary Ann Gower, her husband Herb was one of them. She states, "By the time Herb learned of the Hallelujah diet, he had already had very advanced, metastasized prostate cancer."[15] Although Herb didn't subject himself to chemotherapy, he did participate in several series of radiation therapy, and according to his wife, it severely weakened him. By the time he had started the Hallelujah diet, the cancer had already spread, a typical conclusion. Cancer is cancer, and it doesn't matter what body part it is in, it's still cancer with all the same causes. It's the last stage of disease, and it rules over a terribly depleted and damaged body.

Cancer patients never die from the original cancer because it continues to spread even if one gets surgery to remove the cancer. It will continue to return somewhere else, and the cancer treatment will only make a quick casualty. It kills and destroys the function of the organism. Rev. George Malkmus has an amazing testimony about his own recovery from colon cancer. He declined all medical treatments and adapted to a pure vegan diet. He drank a lot of raw vegetable juices and just maintained a raw plant diet, rejecting all processed and refined foods, and within a year, his body recovered and healed from the cancer. He continues to stay healthy and disease-free because he remains diligent and determined, not chained to the past in any way. His goal is for continued healing and to teach others to do the same.

It may take years for cancer cells to become cancerous tumors, sometimes ten–fifteen years until the discovery and diagnosis of cancer. Based on this lag of time, people do have time to take an action of creating a new environment, one of cancer-defeating, not cancer-promoting.

People think that they can consume anything they want. They can, but most of these consumed items are not good for the health of the human body. Alcohol, tobacco, preservatives, and additives in the food products are poisonous chemicals that pollute, contaminate, and kill the body. Caffeine and sugar are addictive drugs that lure people into their webs of destruction.

The causes of cancer start with enervation, a weakened state and low nerve energy. Therefore, these toxic substances, when internally ingested, weaken the immune system; the toxins accumulate and build up. At this point, the cellular destruction begins to take place. On the cellular level, cancers begin right here. The nervous system begins to become irritated, initiating the inflammation and pain within the body, especially in the muscles and joints. The nerve endings and muscles become even more saturated. The cellular destruction is becoming more abundant and acute. The body is still trying to relieve itself of the burden of the poisons by creating an ulcerous outlet. When people use drugs to reduce the body's symptoms, it only aggravates the body's cleansing process and just makes things worse. The body in this compromised and unrelieved state will continue to harden the tissue in specific areas to quarantine the toxic poisons into one area for the body's protection. If one continues to ignore the body's message, these cancer cells continue to migrate and mutate. They are now totally out of control! According to TC Fry, "Cancer cells live in a hostile environment but still divide and flourish as long as nutrients are available to them…People sometimes ask when cancer begins. Hygienists or life scientists say that it begins with the first cold or rash of childhood."[16] Well, stated that cancers occur long before the diagnosis; they just don't happen suddenly like most people believe.

Olin Idol states in his Hallelujah Acres health tip, "Way back in 1971, the president of the United States, Richard Nixon, declared a national War on Cancer by signing the Conquest of Cancer Act, thereby officially inaugurating what has become known as the War on Cancer."[17] That was thirty-eight years ago, and many organizations spend billions of dollars on cancer research, and we are not any closer to the cure for cancer. In fact, there are more people dying of cancer now more than there were back then. It is a big scam and a grave lie. The cancer treatment industry is a *huge* business. They all say that no one knows the cause of cancer and are still researching, but look at those who have made a dietary change with the healing of their bodies. Unfortunately, no one wants to listen to them. They are shut up because of the companies that are making money from the illnesses of the people.

According to Olin Idol, "Every 55 minutes, another American dies of cancer."[18] The animal proteins, animal fats, processed foods, processed and refined sugars, white flour increase the levels of insulin in the bloodstream, thus stimulating the growth of cancers. The processed foods are even more damaging to the human body than normal animal flesh. These types increase the risk of cancer when eaten on a daily basis by 49 percent, according to Michael Donaldson, PhD. He goes on to say that in a "study reported in 1994, it found that children who typically ate twelve hot dogs or more a month had a 9.5 times the risk for childhood leukemia as those who ate less than four per month. Households where the dad and child both ate twelve or more hot dogs per month had a 19.8 fold increase in childhood leukemia. Other studies have confirmed a link between processed meats and childhood cancer." [19] The medical profession in its sheer ignorance does not have any knowledge of nutrition or understanding of how the body's self-healing and properly combined foods can allow recovery beyond what the medical doctors think is the only way. Cancer is a matter of nutritional deficiency. Doctors only give the options of drugs, surgery, and traditional medical interventions while telling the patient to eat whatever they want because, after all, "it really has nothing to do with it," I have heard doctors say.

The conventional cancer therapies have too many dangerous and damaging side effects. The chemotherapy affects the whole body. It damages the healthy cells as well as the cancer cells, and the body cannot fight off and defend itself against this abusive trauma. These procedures do not even kill all the cancer cells; that is why doctors insist getting a specific number of rounds/treatments done. It also impairs the immune system, impairs the liver detoxification, and the body's ability for nutrition. It also alters the DNA code of the body's cells. According to Anne Frahm, it can "permanently damage the kidneys, the heart, and the gallbladder."[20] Radiation therapy can affect the healthy cells in the treated areas and will impair the body's ability to tolerate the treatment and to maintain overall health. It weakens the body and makes the body's self-healing mechanisms ineffective. Radiation creates cancers and in itself is extremely dangerous. Surgery can be a useful treatment at times, but how often does one hear some say, "We think we got it all, but we better do chemotherapy just in case."

"Cutting, burning, and poisoning may help for a time, but they don't get to the cause of the disease,"[21] says the Frahms. People are in a drug-oriented society; they look for a quick fix and a cure to get rid of the symptoms but never dealt with the cause. They do not seek the cause because they think that the drugs and treatments are the cure. If it doesn't work, they will go in more aggressively, which includes more surgery, drugs, etc. If that fails, and most certainly it will because they aren't dealing with the cause, the doctors blame the patient and hand them the death sentence, "You have such and such time left. There is nothing more that we can do." Sometimes they don't even say "I'm sorry."

The cancerous tumor is not the disease; it is just the symptom of a deep underlying cause. What needs to happen is to remove the cause and to restore the body to regenerate and heal itself instead of aiming to remove the tumor.

Frahms claim that "cancer grows when the immune system has been compromised, either an inherited compromise passed from mother to child, or developed compromise acquired over a number of years from diet, lifestyle, and environmental exposures."[22] Cancers will continue to return with a vengeance unless the immune system is strengthened and the body is regenerated and healed by good nutrition.

Another casualty to cancer was a journalist named Tony Snow, who died at fifty-three following a series of chemotherapy treatments for colon cancer. His colon was removed followed by chemotherapy. Two years later, he had surgery again after a tumor had grown in his abdominal area, near the original site. According to Andreas Moritz, "The previous series of chemotherapy treatments inflamed and irreversibly damaged a large number of cells in his body and also impaired his immune system, a perfect recipe for growing new cancers. Now, unable to heal the causes of the original cancer (in addition to the newly created ones), Snow's body developed new cancers in the liver and other parts of the body."[23] He died from the effects of chemotherapy, not from the disease itself. Chemotherapy doesn't kill the cancer, it kills the body itself. It has never been shown to kill any cancers. The disease is the body's attempt to heal itself, which it actually tries to by developing the cancer.

According to statistics on breast cancers, in 1950, 264 out of one million white American women died of breast cancer. Twenty-five years later, the death rate was exactly the same, but by 1985, it had risen to 275. In the 1990s, it began falling slightly. By 1995, the rate dropped to 248, 6 percent less than forty-five years earlier. But the picture for African Americans is even more discouraging. In 1973, the first year government records were compiled, the death rate for black women were 263 for every 10,000. By 1993, it had soared to 319.[24] Robert Bazell wrote a book on the making of a cancer drug in 1998 and I am sure the statistics are insurmountable by now. Google Internet Research states, "In 1960, 1 out of every 20 women was affected with breast cancer. Now in 2010, one out of eight women will be afflicted with this disease. It is now estimated that 207,090 women will be diagnosed with breast cancer this year, and 39,840 will die of it this year."[25] These are very sad and grave statistics when they don't have to be this way, based on ignorance, stubbornness, and sometimes sheer laziness rather than to conform to a healthier diet and lifestyle. Many women will look to all of the drugs, chemo, surgeries, and other medical treatments for a cure. They are looking for outside sources to blame and fix them rather than taking responsibility for their own body's disease and recovery. These are desperate women living in a hopeless and desperate society. Living this way, the causes aren't dealt with, and cancer always returns to kill the person.

Women live in fear of breast cancer. Many will even have both of their breasts removed surgically rather than face the risk of getting breast cancer. Hormones are to blame, but what are even more to blame are the synthetic hormones that the doctors prescribe to their female patients, including birth control pills. The causes in young woman under the age of fifty who are diagnosed with breast cancer are poor diet, lifestyles, and birth control pills. But what people fail to realize is that cancer *is* cancer. It doesn't matter where in the body it is located, it's still cancer. Surgeons will cut it out, oncologists will offer chemotherapy and radiation therapies, but it will always return, unless the cause is removed. Surgery does not always excise the cancer entirely. Chemotherapy and radiation therapy are often just more of a problem, destroying much but not necessarily all of the cancer, and usually harming the healthy tissue in the process.

Breast cancer is unpredictable, sometimes it is wholly contained in a tumor and spreads from the tiniest tumor long before it can be detected or removed. A mammogram only X-rays the detected cancer, but it is there long before it is seen. Cancers are forming ten–twenty years before they can be detected. Women can have had a clean bill of health, and then six months later, they will have a very aggressive form of cancer and will be dead in less than a year. The radiologist is to blame for not detecting it on the previous X-ray. This is a true statement. I know personally of one case involved. It was sad; the victim was a doctor's wife. Cancer shows no favoritism. People need to understand that what they put into their bodies can, and oftentimes will, kill them.

The cancer may occur in a different body part, and people will say they are still cancer-free survivor of breast, prostate, and other cancers. People don't see that they are still getting their disease back with a vengeance. A person with cancer must be very aggressive in his/her reform to a new diet and lifestyle.

I have a friend who is ecstatic that she is an eleven-year breast cancer survivor, but a few months back she went through a surgery without chemo to have half of her cancerous thyroid gland removed. She's on heart medicine and blood pressure drugs and also has problems with acid reflux. She said she does eat some fruits and vegetables, some raw and some cooked. She claims she eats healthy, but one begins to wonder especially with the acid reflux disease. She is an obsessive housecleaner whose daily usage of caustic bleaches and cleaners had caused her family to sleep in the garage because of the excessive bleach fumes. Her family members all suffer severe health challenges but fail to realize that the improper food combinations and toxic household chemicals are killing them. People stubbornly hold onto their beliefs and feel they are living healthy lives. This family does strongly resist change even though they've been told that it's harmful to their health.

My own husband almost died because of what the medical system was doing to cure him from chronic lymphocytic leukemia. He had to become more determined to follow the nutritional pathway to health, stop listening to the doctors, and start making wise decisions by taking responsibility for his own health. His is a long, sad story, but it may have a happy ending. We are still on the journey.

Cancer is the number one cause of death today, and it needs not to be feared because the cause of cancer is known and prevention can stop it in its tracks before it even occurs in the first place. There is a better way of dealing with cancer than the world's way.

David Servan-Schreiber states that "eighty-five percent are caused by environmental and lifestyle factors. People can control what they eat. Diet is the key factor that determines who gets cancer and who doesn't."[26] Strong food therapy is the best and only way to have a victory over cancer.

It is hard to change. People especially resist change when it comes to their diet. Many people may find it easier to change their religion than changing their diet. People will cling most fiercely to their foods because they use foods for their comfort and pleasure. Those who do change without looking back at what they think they are missing have developed a change in their thinking and attitude, keeping them determined even when the body does get well. Many people may fall back because their thinking remains bad and they continue to be chained to the past. This is called stinking thinking. They have just gone on a diet to relieve the symptoms but not for a consistent and lifelong change. As I heard someone say, "I can help you if you are the person who eats to live, but not if you live to eat." People must be held accountable and responsible for themselves. Disease is a person who selfishly doesn't care about anyone except him/herself. Our lives affect others around us. We are not entities unto ourselves. We have been deceived in the past, but like Jesus said, "And the truth shall set you free!"[27] Physical healing begins and starts from within.

Endnotes

1.   Harvey Diamond, *Living without Pain* (VP Nutrition, 2005), 48.

2.   Diamond, *Living without Pain*, 57.

3.   Chris Padgett, "Silent Attack: Depression The Other Type of SAD," *Hallelujah Acres Health News Magazine* 58 (November–December 2009): 14–15.

4.   George Malkmus, "Grain Does the Body Bad Part 2," *Hallelujah Acres* Internet Health Tip 552, June 17, 2008.

5.   Malkmus, "Grain Does."

6. John R. Lee with Virginia Hopkins, *What Your Doctor May Not Tell You about Menopause"* (Warner Books, 1996), 152.

7. Lee et al., *What Your Doctor*, 153–154.

8. Leon Root and Betty Kelly Sargent, *Beautiful Bones without Hormones* (Gotham Books, 2004), 131.

9. Galatians 6:7 (NKJV).

10. Kristina Anderson, "Gastroesophageal Reflux Disease," *Radiologic Technology* 18, no. 3 (January/February 2010): 251.

11. Anderson, "Gastroesophageal Reflux Disease," 256.

12. Ibid., 252.

13. David Frahm and Anne Frahm, *Reclaim Your Health*, (Putnam, 1995), 82.

14. Malkmus, Hallelujah Acres Diet and Lifestyle Health Tip 566, September 23, 2010.

15. Mary Ann Gower, "Hallelujah Diet Too Late," *Hallelujah Acres Health News Magazine* 54 (March/April 2009): 4.

16. T. C. Fry, "Nature and Purpose of Disease" (lesson 2, a course in Natural Health, Fit for Life Sciences Institute) 2, 37.

17. Olin Idol, "The Cause of Most Cancers Revealed," Hallelujah Acres Diet and Lifestyle Health Tip 598, May 5, 2009.

18. Hallelujah Acres Diet and Lifestyle Health Tip.

19. Michael Donaldson, "Will Johnny Get Cancer…," *Hallelujah Acres Health News* 54 (March/April 2009): 6.

20. Frahm et al., *Reclaim Your Health*, 92.

21. Ibid., 94.

22. Ibid.

23. Andreas Moritz, Hallelujah Acres Diet and Lifestyle Health Tip 567, Sept 30, 2008.

24. Robert Bazell, *Her-2: The Making of Herceptin, A Revolutionary Treatment for Breast Cancer* (Random House, 1998), 11.

25. Google Internet Research, 2010

26. David Servan-Schreiber, "The Anti-Cancer Diet from A Doctor Who Survived Cancer," *Bottom Line Personal* (February 2009): 1–3.

27. John 8:32 (NKJV).

CHAPTER 8

Common Human Illnesses and Diseases

In the past years, there was, in medical terms, diabetes. One kind only. Now there are prediabetic syndrome/condition, type 1, type 2, juvenile, and adult; the list goes on and on. The intake of refined and fragmented junk foods, animal proteins, sodas, and fast foods just continues to add to their problems.

Type 1 diabetes is a condition in which the pancreas fails to produce insulin, and type 2 diabetes, which is more common, is the failure of the cells to respond to insulin. Medical doctors state that these diseases are hereditary, but all that is hereditary is the learned behaviors and patterns of diet and lifestyle, not DNA.

In the normal healthy body, the insulin levels normally rise after eating and then lower again after the digestion of foods. But in the standard American diet, the continued snacking of these junk foods, fats, processed/fragmented foods, sodas, sugars, and the eating of the animal proteins, etc., caused the insulin levels to rise and stay high throughout the day, causing all types of metabolic problems including insulin-resistance in the cells that falls into the range of type 2 diabetes. According to Andrew F. Smith, author of *Encyclopedia of Junk Food and Fast Food*, "an estimated 2.6 percent of Americans are known to have diabetes, and more than 600,000 new cases are diagnosed each year." He states, "According to the Center for Disease Control (CDC) in 2001, 71,372 deaths were attributed to diabetes."[1]

Diabetics have impaired bodies whose circulatory systems are weakened and faulty. They are candidates for amputations, blindness, strokes, heart disease, and other maladies, all because of death by their forks. "According to medical researchers," Elizabeth Church states in her article "'Imaging Diabetes,' the distribution of fat or adipose tissue within the body, where it is deposited, how much, what type of fat is involved, and whether or not this fat has infiltrated the organs plays an important role in the aspect of disease, present and future. Fat or adipose tissue is an active organ that releases various substances into the bloodstream."[2] She cites as an example that liver fat content is associated with insulin resistance. "Liver fat is probably the most dangerous; it creates hypertension, high blood sugar, high triglycerides and low HDL."[2] Belly fat, as seen in a growing number of obese people, predicts cardiovascular disease while an excessive waist circumference with central fat deposits are indicator that the individuals are more prone to type 2 diabetes, metabolic syndrome along with cardiovascular disease. Subcutaneous fat is more prone to preventing the flow of lipids to other areas of the body.

The heart is an adaptable organ, capable of gaining if needed, energy from various sources from the resilient body. But in people who are obese and diabetic, it tends to become burdened; and as fat tends to also surround the organ, its vessels may tend to squeeze the heart, cutting off its circulation. It thus creates heart attacks and enlargement of the heart, thereby shrinking the vessels. Arteriosclerosis, which is a weakening and hardening of the arteries, is also more prevalent in the obese and diabetic person.

The children whose lifestyles mimic their parents by fault will end up with the same diseases, if not worse, because theirs started at a young age. Obesity and diabetes, is so much more prevalent in the youth of today. "Today's teens," states Andrew Smith, "drink twice as much carbonated sodas as milk and as a result only 19 percent of girls get the recommended amount of calcium."[3] Many people prefer high sugar and high fat diets to the healthier ones and favored sodas instead of fruit juice, fruit or pure water. These healthier foods that reduce cancer, heart disease, and osteoporosis tend to be ignored. The children prefer to fill up on junk foods; therefore, they will eat far fewer healthier foods. The parents are not teaching their children good health behaviors but unhealthy ones that destroy their bodies. Obesity in children, as well as adults, is on the rise. George Malkmus, *Hallelujah Acres* author and founder, states, "Our general indicator of overall health of the people of any nation is the percentage of the overweight and obese population as compared to the population that is in the healthy weight range."[4] The US Department of Health and Human Services maintains, claims Olin Idol in his research, that "sixty-five percent of the population between the ages of 20–74 were overweight in the years of 1999–2002, and 31.1 percent were considered obese. Also, among children 6–11, 15.8 percent were overweight, and according to a report from MSNBC.com, it was recently reported that 2 million US children 12–19 have a prediabetic condition linked to obesity."[5] This obesity is due to inactivity, sitting before computers, playing video, computer games instead of getting active and running around and playing outdoors. This condition is a risk to diabetes and cardiovascular problems. This generation of children seems to have more serious health challenges that those say forty–fifty years ago. In fact, leukemia is the number one killer of our children because of the drugs, vaccines, and chemicals in the diet of junk foods. Andrew Smith states, "For the first time in history, the number of overweight people in the world rivals that of the underfed."[6] Other countries' obesity rates are increasing rapidly. In China, Andrew Smith continues as an example, "Their overweight population increased from 10–15 percent of the population in just three years. In Brazil and Colombia, the obesity rate is now about 40 percent of their entire population. In the United States during the last fifty years, the Americans are continuously gaining weight; 61 percent of Americans are now judged overweight. And even more alarming is that 25 percent of American children are now considered overweight. Some medical statistics now show that 248,000 Americans die prematurely because of obesity."[6] The primary cause of death is smoking and the secondary cause of death is obesity.

The rise in obesity is due to the rise in the fast food/junk food industries. These companies have been targeted as responsible for the increase in obesity. The government is getting involved with having these companies come up with healthier foods like they really can and should. They have been ordered to cut the trans fats, MSG, and extreme high sugars, but cutting isn't deleting. The government says a minimum certain amount is okay and may or may not be added onto the label. The problem is all of these foods contribute to the increasing cases of this disease or the development of this disease. These companies make this inexpensive, high-calorie, and high-fat food very accessible through their advertising agents, especially targeting the children who watch TV. Even more alarming statistics are coming forth. Andrew Smith writes, "Over the past three decades, the rate of obesity has more than doubled among preschool children and adolescents and tripled among school age children. And certain nationalities are more prevalent than others with high obesity rates, but all are affected."[6]

Statistics now indicate that 65–70 percent of Americans are now overweight or obese with more than 25 percent of children and adolescents being overweight. Children should not be overweight because that is considered child abuse. Inactivity is the main cause for obesity. No one wants to exercise, take walks or engage in any activity except to be driven somewhere, play on computers, or watch TV. It is so sad to see all of this happening. The inactivity, along with the effects of the fast food diet, are damaging to these young people. According to the Hallelujah Acres (3/2/04) Archives Health Tip number 328, "In 1996 children ate only one in 10 meals from fast foods restaurants. By 1997, that ratio was one to three. Overweight is now the most common medical condition of childhood."[7] It seems that these young people are now getting "old people's diseases."

I had a patient, a thirty-three-year-old male who had his colon surgically removed because of diverticulitis and irritable bowel syndrome. A meat-and-potatoes, soda-and-beer-drinking guy, He didn't eat any fruits and vegetables. "You are what you eat," as the saying goes, and he definitely was an image of poor and damaged health. All he had to do instead of the surgery would be to change his diet and lifestyle. The mother of a work associate of mine also had the same disease as this young man, but she did change her diet to a much healthier one and is free of the effects and symptoms of her disease, and best of all, she still has her colon.

With all the diet books, surgeries, drugs for weight loss, and low-fat foods, why are people continuing to become even fatter and sicker? People want their cake and eat it too. Diets are only a temporary fix. If a person wants to gain weight, just go on a diet, especially a yo-yo diet. One will most definitely gain weight. I did it for years before I adopted the natural hygiene lifestyle.

Weight-loss is a big moneymaker. Everyone has a new diet book out, but of course, none of it works, and everyone has failed to inform the public. The only way anyone will lose weight and keep it off is by getting rid of *all* of the processed foods in their diets and eat a diet of whole, raw, healthy fruit, vegetable, sprouts, seeds, and nuts and also include exercise in their lifestyle. When the cause of obesity and disease is taken away, a person will be trim and healthy and continue to stay that way.

Andrew Smith and Scripps Health System in San Diego, California, both state that of the American population, 61 percent are judged to be overweight.[8] Children are suffering even more today than their parents with the rise of fast food and junk food industries. According to Andrew Smith, obesity in children and adolescents in the past twenty years has doubled with 25 percent of the children considered overweight.[9]

It is insanity. Those who are severely obese will have even more weight-related diseases and require more expensive treatments in comparison to people who are just fat.

Endnotes

1. Andrew F. Smith, *Encyclopedia of Junk Food and Fast Food,* (Greenwood, 2006), 5.
2. Elizabeth Church, "Imaging Diabetes," *Radiologic Technology* 80, no. 4 (March/April 2009): 350.
3. Smith, *Encyclopedia of Junk,* 4.

4. George Malkmus, "Hallelujah Diet—America's Best Weight Loss Program," Hallelujah Acres Health Tip, January 5, 2010.

5. Olin Idol, "The Solution to the SAD State of America's Declining Health," *Back to the Garden Health News* 40 (September/October 2006).

6. Smith, *Encyclopedia of Junk*, 201–202.

7. George Malkmus, "Sixty-four Percent Are Overweight or Obese," Hallelujah Acres Health Tip 328, March 2, 2004.

8. Daniella Blau and Alisa Scherban, Scripps Hospital website, Internal internet page for employees for health and wellness. Wellness.com, 1–3.

9. Smith, *Encyclopedia of Junk*, 17.

CHAPTER 9

Diabetes

According to Beverly McMillian, "Diabetes is one of the most common and serious endocrine disorders."[1] Elizabeth J. Church stated, "Diabetes is a metabolic disorder in which the body fails to produce or properly use insulin, a hormone needed to convert sugar, starches, and other foods into energy."[2] The body will break down the majority of the food that we eat into glucose to be poured out into the bloodstream as the body's main source of fuel for cellular energy. For the body to make energy, its one hundred trillion cells must get their fuel from a very simple food source (glucose), something that can be quickly broken down to be utilized efficiently. The simplest form is from a raw plant-based diet of living foods that are very simple to digest and assimilate. These foods should form the main portion of the diet because they include all of the important nutrients for the optimal health of the body.

Glucose levels of the blood are regulated by the hormone insulin, released by the pancreas in small amounts as needed. The liver helps in removing about two-thirds of the glucose from the blood circulation and stores the glucose and converts it to glycogen for later use. The blood glucose levels rise to an increased level that stimulates the pancreas to release insulin that allows the glucose to enter in and to fuel the cells of the body. The insulin permits glucose to leave the bloodstream and rapidly fuel and feed the cells for energy, bringing the blood sugar levels back to normal. "When insulin is insufficient or the body is unable to use it properly, the amount of glucose in the blood increases to unhealthy levels (hyperglycemia), and cells are starved for energy," concludes Church.[2] Over time, the high blood glucose levels will damage the blood vessels and capillaries and nerves. When the pancreas stimulates too much insulin, too much blood sugar enters the cells, causing the blood glucose levels to become too low, resulting in low blood sugar or hypoglycemia. Diabetics do have an increased risk of arteriosclerosis and calcifications of the arteries and other large blood vessels. More fats are broken down when insulin blood levels are low and these accumulate in the vessels and heart. The capillaries are thickened especially in the areas of skin and skeletal muscles; the most evident being the renal glomerulus cells; (these are the blood filtering areas of the kidney) and of the eye. Neuropathy, which is injury to the nerves and, according to Susan Hazard, is "associated with destruction of the myelin sheath of nerve tissue and nerve cell degeneration. This involves sensory and motor nerves, nerve roots, the spinal cord, and the autonomic nervous system. Affected nerves show basal membrane thickening similar to the capillary abnormalities."[3] Those with diabetes will suffer the trauma of a damaged body with poor circulation; amputations, blindness, kidney failure, and neuropathy. Diabetics whose conditions are not controlled will also suffer from very impaired healing with persistent sores and foot ulcers. If the blood sugar drops too low, for example, with an insulin overdose, the nervous system is severely affected. The brain, which relies on the glucose, has been deprived of it and cannot continue on with its functions. All the sugar has entered into the cells and the brain is depleted; thus, the person lapses into a coma. The person is given a candy bar or some pasteurized juice and all is well. Or is it really? There isn't any established cure. Did the diabetes cause the damage or was the body already in a compromised state enough to accept another disease, diabetes?

This is not just a one-organ disease; it affects the entire body. For example, treating hyperglycemia does not produce health in any way. The treatment of insulin does nothing to take away the causes, heal, or cure the damaged body "The real cause of diabetes came before the deficiency of insulin," says, Susan Hazard. "It's the excesses, deficiencies and poisonous habits."[3] The excesses include stress, worrying, overeating, overworking, etc. The deficiencies are lack of exercise, lack of sleep, improper foods, lack of sunshine and fresh air, lack of emotional serenity, etc. Lastly, the poisonous habits add the rest of the lethal burden to the already toxic load of the body. These include the poisons of overabundance of animal proteins and fats, alcohol, sodas, coffee, refined sugars, and flours, processed foods with the chemical additives and preservatives, cigarettes and the drugs to mask the symptoms of the already damaged health.

There are various forms of diabetes, and the most common ones are Type 1 and Type 2 diabetes. Type 1 is known as "juvenile" and "insulin-dependent" diabetes. Church accounts that there are "an estimated 5 percent to 10 percent of all diabetic Americans."[4] The medical professionals claim it is genetically-inclined. The most preventable, Type 2 diabetes, is referred to as "adult-onset" or "non-insulin dependent" diabetes, and this one accounts for the most often diagnosed of the diabetic population. Church stated that "at least 246 million of the world's adult population have diabetes mellitus. In 2025, that figure is expected to reach 380 million. Presently, approximately 6 percent of global deaths are due to diabetes. This all too often represent 'lifestyle related disease' and its consequences are largely preventable." [4] Stressful situations may also affect the blood glucose levels. In fact, adrenaline and other adrenal hormones boost blood sugar levels.

The medical community has indeed understood that Western lifestyle, in its sedentary ways, processed foods and fat-related foods can and will lead to certain types of diabetes and the consequent pathologies and diseases. Medical costs are soaring but, people still are not being educated or given any direction how to prevent their diseases or how to experience healthy and symptom-free living. Patients go to the doctors with specific symptoms and, instead of education on nutritional and health aspects, the doctors use the opposite, "What is your symptom? We have a drug for that!" Most doctors do not believe that food or the change of diet has anything to do with diseases, and will convey that to their patients. People are not encouraged at all. Patients are told to consume a lot of protein-enriched foods, burdening the digestive system and creating more of a toxic overload. The digestion of proteins is the most difficult for the body to accomplish. It is very important for the diabetic person to consume foods that do not require significant energy and must contain little, if any, toxins or chemicals. The standard American diet doesn't provide any nutrients or healthy fats that are necessary to maintain healthy cell membranes. These diets consist of the overabundance of unhealthy animal proteins and hydrogenated fats that just slowly block the membranes of the cells, blocking the nutrients from entering the cell and the wastes from exiting the cells.

Energy is needed for healing processes of the body, and the higher the toxicity, the more impaired the body becomes. All refined foods must be avoided because of the chemical content, which only creates more of a problem on the already challenged body. The required fat in the diet would be found in nuts and avocados, which are to be eaten moderately a few times a week. The carbohydrates found in fresh raw fruits and vegetables are easily digested and assimilated; they also contain all the base minerals and other nutrients so important for the healing of the body. It may be necessary at first to eliminate sweet fruits such as bananas and dried fruits at least until a higher degree of heath is achieved. According to Rev. George Malkmus, "In order to construct healthy cell membranes, the cells need the nutrients and omega 3 fatty acids found in plant-source foods. These foods keep the insulin-glucose pathways into the cell functioning normally so the insulin can easily slip just the right amount of sugar into the cell to satisfy its energy needs."[5]

The key to ridding the body of the symptoms is to eliminate the causes of diabetes and disease: the chemicals, the poor diets, and destructive lifestyles. Rev. George Malkmus states, "As the person stops placing all that fat into their body and starts a 100 percent raw plant-based diet, the fat that was blocking the insulin begins to fall off the cells. Almost like magic, within a few days to a few months, blood sugar levels for most type 2 diabetics will begin to normalize, and soon there will be no more need for additional insulin."[5] The insulin levels must be monitored, and when there is a need to cut down, it must be done very gradually.

When given the proper conditions, the body will begin the natural healing processes if the body is not beyond the point of destruction; health can then be restored. When a healthier lifestyle is adhered to, people will be able to eradicate/eliminate from their disease. A diet that is biologically adapted to the body is best for disease-free, optimal health. Our bodies are fearfully and wonderfully made, so let's take care of them! A word of caution. It is best if a diabetic, when desiring a change of diet, to have the insulin levels monitored carefully by a healthcare professional. If the previous levels of insulin continue with the new diet change and beginning an exercise program, the blood sugar levels may drop too low. It is important that the insulin be adjusted accordingly as the blood sugar levels fall.

Despite the ominous increase of diabetes in the world, there is one success story that may set the standard in the future. Cuba has instituted an organic farming program that has led to a tremendous decrease in diabetes on the island.

In the early 1990s, Cuba lost a lot of money once given by the Soviet Union as subsidies. The nation once imported most of its food but could no longer afford to. Then the Cuban government came up with the idea of promoting local organic farms.

Today, the Cuban organic farms are a complete success. There are thousands of these all over the country from rural areas to central Havana. The government purchases a certain amount of crops and allows the farmers to sell anything over that amount privately. What once began as an economic necessity has turned into the finest anti-diabetes activity in the world. Today, Cubans have only ⅛ the cases of diabetes as Americans. And that number is decreasing. From the first grade on, Cuban students are made aware of the deadly effects of diabetes. Venezuela has begun a program based on the Cuban model, and that country is starting to see a decrease in the number of diabetes cases.

Endnotes

1. Beverly McMillian, "Diabetes," in *The Illustrated Atlas of the Human Body* (Argosy, 2008), 122.
2. Elizabeth J. Church, "Imaging Diabetes," *Radiologic Technology* 80, no. 4 (2009): 341.
3. Susan Hazard, "Sugar and Carbohydrate Metabolism Disease" (lesson 73, a course in Natural Health, Fit for Life Sciences Institute), 1534.
4. Church, "Imaging Diabetes," 341, 344.
5. George Malkmus, "Diabetes—A Natural Approach," Health Tip, *The Hallelujah Acres News Magazine* 706 (2011): 3–4.

CHAPTER 10

Obesity

In her article, "Medical Imaging's Role in Bariatric Surgery," Anne Mattarella, BS, ELS, states, "Obesity is now declared a national epidemic in the United States, which is now the fattest country in the world. Obesity has become the biggest threat to one's health. It causes more health problems than either smoking or alcohol use." April Reynolds also indicates that it has become the number one health malady in her article, "Obesity and Medical Imaging Challenges." She states "that *68 percent* of Americans are overweight and nearly half are obese." She added the dire statistics that "obesity is thought now to be the second-leading cause of preventable death in the United States, claiming an estimated 300,000 lives each year; smoking and alcohol abuse rank just one step higher."[2] Obesity has now increased from 60 percent–70 percent between 1991 and 2000, these authors claim. The "normal BMI (body mass index) is 18.5–24.9, with overweight at 25.9–29.9, while obese is 30.0–39.9 and morbidly obese is greater than 40." [2]

According to April Reynolds, "Although much has been done—especially in the United States—to raise awareness about the dangers of smoking and alcohol abuse, little has been done to publicly combat the problem of obesity,"[2] She also questions the concept that "according to research, there is a disconnect between the rising obesity rate and the strain on the medical resources, and the obesity education available to health care practitioners."[2] It has now been estimated, claims Reynolds, "that one-third of the adult population is classified as obese, and there are no signs of slowing down."[2]

These doctors are at a standstill concerning health education to the public. It seems that the food manufacturers, made up of the junk good/fast food industries, have hindered the education because they would lose out in their profits. One cannot make these food-stuffs healthy for consumption and nutrient assimilation into the human body. It is *impossible*. The processing alone kills all possible nutrition even if it started off as a real food item. Inserting chemicals only adds more to the toxic value. Then a continued lifestyle of these products will only interfere with the chemical and hormone balance, thereby, this accumulation will not only add to the weight problem, but also to the disease issue.

The excess burden on the body only contributes to the diseases of diabetes, heart disease, hypertension, strokes, cancers, gout, sleep apnea, as well as sleep deprivation, respiratory problems, gastrointestinal problems, and excessive weight gain. Today, obesity ranks along smoking and chronic alcoholism as the major contributors of chronic and impaired health conditions, and is thought to age the body roughly twenty–thirty years. Even obese children have the arteries of adults, and they are only kids. How sad and abusive for these victims. Obesity in childhood contributes to the same health challenges as adults who are obese—type 2 diabetes, asthma, sleep apnea, and cardiovascular disease. April Reynolds states, "Considering that only 5 percent of obese adolescents will be able to lose weight successfully as adults if weight loss is not achieved during adolescence,"[2] therefore young people run the risk of carrying weight-related issues into adulthood.

These young people will also carry psychological problems related to childhood obesity in their adult years. Children can be cruel and peer abuse can indeed traumatize the obese child, thereby making him/her lose their self-esteem. This could develop into depression issues later on. There can be a lot of lifetime struggles that could have been prevented by developing healthier diets and lifestyles. Because the fault lies with the parents, it is considered a form of child abuse.

April Reynolds, states, "It is estimated that 25 to 30 percent of adults in the United States are completely sedentary."[2] Because of this fast food lifestyle with the cheap processed foods/junk foods, the toxins accumulate within the body. The body's cleansing process is hindered, the body's systems slow down, and the person becomes even more tired and sedentary, thus the squirrel cage effect. Consequently, the weight of the obese child will also increase. The fatter one becomes, the more good health reduces and diseases develop. You've got the picture, and it's a very sad one indeed.

The inner respiratory system is pushed around because of the excess accumulated fat; therefore the obese person will end up suffering from sleep apnea. Sleep deprivation alters the body's hormones, resulting in amplifying one's appetite, especially for high carbohydrate foods. The lack of sleep and poor eating creates a loss of nerve energy, therefore compounding the sedentary lifestyle even more. Some of the ways of gaining *adequate sleep* would be to start an exercise program, and walking is the simplest way to begin. In fact, even the wheelchair bound (those with improper diet and destructive lifestyle, not traumatic injuries) can devise an exercise regimen into their lives. Proper cleansing of the body is to be done throughout the mornings by eating only fruit from 4:00 a.m. until 12:00 noon. Fruits only. It can be eaten whole or in freshly made smoothies. Lunches should consist of fresh raw produce salads and dinners should be a large salad with a limited amount of cooked food, nothing processed just fresh foods. The last meal of the day should be consumed at least two to three hours before bedtime.

There are many individuals who believe the hygienic system with its fresh raw fruits, vegetables, nuts, and seeds and self-discipline are just way too difficult; but someday, they will have to wake up because their way is taking their bodies into the depths of destruction with all of their diseases. Many will continue to regain their lost weight because they can't give up the lifestyle that shackles them to it.

"Studies have shown similarities in the brain chemistry of people who are obese and those addicted to drugs. A compulsion to eat and a loss of control are core factors in obesity. The reason is the imbalance of dopamine in the brain," claims April Reynolds.[2] Dopamine is the "feel good center of the brain," Pierce J. Howard, PhD, states in his book *The Owner's Manual to the Brain*. "Drugs now available for appetite control treat symptoms, not causes. They do not address the root causes of craving and satiety, but rather provide the effect of pleasure from having eaten, and exciting these pleasure centers, thereby covering up the cravings."[3] Most of the processed foods consumed on the standard American diet are so filled with chemicals, preservatives, and additives; and these are the bandits that rob the body of its nutrients, adding toxins that play havoc with the body's hormones, which create the horrible addictions and cravings, intensifying the dilemma even further. Chemicals are drugs to the body and are treated as a poison.

If the body loses chemicals, as with any drug, it loses control, and the addiction heightens. It's a lost cause. The irresistible cravings will continue to take over and overwhelm then the person loses, but not weight; that just keeps on gaining. Drs. Robert and Elizabeth McCarter claim, "Overeating is probably the most difficult bad habit to overcome. In fact, it is said that only about 5 percent of the obese are successful in reducing their weight to what it should be."[4]

"Overeating is the chief cause of all diseases," states Hannah Allen. "And disease shortens and destroys life."[5]

Obesity is not only damaging for the people and their health but also within the medical realm. It will be improbable to get proper treatment because of the extra pounds of fat that get in the way. For example, there are weight limits for hospital equipment, and often times, people will exceed them. In our hospital, there was a particular patient whose weight surpassed the equipment limits, and to get the exam ordered by his doctor, he had to be transferred to the city zoo.

In radiology departments there are severe challenges with the diagnostic imaging, such as, under-penetration of X-rays and having to do X-rays in quadrants to get all the areas to view, which means extra radiation for the patient, and radiologists who are unable to give an adequate correct diagnosis, also a body habitus unable to fit into the CT or MRI machines.

People don't seem to realize that obesity is a consequence of one's own destructive diet and lifestyle. The body is rebelling against all of the foreign and destructive chemicals and substances. The processed foods with all of the chemicals and additives that are a part of the standard American diet are very addictive; thus, this way of eating will continue to add on the pounds. People just don't become fat; it's a process, quite like the statistics of "one will gain five pounds a year." Living the standard American diet will make that a reality. The fortunate part in my own case was I did not gain hundreds before I woke up to what I was doing to myself, but it was still too much for me. I hated myself the way I was, and that was my dilemma, my turning point.

The treatment of obesity is a big business at the expense of too many desperate and hopeless people. Everything has been tried, and they are still left wanting. Nothing they have tried has made them any thinner, only fatter. I came to the sad conclusion in my dilemma that if I had never dieted in the first place, I wouldn't be as fat as I was; and all the preservatives, additives, and processed foods not only kept me from losing weight, but they were all making me fatter. I gained weight not necessarily because of how much I ate but because of what I ate. I do know that the Weight Watcher's program now has accepted that all raw fresh fruits and vegetables are free foods: have no points or calories. Eat as much of these as one wants, and weight won't be an issue. But eat manmade products or cooked foods and one will be destined to always be fat and will remain that way, maybe even fatter. The hardcore truth is that it has to become a determined discipline to come out of the prison of obesity.

Susan Hazard, PhD, states, "A person who habitually overeats is no less an addict than the alcoholic."[6] Overeating wears out the vital energy of the body through overstimulation because of the chemicals that the body is trying to eliminate as well as the overworking of the digestive system, the organs, the heart, and the endocrine system. These additives, colorings, preservatives, and other toxic chemicals generated by these foods, which are consumed, put a strain on the entire body, as well as depleting the health and vitality of the individual. Most people are addicted to these chemically-induced foods, thus the problem of overconsumption. The overeating of these food types disables most of those who indulge; tending to make them gluttons who will die prematurely from their teeth. "Constant overeating," insists Hannah Allen, "will gradually distend the stomach, after which the person does not feel satisfied until he eats to fill the distended stomach. Constant overeating may also delay the restoration of the body's normal ability to digest the food comfortably."[7]

Clent Manich was one of these people who continued to gain more and more. He topped off at 447 pounds when he was measured for his wedding tuxedo in 2005. He suffered many health challenges that were related to his weight. He wrote in his article, "The Incredible Shrinking Man" that his pancreas was shutting down, he was suffering from chest pains, and he thought he was dying. Then Manich says, "In 2006, my triglycerides were over 6,000, and the doctors couldn't even register my sugars because they were over 600. My AI-C (a test that measures glucose levels over several months) was 13.5 and normal range is between 4 and 7."[8] He also had type 2 diabetes and was told that if he didn't change his eating habits, he would be lucky to be alive in four years. The more he tried to diet or exercise, the more weight he gained, and he became very depressed. His turning point came when he injured himself on his treadmill and he needed to see a physical therapist and chiropractor who happened to be a Hallelujah Acres health minister. The Hallelujah diet and exercise program helped to motivate Clent to lose fifty-two pounds in eight weeks. He went back up more than four hundred pounds. Feeling like he not only let himself and his family down but also the doctor, he didn't go back for about a year because he was too embarrassed. He then was told by the doctor about a 525-pound woman who was successful at her weight loss with green smoothies (see recipes). "She lost 127 pounds in about six months." Speaking on behalf of his own journey and experience, Clent concluded, "If she could do it, I can do it."[8] The smoothies helped him to get beyond the cravings for meat, and he did lose one hundred pounds in fourteen weeks. He also uses BarleyMax (see resources) as a part of the Hallelujah Acres diet. (See www.hacres.com for diet information and BarleyMax information). He claims that his skin shrank along with him by following these regimen. He had no hanging skin even after he lost two hundred pounds. He concluded, "When you combine BarleyMax with the green smoothies—all that chlorophyll—I'm telling you, it really does make your skin shrink."[8] He is his own testimony.

Exercising as well as implementing the new eating program are the only ways the weight will come off and continue to stay off. Clent himself decided to eat only a 100 percent raw plant diet for generally eating 15 percent cooked food for the evening meal is less stressful to the body, but he wanted the weight to come off faster. Clent explained the big problem: "When you unload that amount of fat, that fast, it's really hard on your liver because fat is stored up acid. So when you lose the fat, all this acid is released into your bloodstream—I needed to take digestive enzymes to support my liver."[8] This man's approach had its challenges, but it was a natural approach. The decision to stick with this lifestyle was his alone, and a person can and will fight all the demons along the way: demons of old habits, built-up toxins, the psychological cravings, the addictions to the self-destructive foods, no motivation, and the desire to quit. The strong will survive, and sticking with it becomes an achievement of total and optimal health.

Hannah Allen states, "Frost and Sullivan Inc., a national market research company, noted that 70 million overweight individuals are willing to do almost anything to shed some weight. They use appetite suppressants, obesity prescriptions, reducing pills, diet books, mechanical devices, health spas, and even surgery, such as intestinal bypass operations, cutting of the vagus nerve, and gastric stapling."[9] Yes, anything except changing their diet and lifestyle from the processed, junk foods/fast foods diet to a healthier one of fresh raw produce and daily exercise.

There are many different treatments for obese people to give them a glimmer of hope of weight reduction. There are many that are not wise pathways to follow, and some will lead to serious consequences.

There are medications for weight loss. "The estimated annual total cost for these in the United States alone has been $33 billion," states April Reynolds. "Their safety has not been established. Many in the past years have died due to their serious side effects."[10]

There are about three types of bariatric surgical techniques that many will opt for. They are restrictive, malabsorptive, and a combination taken from both the restrictive and the malabsorptive. These surgical procedures are said to be the most effective way in controlling weight because dieting alone can be ineffective. Most of the time it's because it conforms to the ways of the world since the standard American diet will make one gain weight on a continual basis. The diet the world lives on overfeeds and doesn't nourish the human body. The cravings that are experienced indicate that the body needs proper nourishment and is not getting it. These cravings will continue until the body is fed whole raw living foods that God created, not man's invention. We will go more into this later.

Gastric banding was first introduced in 1993 as a less-invasive surgical procedure for morbid obesity. During a laparoscopic procedure, a silicone band is placed around the gastric fundus of the stomach. This band can be tightened or loosened to control the size of the food passage via a subcutaneous port. The band is adjusted by an injection of sodium chloride through the skin into the port. These band procedures are not without risks.

This band has been designed to create a full-feeling from slowly eating small amounts of food and thereby learning new eating patterns. The main idea behind the band initially was behavior modification. This was a way that is meant to teach/train an individual to eat less, thereby losing weight and developing new habits for a lifetime of health.

The person who has a gastric band needs to chew the foods slowly to an almost liquid state for this bolus to enter into the stomach without any mishap. After all, the band does not expand like the esophagus does. This practice will prevent foods from getting caught and creating an obstruction. Breads and meats should not be eaten, as these types of foods cannot be chewed until liquid as raw produce can. Vegetables can be juiced or blended if needed to gain nutrients, because the eating of raw carrots or other hard vegetables may prove to be challenging. Many times, doctors may suggest to their gastric patients eat cooked foods as these are softer foods that can easily go through the band. The only problem is that the person will tend to overeat for lack of nutrition. The body will continue to set up cravings for more food until the body has its nutritional levels satisfied with living foods. Only fresh raw produce; seeds; nuts; fresh, distilled water fit the bill.

Once the amount of food is decreased, the body weight will also decrease. The band will need adjustments occasionally as it will tend to loosen, creating more food intake and weight gain. This type of procedure was created as a crutch device to help people learn to control their food intake and to become aware of their body's feeling of satiety.

It does have some risks or complications. The one that can create the most dangerous mechanical malfunction is the band itself slipping out of place. Another complication may include too tight of an adjustment, stopping the food from entering the stomach. The one that most people do not seem to understand is that their food choices must be altered. People think that they can continue eating the same foods as they were eating before their surgery, only in smaller portions. The foods that are consumed need to be chewed very well, almost to a liquid state not to be caught and stuck in the tightened band. Some foods, animal proteins for example, cannot be chewed well enough to liquefy and swallow to pass through the restricted area of the stomach. The meats can then become caught in the esophagus and can be detrimental to the person's wellbeing. The person must be very careful and slowly eat his/her food and be aware that the body is going to be limited in some ways. The learning of new ways of eating, the way the body responds, and also becoming aware of the satiety of the stomach are to be included in the new way of life.

According to *Radiologic Technology Journal*, gastric bypass is the most effective and the most common of the gastric procedures.[11] It can also be the most dangerous for the human body. The bypass procedure can be performed via open surgery or the laparoscopic method, thereby bypassing the stomach, the duodenum, and a small portion of the jejunum, thus reducing the area in contact with food and the time it takes to absorb food, resulting in a decrease in the amount of calories and the nutrients that are absorbed. There are several variations to this, but all these achieve the same result: bypass the stomach. This is malabsorptive because the stomach is made smaller or bypassed entirely. Therefore, no enzymes or nutrients are gained at all during the digestive process. The body is not going to be fed properly.

The digestion of starches and glucose begins in the mouth with the mastication and insalivation of the food. This process then signals for the digestive juices, which are present in the saliva and in the gastric secretions and in the walls of the stomach, to begin their work. These digestive glands supply the different enzymes needed for the foods to digest and pass through the rest of the alimentary canal. The stomach allows for the digestion of proteins and fats. Hannah Allen gives a brief review of an important aspect of the digestive process. "Gastric secretion is continuous (except during fevers, gastric inflammation, pain, or strong emotions; fasting is indicated when any of these conditions are present)." She concludes, "Hunger and the sight, smell, taste or thought of food stimulates gastric secretion."[12] The stomach secretes about three pints of gastric juice every twenty-four hours and usually half is required for a hearty meal. So if a person eats more than two big meals a day, the body is going to be depleted, and in the case of those who underwent a bypass procedure where there isn't any stomach, the body becomes seriously depleted.

The cellulose (fiber of the raw produce) provides the bulk to move the foods through the elimination of food residues. Processed foods and cooked foods do not contain any cellulose or nutrients of any kind.

As the stomach empties its liquid portion into the duodenum, it meets with a very acid fluid. This semiliquid mixture then proceeds further into the small intestine where it meets up with an alkaline mixture consisting of pancreatic juice along with bile and other digestive enzymes. (The bile is secreted by the liver and stored in the gallbladder for the emulsion of fats.) Hannah Allen states, "All of the absorption should occur by the time the food passes through the small intestine, and the residue proceeds into the large intestine (the colon)."[12]

This is a very brief overview of the physiological course of the digestive process. From this, one can see the importance of having all the organs of the body's processes. In fact, when any organs are removed, the body will suffer severe challenges. It all works together for optimal digestion. Malabsorption occurs, resulting in loss of nutrients, diarrhea, and severe toxicosis. Loss of health is a result. Dumping syndrome is an occurrence of any surgical procedure particularity with a gastrectomy. The symptoms include weakness, nausea, vomiting, sweating, and palpitation soon after eating. Doctors may recommend a high protein diet and eating many small meals throughout the day consisting of dry foods such as breads and crackers. This generally makes a person feel worse. A wiser, more natural approach would be to eat frequently meals of juicy fruits, chewing them until liquefied, blended salads (these are the usual salad fixings put into a blender and sipped very slowly, allowing the mixture to mix with the saliva), and freshly extracted raw vegetable juices, made daily in a juicer (see recipe for salads and vegetable juices). (Mostly organic carrot juice with leafy green vegetables, celery, tomatoes, beets, etc.) This is to be consumed at least twice daily, eight–sixteen ounces each time, sipped very slowly. These raw fruits and vegetables will allow the body to gain nutrients and optimal health. After a while, the body will compensate for its loss, but ideal health generally is not obtained after organs have been removed. If the nutrients aren't given through the raw produce, the person may end up suffering a lifetime as a digestive cripple all for the sake of losing weight.

I had a client to whom I suggested the nutrient value of the raw juicing after his bypass procedure. He followed it faithfully (hope he continues) and claimed that he felt great and was healing well when I saw him two weeks later. The fresh raw juicing is the only way the body will receive any nutrients, continue to heal, and experience any kind of health and wellness.

Most people who have these procedures want to continue eating their previous diet and will end up with a different set of problems. They may lose a little weight because of the decrease in the food intake, but then some have gained it back and more by not following and adhering to the guidelines. One must be willing to change his/her diet and lifestyle that continue to add unwanted pounds. That will be the only way to lose weight and, most importantly, keep it off. In my own experience, my weight would yo-yo every time I started to eat any processed foods. I didn't get it right away until I gained ten pounds in a short period. It's an important awareness that helps keep me diligent. After all, I can't afford to keep several sizes of clothes. I'll stick with just one.

Once the additives, refined sugars, and flours and chemicals are stopped, the toxins that the processed foods produced will still need to be eliminated, and until these poisons are gone, a person may continue to experience the cravings and addictions as part of the withdrawal process. To expedite the healing process, the drinking of fresh vegetable juices will be very important as well as having a stick-to-it attitude. Do not quit! When one begins to lose the excess weight besides dealing with the cravings and withdrawals, all the psychological issues just don't go away. There is also the lifetime of demons that may intensify and will have to be combated. No one wants to confront withdrawals, the physiological ones as well as the emotional baggage that has also been carried along. It's going to be a process, a continued one. It's wise to begin to look at it as a journey. A person will begin to get in touch with his/her body and the emotions that have been continually buried under the pounds of food that have been stuffed to quiet them. Just take it one day at a time. After all, the fat didn't just happen, and it's not going to come off overnight. The fears will go away. After all, this too shall pass. The time is now to be in awe and revere the body that was made by God. After all, I have given Him my eating problem, and he's in charge of the journey.

Endnotes

1. Anne Mattarella, "Medical Imaging's Role in Bariatric Surgery," *Radiologic Technology* 82, no. 4 (2011): 348.
2. April Reynolds, "Obesity and Medical Imaging Challenges," *Radiologic Technology* 82, no. 3 (2011): 219.

3. Pierce J. Howard, *Owner's Manual to the Brain* (Bard, 2006), 142.

4. Robert and Elizabeth McCarter, "Methods for Inducing a Lifestyle Change" (lesson 91, Natural Health course, Fit for Life Sciences Institute, 1899.

5. Hannah Allen, "Overeating, Fasting Fanaticism and Diet Fanaticism" (lesson 44, Natural Health course, Fit for Life Sciences Institute), 1001.

6. Susan Hazard, "Natural Approach to Overcoming Addictions" (lesson 69, Natural Health course, Fit for Life Sciences Institute), 1458.

7. Hannah Allen, "How to Break a Fast/After a Fast" (lesson 48, Natural Health course, Fit for Life Sciences Institute), 1067.

8. Clent Manich, "The Incredible Shrinking Man," *Hallelujah Acres Health News Magazine* 53, 1–2.

CHAPTER 11

Life's Lessons

The Serenity Prayer

God grant me the serenity to accept the things
I cannot change,
Courage to change the things I can,
And the wisdom to know the difference.

The Twelve Steps of the Alcoholics Anonymous Program[1]

1. We admitted we were powerless over alcohol and that our lives had become unmanageable.
2. Came to believe that a Power greater than ourselves could restore us to sanity.
3. Made a decision to turn our will and lives over to the care of God as we understood Him.
4. Made a searching and fearless inventory of ourselves.
5. Admitted to God, to ourselves, and to another human being the exact nature of our wrongs.
6. Were entirely ready to have God remove all these defects of character.
7. Humbly asked Him to remove our shortcomings.

8. Made a list of all persons we had harmed, and became willing to make amends to them all.
9. Made direct amends to such people wherever possible, except when to do so would injure them or others.
10. Continued to take personal inventory and when we were wrong promptly admitted it.
11. Sought through prayer and meditation to improve our conscious contact with God as we understood Him, praying only for knowledge of His will for us, and the power to carry that out.
12. Having a spiritual awakening as the result of these steps, we tried to carry this message to alcoholics and to practice these principles in all our affairs.

My life lessons are based on the Serenity Prayer and the principles of the Twelve Steps of AA. I know you are going to ask, "Why did you include *this* chapter in your book?" Good question. Because this is the *only way* I've gotten through the last thirty-two years of my life without quitting. Yes, I have wanted to dive off the face of the Earth when things got tough and the addictions were getting the best of me. I had the advantage of going through the doors of AA and looking from the bottom up, the only way one can see any sanity or insanity for that matter. I learned never to look back with any longing for anything but to look forward to a new life one moment at a time.

Life is serious enough without taking it too seriously. I had to learn to be free of *all* of my addictions and the only way that would happen is to continually go back to step 1: I am powerless and *only* God could help me. Therefore, I had to face Life's Lesson One—my powerlessness. I am powerless and cannot change me or anyone else.

I am powerless over alcohol.
I am powerless over all drugs.
I am powerless over caffeine.
I am powerless over nicotine.
I am powerless over refined sugars and flours.
I am powerless over preservatives and additives.

I am powerless over processed foods/fast foods/junk foods.
I am powerless over all chemicals.

And I *was* powerless over the effects that all of these things had on me. I was addicted to them. They all would take control of my body and would render me powerless. They would all create disease, weight gain, and insanity along with death (in the cases of alcohol and drugs). Did I want these things in my life? Did I really need these things in my life? For my body and me to function optimally, I said no to both of those questions. I had learned to compromise throughout the years to fulfill a "craving" of food or drink. I make my own without the entire chemical poisons, using ingredients that my body can handle.

I have struggled over the years with my passion to eat. That is the one I still struggle with. One can let go of the other addictions. After all, not even one of my past addictions shall pass my lips because my body will lose control and I will demand more. But what about food? We don't stop eating; after all, food is what sustains our body and our lives. The only way that I can maintain any kind of control is to be careful of what I eat. I had to change my entire diet and lifestyle radically. I then do not have to deal with any cravings, at least not the physical ones. As a recovering food addict, and I don't say that lightly because I am still in the process, the cravings would come through the stinking thinking process, that is, the psychological cravings. This is why I still rely on the principles of the Twelve-Step program (One Day at a Time) to control the thinking. My personal journey on that continues to this day.

So it now becomes another one of life's lessons, and this is just the tip of the iceberg. I am in the process of this part of the journey and learning what it will involve. It takes pulling away from the table to learn what satiated is. It can be a silent emotional struggle. What I mean by silent is there isn't any spoken dialogue. But the dialogue is between my body and me. The rule of the body is not to overeat. Another of life's lessons is to listen to our bodies. There is a fine line between being satisfied and feeling full. Many others know it they eat until they are satisfied, but food addicts don't do that. If it tastes good, they keep on eating until it's gone. I only have two choices—

sickness or health—that lead to life or death. I want to be and feel more alive than anything else. It will take determination, persistence, patience, and most of all, a desire to become an overcomer. Let's stick to this goal together. Let's not quit before it happens. After all, it is a journey not a destination. *One day* at a time.

The other steps of the program are for the sanity portion of our lives. We must not remain in the victim role any longer by blaming others for our wrong choices, stinking thinking, and the consequences of destructive living. We must take responsibility for ourselves. I can and will admit my wrongs, so I don't have to carry a sea of guilt. The bottom line of what I learned in AA is to learn to be *gut-level* honest with ourselves and with God. We stand naked before our Creator, completely vulnerable, something most of us do not want to do. I had to learn to look myself in the eye each and every day. After all, I live with myself twenty-four hours each day. I had to not only learn to like myself but to learn to love myself as God loves me. When I learned that, I did not want to continue to destroy my body and myself any longer. I learned to respect and cherish the one and only me. It is time to be in awe and in reverence of the body that was made beautiful, God's perfect creation. I guess you could say that I finally am growing up, and thus, I am gaining freedom and peace of mind. Life's lessons can hit you like a brick wall. They may hurt for a while as we learn from them because we are never prepared for them when they do come. Life has its lessons to learn and I would rather learn them once than have to keep repeating them over and over until I do get it.

There's joy in the journey because someday I am going to get it and be an overcomer.

Endnotes

1. Alcoholics Anonymous, *How It Works* (Alcoholics Anonymous World Services, 1976), 59.

CHAPTER 12

Eating Disorders

Millions of people in this society use and abuse food in the same way that the alcoholic abuses liquor. This is called addictive eating and is the major characteristic of all eating disorders. It is a result of biological, psychological, and sociological factors. The ones that will be addressed are anorexia nervosa, bulimia, and binge eating/compulsive overeating. These are all compulsions and obsessions concerning food and a loss of control or a fear of losing control.

We are all given free will to make choices that lead to consequences that can be for our good or can seriously harm us. The choices we make determine the consequences of our life. Many of us seem to make destructive choices. I did, and they locked me into a prison of despair for years.

Anorexia nervosa consists of dieting to the point of starvation. It focuses on eating as little as possible regardless of hunger, generally with the use of self-starvation, laxatives, and diuretics. The body becomes deprived of food energy and lack of nutrients. Young women generally may use drastic measures for weight loss or to avoid gaining weight. It can, and sometimes is, incline toward control issue, undereating often as an attempt to punish oneself or other people. It will often be a reflection on how people see themselves and their misconceived image of how others view them. There are severe nutritional deficiencies related to this type of lifestyle, which may have started off as a diet. This will then turn into the worst nightmare imaginable because, at one point through this grueling existence, one may try and eat and the body will rebel. The body will not know how to respond normally to food; it will not allow the foods to stay down and also will be unable to utilize any necessary food elements.

The body's endocrine system needs proper nutrition to aid in the body's proper functioning. When the hormones are disrupted, menses stops, making the reproductive function cease. This is dangerous because when menstruation ceases, the risk of osteoporosis starting increases. The bones become more fragile and are at greater risk for fractures.

The muscles begin to atrophy and weaken from loss of essential nutrients and lack of exercise. The joints begin to become unstable because of muscle weakness. The repeated self-starvation and laxative abuse severely upset the fluid and electrolyte balance required for the nerve impulses and muscular contraction. The muscles of the heart and brain are gravely affected. Beverly McMillian, author of the *Atlas of the Human Body*, writes, "The heart muscles weaken, heartbeat slows or becomes erratic and blood pressure falls abnormally."[1] The brain, with the lack of the optimal electrolyte function, slows the reflexes, impairs the thought processes and the nervous system becomes faulty. The hypothalamus region of the brain secretes the hormone orexin to the receptors within the brain to stimulate appetite. Those who suffer from eating disorders ignore the important built-in messages within the body that urge one to eat. There is a constant battle trying to defeat the body, and becoming its master. This only deteriorates it further, sometimes to the point of death. The skin becomes dry because of malnutrition. The dehydration of the body occurs from the loss of fluids, which complicates the functioning of the kidneys, thus increasing the risk of kidney failure. The motility rate of the digestive system slows, and the intestines have a difficult time with their attempt to absorb nutrients properly.

Bulimia "is a binge-purge syndrome in which the individual drastically overeats several times a week,"[1] and according to the *Atlas of the Human Body*, there is an obsession with eating but at the same time a desire to be thin. The bulimic person has an extreme fear of becoming fat or overweight. One feels like an emotional basketball and can never be happy living in this condition. One's life seems to constantly revolve around food. The scale which is the main control of how much and what kind of foods are eaten, when to eat, and the amount of exercise is to be done each day. Other measures, such as the use of vomiting, laxatives, and/or diuretics, are also used to purge the overeaten foods from the digestive tract. Some foods, such as refined sugars, will exit through the walls of the stomach within minutes, so the vomiting and other avenues used will just be in vain. The consequences of our behavior many times are out of ignorance, but the suffering continues nonetheless.

Vomiting starts off to be self-induced, but later as this practice continues, it becomes involuntary. Some bulimics may binge and vomit up to ten times during the day and may also consume laxatives and/or diuretics daily to prevent weight gain, all in an attempt to desperately reduce weight, and one's overwhelming sense of guilt as well as disgust with themselves and their behavior. They generally live with monumental guilt, depression, hopelessness, and stress. As the guilt mounts, so do the binges. It seems like an endless cycle of despair. The abuse of the body never takes away the destructive emotions.

Some may over-exercise for hours to the point of damage to the body, injury to the joints, and muscles, stress fractures from excessive jogging and the like. Many will recoup for short periods only to go right back out and hurt themselves even more because there wasn't enough healing time. They perceived that they would gain weight if they rested too long.

Over-exercising was my way out. I couldn't vomit or do laxatives, but I would exercise for hours, weight training, jazzercise classes, jogging, and long bike rides. This was done six or seven days a week. The joints and muscles are more prone to injuries with this type of regimen. Even so, I continued and experienced many injuries because of this type of behavior, including those that would haunt me as I aged. Strenuous exercise also depletes the electrolytes that are crucial to the heart's functioning, which is getting eliminated through sweat.

It seems that every time one sits down for a meal, it may end up as a binge. These binges will seem to become closer and closer together. Eventually the bulimic is so out of control that every time something is eaten, it turns into a binge. Bulimic people seem helpless to push away from the table until they are overly stuffed and disgusted once again because of another failure. The pleasure is gone from eating. There isn't any enjoyment; it's just a strategy and conquest over the body, the scale, and to win the battle with food. It becomes a compulsive addiction and a control issue that plunges a person into the depths of despair and hopelessness. They are never cured, never happy, and never satisfied. A dark cloud of doom continually hangs over their heads and controls their lives. The depression seems to become deeper and darker; the guilt never ceases to end. Everything is out of control; life is built around food, thinking of it, eating of it, and trying to get rid of it once it's ingested. Not only is there a loss of control but also a loss of freedom. It has become a prison without any escape.

According to Hannah Allen, a natural hygienist and professor at the Fit for Life Sciences Institute in Winnepegg, Canada, "Binge eating becomes very dangerous and can result in metabolic alkalosis, a destruction of the body's ability to maintain its acid-alkaline balance. It can damage the liver and the kidneys and can be life threatening. The constant eating (food in their mouths for hours at a time) also results in tooth decay."[2]

For many people, food is their only source of pleasure and comfort. The foods that we consume can and will be the main sources of the cravings and addictions, especially the processed foods with all of their addictive chemicals. Most foods binged on are the addictive foods, the processed and junk foods. The cravings from these foods can get monumental and uncontrollable, compelling the body to plunges downward into overeating and, in severe cases, binge eating and compulsive overeating. The binges become closer together. The guilt trips start up again, overwhelming the emotions, and negative thought processes continue to burden the individual. The cycle then continues to start over again, sometimes with fever pitch, and there doesn't seem to be any relief in sight, just hopelessness and despair.

"I am *powerless*," they think. We must remember that. It turns from a physical addiction into a psychological disorder.

Binge eating is a way of coping with the problems of life or for that matter, not coping with them. "Binge eaters can pile on the calories by the thousands compulsively and not even realize what they are doing."[3]

They have not enjoyed or were satisfied with their spree. It was just a way of running from reality. They may even say, "I don't know when to quit, but neither do I want to quit." At least no one may go out of their way to say so, but the actions seem to take over the thoughts and emotions. It then turns its ugly head into a control issue, which goes from there to an addiction or loss of control. "Leave me alone. I just want to eat myself into oblivion, and never come out of it," a bulimic will say. It's during this time when one's life is now out of control. Some use alcohol, drugs, or shopping while others just silently eat their way into oblivion.

It doesn't matter which came first, the destructive thinking process, the wounded spirit and painful emotions, or the damaging lifestyle and diet. In the case of eating disorders, they all work together to help us or to harm us. What are we doing to ourselves? The addict is a runner and a hider just desperately seeking relief from pain.

Jane Fonda admitted to her bulimia and eventually realized what she was doing to herself. She was determined to stop with will power and exercise. Her pattern took sixteen years to break. I dug a grave to protect myself from pain—emotional, mental, and spiritual—which wasn't going away, and I always felt dead inside. I just continued digging the grave deeper and deeper with all of my addictions. It is easier to blame everyone else for me being the way I was so I didn't have to change anything, but I was still hurting and still miserable. I let food be my only comfort and distraction. I am in the recovery process after living in the depths of my last addiction for at least thirty years.

Hannah Allen states, "The body chemistry is influenced by the foods that are eaten. When the diet is altered and the new diet is maintained for a given length of time, the enzymes, body fluids, and glandular secretions become increasingly adapted to the influences and requirements of the new food program."[2] The body will struggle to adapt to the overabundance of junk food or too much of any food for that matter.

By reducing one's intake of foods but continuously consuming the processed and junk foods, the cravings will continue to accelerate. Once the nutritional needs of the body are met with a wholesome diet, the perverted tastes and cravings will reduce and vanish. Hannah Allen discusses John M. Douglass, MD, internal medicine specialist at Southern California Permanente Medical Group (in his reports in the *Medical World News* and the *Annals of Internal Medicine*) saying that raw food diets reduce or eliminate the need for insulin in many diabetics, reduce blood pressure, and develop an inner feeling of cleanness that causes people to want to reject such habits as smoking, drinking, and overeating.[3] Susan Hazard also states, "Beware—the purer your body, the more aware and sensitive you are to the things that are harmful."[4] Your body will react violently to the poisons consumed after you have not partaken them for some time. It's best after you have rendered yourself clean then stay clean. It really isn't worth it to get sick again because each time will only be worse.

Natural hygiene is a way of life, not just a temporary diet to feel good at the time. It is a way to having optimal health. It is a simple lifestyle, definitely not easy; the simple way to overcome the problem of overeating and cravings is to eliminate the cooked and processed foods.

It is difficult to break old habits, for it may feel like going through withdrawals, basically leaving one's comfort zones. It's best to remain diligent and focused because habits come automatically without thinking. It takes determined thinking to change to new behaviors. Remain focused and resolute because the only failure is giving up. Once the new behaviors are repeated often enough, it will become the new habit. Protect your body and all of its organs. To be sick or not, it is your own choice. Be responsible for your own body.

Endnotes

1. Beverly McMillian, "Eating Disorders," in *Atlas of the Human Body* (Weldon Owens, 2008), 192–193.
2. Hannah Allen, "Overeating, Fasting Fanaticism and Diet Fanaticism" (lesson 44, Natural Health course, Fit for Life Sciences Institute), 992, 1000.
3. Susan Hazard, "Natural Approach to Overcoming Addictions" (lesson 69, Natural Health course, Fit for Life Sciences Institute), 1460.

CHAPTER 13

Infertility

There never used to be as much a problem with infertility as there is in this day and age. A few decades ago, no one ever heard of fertility clinics. Now, there are many types and procedures for the infertile couple who desires to have children but can't.

The problem can lie in the woman or the man or both. It can be with an imbalance and/or reduction of the levels of hormones. The use of IUDs, birth control pills, and previous abortions has set a dangerous condition for the body to comprehend. They can put some stress on the woman's body. The stresses of living in a fast-paced society in this generation will also take its toll on the body because the woman's body needs to be relaxed, calm, and in good working order to become pregnant.

Probably the biggest contributor to infertility is the amount of chemicals in this environment, especially in one's diet. These chemicals are breathed and eaten. They are in our home environment, absorbed into our skin through all of the bath and beauty products, laundry detergents, pesticides, and insecticide sprays, etc. The chemicals are the main cause of the overall body pollution. Conception may not be an occurrence if both the male and the female reproductive cells are saturated with an overwhelming amount of chemicals.

The body seeks health and proper functioning. The couple that desires to conceive a child and is finding it difficult will need to clean up their bodies and their environment. It is important to relieve the stresses in their lives and just learn to relax. All this needs to start *before* conception.

The prospective parents need to start eating fresh, raw whole fruits; vegetables; small amounts of seeds and nuts, sprouts and to start drinking distilled water. The mother needs to be diligent about getting regular exercise; developing a good, positive, healthy attitude; getting regular sunshine, and getting enough sleep and rest. It is also imperative to live in a clean environment, also bathing herself regularly. If her body has been a toxic dump, she may need to fast for a short time to eliminate these toxic wastes, encouraging her body to regenerate and heal itself. The foods she eats will begin to be assimilated; therefore, she will have much better nutrition and functioning of the cells and organs, especially the reproductive system. The body needs to be pure and free of chemicals to conceive and bear a healthy baby.

Alcohol, cigarettes, and caffeine are also adding too many poisons and must be eliminated. "The meats, animal proteins, will need to be gradually eliminated as they have created a lot of estrogen dominance," according to Dr. John R. Lee. This is an excess amount of estrogen. He states that not only the animal flesh contains too many hormones, but processed foods as well.[1] The cooked foods, grains and all refined products need to also be eliminated whether by starting gradually or by going cold turkey. It depends on one's desire to start a healthy lifestyle for that healthy body to conceive that healthy baby.

Endnotes

1.   John R. Lee with Virginia Hopkins, *What Your Doctor May Not Tell You about Menopause* (Warner Books., 1996), 258.

CHAPTER 14

What's Happened to
Our Children?

Our children are suffering from the devastating effects of our nation's diseases. The children are victims of their parent's poor diets and perverted lifestyles. This can be and is a tragedy. These learned behaviors, not genetics, are continuously passed down from generation to generation with each generation becoming sicker and more diseased. Good behavior, proper and healthy diets and lifestyles are to be passed down to help our children and subsequent generations and the future of the nation. What are we doing to our children?

Unfortunately, all that has been taught has not been helpful but damaging in the worst way. I consider this as abusing our children. It all begins before conception. A proper healthy diet and lifestyle need to be lived and taught by example, the example of the parents. I could go on and on about all the things that are wrong. These wrongs are from each generation and have only become worse. But I will just speak about the perverse diets and destructive lifestyles.

Childhood is to be a time of innocence, learning, and experiencing. Children need to be fed properly for their growing bodies to develop properly, free from sickness and disease. There are the minor childhood diseases that come and go as the body cleanse out its toxic wastes, but now children are becoming plagued with adult diseases as well. That's the tragic part.

More children than ever are experiencing asthma, allergies of all sorts (food and environmental) ADD/ADHD, autism, leukemia, and now they are becoming a part of the adult generation diseases with obesity, high blood pressure, diabetes, high cholesterol, juvenile arthritis, colitis, chronic fatigue depression, and juvenile fibromyalgia.[1]

According to Marilynn Marchione, AP medical writer, as of November 11, 2008, "Obese children as young as 10 had the arteries of 45-year-olds and other heart abnormalities that greatly raise the risk of heart disease. About a third of the American children are overweight and one-fifth are obese."[2] In fact, some doctors are recommending cholesterol-lowering drugs for some kids.

Ultrasound studies were used to test the thickness of the major neck artery of the children ten–sixteen years old. There were seventy volunteers as stated by Marilynn, who participated in the study. These children's vascular age was at least thirty years older than their actual age. Their arteries are starting to stiffen due to adult plaque diseases. The breakfast and lunch meals offer no surprises in parallel to their heart and artery challenges. This is more evidence that fat causes premature aging. Children are too young to have these serious problems, and it is all the fault of their parents.

The life of a child is tough enough because they do not understand the world through their immature thoughts and emotions; they need to be guided lovingly through life, not dragged through hell as many of them are with these health challenges created by their parents.

Obesity is not due to genetics, according to Michael Donaldson. "Our genes don't change that fast."[3] Healthy lifestyles and living need to be taught by example and practiced early in one's life from infancy on. In fact, women need to eat very healthy before becoming pregnant and while nursing for the future benefits of their children.

The parents are in control of their child's learning experiences, especially very early in life. These learning experiences include their health and lifestyles. If a parent is eating and living unhealthy, so will the child. If the parent is obese, so will the child because of the learned behavior. No one is stuck being overweight, especially children. Parents need to provide and assimilate activities to do on a family basis other than playing computer games and TV-watching. Eating healthy raw produce meals, not the junk foods/fast foods, help in keeping family meal times on a calm basis. Train the child in the way he/she should go, including healthy attitudes and good eating habits.

We need to teach our children discernment about the world's standards of eating and living. It's also about ridding these young bodies of all the pollutants, especially sodas and sugary drinks. These sodas are just garbage foods. It's better to eat a piece of fresh fruit rather than a box of pasteurized (cooked) fruit drinks or juices. Children need to learn to snack on fresh, raw fruits and vegetables and to know they do not need to eat all day long. The meals need to start with raw fresh foods. This is a very important concept for children to get used to. These raw foods will feed and fill the body with more nutrients than too much of other cooked foods. The most important thing to teach children is the consequences of making the wrong food choices.

According to Michael Donaldson, it's best to "use positive and negative examples, citing people they know, in order to teach graceful discernment without self-righteousness or pride."[3] When children go out into the world, they will need to know what are the best choices to eat when they eat at a friend's home so that they will develop good habits throughout their lives.

A friend of mine's son was taught very well and learned a lifetime in his short twelve years of life. When he attended a birthday party, he ate the fruit and vegetables and very determinedly rejected the cake. This young man chose this way even though his parents weren't even there with him. The host father of the party called my friend to find out if that was for real. How any twelve-year-old could avoid cake was beyond this gentleman's boggled mind. So he had to check this out himself. My friend was very proud of his son and knew that he had passed with honors. He learned well. That's what it's all about, preparing our children for a very healthy and productive future where they can take good care of themselves and pass the message and example to others. No, children do not need to be fat.

Our nation is very sick. Michael Donaldson, PhD, in his article "Why Are We So Sick?" writes, "We spent $1.5 trillion on disease care in 2002.

- One out of 150 children has autistic spectrum disorder.
- In some cities, 105 of the children have ADHD, more than four million children have this diagnosis in the USA
- Fourteen percent of Caucasian children ages 6–11 are overweight; 21 percent of African American and 23 percent of Hispanic children are overweight.
- Leukemia is the number one killer of our children today. This is probably due to the tremendous amount of childhood vaccines."[4]

Prevention is easier than recovery in many or all of these complicated diseases that plague our young children. Fortunately, my husband and I have been blessed with three healthy sons without any physical challenges. We do have one grandson who has sensory issues that could be related to autism. My daughter-in-law, bless her heart, is dealing with these issues with God's grace in the most honorable ways, including nutrition.

In his article, "Help! Autism Stole Johnny!" Michael Donaldson, PhD, states, "One out of every 95 boys has an autistic spectrum disorder, and one out of every 400 girls is likewise struck. One out of every nine boys is diagnosed with ADHD, as well as one out of every 23 girls. Many more have subtle, less well-defined problems." When people can understand autism and reverse it, then they possess the key to every other disease that plagues mankind. Dr. Donaldson continued, "Causes for autism and every other chronic disease are quite similar, but are expressed differently, depending on genetic weaknesses and specific environmental exposures. Some are more severe, some are mild, some sooner, some later. But they all have the same roots: *toxicity* and *deficiency*."[4]

Dietary intervention is necessary to combat this very complicated disease. The autistic child's body usually is quite sensitive and has difficulty detoxifying pesticides and insecticides, bacterial toxins, molds, and heavy metals, especially mercury. When testing is done on these little bodies, these poisons are found in large amounts. Most of these poisons are neurotoxins and interfere with brain/behavioral development. They react differently and have what's called are sensory sensitivity issues. More often than not, they have allergies, particularly to foods that are toxic to the body in general, such as gluten, casein, and sugars. When they avoid sugars, animal and dairy products, their behavioral problems seem very minimal.

Dr. Michael Donaldson, who has performed extensive research on this subject, has important statements on the causes of autism. He claims there is what is called a leaky gut, an imbalance of bacteria and yeast.[4] That is the connection between the gut to the nervous system that connects to the brain and also creates cellular damage. It is really a whole body issue. If there are in this small body too many accumulated poisons that interfere with the whole body at large, there needs to be a serious detoxification and elimination of all the foods that are poisonous to the body; such foods for example include, animal proteins, dairy, wheat, and other grains that have gluten, sugars, and all refined and processed products. The adjusted diet should consist of a plant-based diet of fruits, vegetables, nuts, seeds, fresh water, lots of sunshine, and exercise. Many children seem to camp in front television and computer screens and remain sedentary. These only hinder any stimulus and creative process. Keep children away from all chemicals, especially dangerous drugs and vaccinations of all kinds because they are dangerous to the developing body.

Donaldson concluded, "Rather than seeing autism defined as a disorder manifested by behavior, socialization, and communication (as if autism caused these things), we need to see that impaired detoxification, overwhelming oxidative stress, and chronic inflammation are the central issues that lead to what is called autism. Heal the body and the brain will get well too. It isn't so much a cure as it is a recovery—a recovery of function, of health, and of relationships."[4]

Another serious health challenge for our children is ADD/ADHD (attention deficit disorder/attention deficit hyperactivity disorder). The schools and medical professionals just prescribe drugs (psychotropic drugs), so these children can go to school and sit quietly as not to be disruptive. The problem, in addition to the toxic issues to the already over-polluted body, is that the brain that will not function and learn properly because of these mood-altering effects. These are stimulating and very powerful drugs that do nothing to help the child learn and develop. Ritalin, a drug of choice to ADD/ADHD-suffering children, is a stimulant similar to amphetamine and cocaine. It is an extremely harmful drug.

Processed foods, additives and food colorings toxify the body in accumulated amounts. These, combined with the drugs, just add fuel to the fire. According to the *ADD/ADHD Are There Alternatives to Drugging Our Children?* authors, "It was found in 1994, each person in the United States was consuming from 8-10 pounds of food additives annually. The entire population of the US consumes approximately 100 million pounds of food colors alone. Several scientific studies have shown a significant correlation between hyperactivity and food additives."[5] Dr. Dan Chesnut claims that behavior disorders, such as ADD/ADHD, are affected by "caffeine, artificial sweeteners and sweets, MSG, dairy products, and food dyes."[6] Others are the preservatives in processed foods and drugs. Aspartame is a very definite danger. When aluminum and mercury or fluorides are combined it becomes a very potent toxin to the brain, an excitotoxin.

Throughout the years, studies and experience have proven that these children do not need these drugs. What they need is a change of diet, just to stop consuming all of the overabundance of sugars, refined flours, and starches and processed foods. When they start to eat more fruits, vegetables, nuts— raw, plant-based diet—then their behaviors improve dramatically. Their bodies become less toxic and chemically free; they begin to regenerate and recover. They can begin to learn and manage to lead a very productive life. Nutrition makes all the difference in the world in changing the statistics of mental health. Most of the imbalances in the brain chemistry are created by what millions of American children are eating. It's sad that neither the government nor the parents are doing anything about it. These children are just digging their own graves with their knives and forks and following in the same pathways as the adults before them. The biggest problem is that each generation seems to get worse than the previous one.

The fats, chemicals, sugars, and additives found in processed foods need to be avoided. The omega 3 fats are essential for a child's developing brain, but these processed foods with the trans fats contribute to attention deficit hyperactivity disorder, dyslexia, and other learning and behavioral disorders. Many teens get almost half of their calories from fat, and these nutritionally-poor diets could permanently damage brain development. The brain thrives on glucose from fresh, raw fruits and vegetables. Without it, the learning and the social behaviors of the brain starts to shut down, according to Olin Idol, because of low blood sugar. The brain, as well as the rest of the body, needs nutrients. In fact, Olin points out that hypoglycemia (low blood sugar) has a major effect on criminal and aggressive behaviors, alcoholism, mental illness, and other drug addictions and allergies.[7]

I personally know of parents who have changed their diets and lifestyles for their children's sake, and it seems like everyone lives in heaven rather than hell. They assess the bad points in the lifestyle and diet to save them from malnutrition. Olin states, "An increasing number of well-nourished children will result in a decrease in delinquency, learning disabilities, aggressive behavior, and criminality."[7] There is hope in nutrition because it saves us from ourselves.

Bronchial asthma is generally created by allergies and/or hypersensitivity to external pollutants or internally-ingested substances. Many children are victims of these attacks and the medical profession seeks to either hospitalize or administer some type of drug therapy to relieve the symptoms.

"The underlying cause of bronchial asthma is a state of toxicosis," states Susan Hazard, PhD. "If asthmatics were not enervated and their tissues were not saturated with toxin, there would be no hypersensitivity."[8] The real causes, Hazard claims, are the overeating of wrong foods and of wrong combinations of foods. The body's elimination processes are overburdened beyond capacity and the "toxins are built up in the cells, tissues, and blood."[8]

Children seem to be more out of control of their situation because they are dependent on their parents and caretakers to take care of them. Before conception and birth, their mothers need to eat a raw plant-based diet, but many of them just fill their bodies via the baby through the placenta with great amounts of processed foods as well as other toxins and poisons. What the infant and growing child need are good, healthy whole foods, first breast-feeding then a raw fruit. If not, they are receiving the wrong diet, one that poisons their bodies. To me, this is abuse in the worst sense. Drugs only make them worse, for it just creates a merry-go-round effect.

The child needs to have a clean, healthy body to function properly, not fed or infected by chemicals, additives, and colorings or processed products, including infant formulas. Fresh whole foods offer the freedom needed. Many believe that it's a hereditary factor. After all, the whole family may have these chronic diseases, but it's only a learned way of living. If the unhealthy ways of living were eliminated and the family changed its living habits and patterns, the hypersensitivity and allergies would cease.

Leukemia seems to be the number one cause of childhood death. Leukemia is a cancer of the bone marrow and blood, creating an overproduction of white blood cells that crowd out the red blood cells and platelets. This activity decreases the circulation and functioning of the body. Acute childhood leukemia from the time of diagnosis to death is less than one year.

The treatment is chemotherapy and other types of drugs, and the prognosis is not good. These children do not have a life outside of the hospital. It is so sad.

Susan Hazard states, "The use of antibiotics has also been proven to result in many blood disorders including leukemia."[8] Children are given many different antibiotics for their constant viruses, ear infections, and other childhood diseases and illnesses. These childhood diseases, colds, flu, respiratory illnesses are due to their improper foods, diets, such as milks causing an overproduction of mucous and meats, processed foods, colorings, and additives. This is another disease that could be prevented if their parents fed them a raw plant-based diet.

Dennis Nelson claims with lack of sunlight, the "fibrin and the red blood corpuscles become diminished in quality while the serum or water portion of the blood increased, including leukemia."[9] Hannah Allen, in her report, states, "The rise in leukemia in cattle calls our attention to the fact that blood cancer, or leukemia, is now a major cause of death among children in the United States."[10] We need to feed our children well to keep their young bodies pure, allowing them to grow into healthy adults.

The other drug problem that keeps popping up is vaccination and the dangers that these drugs pose on our children. Children may get sick from chicken pox, mumps, and measles, but there are not any grave dangers from these diseases. However, there are grave dangers and sometimes serious complications from the drugs that are injected into the bodies of our children for the so-called prevention of these illnesses.

One of the lies given to people by the pharmaceutical companies is, "If you had chicken pox as a child, you are more prone to getting shingles as an adult; therefore, you must get a chicken pox vaccine and a shingles vaccine, for the prevention of these serious illnesses."

Rev. George Malkmus valiantly states, "With vaccines, modern science has actually altered the human genetic code as originally created by God in the human bodies of Adam and Eve. This is a sacrilege; a crime against God, and an evil that must be exposed and resisted."[11] Instead of using drugs and vaccinations with their dangerous side effects, people need to be employing means of self-healing the body that God gave us. By doing this, people will employ a proper diet and lifestyle.

Reverend Malkmus states, before their first birthday, our children, "who have received the recommended vaccinations has 48 times the limit the FDA has set as safe limits for mercury." [111] Dr. Michael Donaldson also claims, "There are 15 vaccines containing 28 different antigens. With multiple dosing, there are now 88 antigenic exposures, most injected before the age of six. In 1985, there were 33."[12] Now the greedy pharmaceutical companies are inventing even more vaccinations.

The ingredients in these vaccines are the contaminants of possible bacterial and viral agents along with bits of saline and thimerosal, a preservative with 50 percent mercury and aluminum. "There is a link though between thimerosal and neurodevelopmental disorders,"[12] states Dr. Michael Donaldson. Dr. Dan Chesnut has stated that the "flu vaccine during pregnancy can dramatically increase the risk for autism and schizophrenia." He claims that these vaccines can increase asthma by 200 percent. In fact, it can suppress immunity for weeks after receiving the flu vaccine.[13] If children receive the flu vaccine, it is very dangerous because children are so much more sensitive to mercury and its effects.

The diseases that used to beget the older people now afflict the young as well, even more aggressively because pollutants, chemicals, and preservatives are becoming stronger and more aggressive to the human body. The youth are being bombarded with these poisons at an earlier age, and it's becoming more apparent with the increasing destruction on the human organism than when their parents were growing up. The toxins in the environment and foods are much more prevalent. This has become the age of "Mandatory Vaccines;" foods that have been altered and turned into hybrids. Thus, the quality of the foods consumed is nowhere near what the body needs to fill its basic needs for nutrition and health. The foods that are gown organically, or bought from reputable organic farmers, would fit the bill. Those who do not have the luxury of fresh gardens and fruit orchards have to rely on these organic and local markets. It is most advantageous to make sure the foods eaten are properly combined for the best possible way to digest it and receive its optimal nutrition. It must be a way of life for health, and the best possible way to get it is through natural hygiene. All of the world's standards of eating, pill-popping, and excessive lifestyles will only lead to the path to destruction.

It can never be said enough that the chemicals that are put into the human body poison and destroy the organism. The body needs to be protected not destroyed. The only protection there is must be a properly-combined raw plant diet and not even one chemical of any kind whether internally or externally consumed. It all starts when we are young. Let's take care of our children who are the next generation of the world.

Endnotes

1. Michael Donaldson, "Johnny, Get Moving!" *Hallelujah Acres Health News* 57 (September/October 2009): 12.
2. Marilynn Marchione, "Fat Kids Found to Have Arteries of 45 Year Olds," November 11, 2008.
3. Michael Donaldson, "Why Is Johnny Fat?" *Hallelujah Acres Health News* 53 (January/February 2009): 5.
4. Michael Donaldson, "Help! Autism Stole Johnny!" *Hallelujah Acres Health News* 55 (May/June 2009): 10–11.
5. Michael Donaldson and Olin Idol, "ADD/ADHD: Are There Alternatives to Drugging Our Children?" *Back to the Garden Health News* 33 (July/August 2005): 26.
6. Dan E. Chesnut, *Lying with Authority* (Restoration Health, 2008), 79.
7. Olin Idol, "Food and Behavior A Natural Connection," *Hallelujah Acres Diet and Lifestyle Magazine* 50 (May– June 2008): 23.
8. Susan Hazard PhD, "Allergies, Hay Fever, and Other Chronic Illness," part XIV, lesson 71, course in Natural Health, Fit for Life Sciences Institute, 1497.
9. Dennis Nelson, "Air, Sunshine, and Light Essential to Health," part III, lesson 13, course in Natural Health, Fit for Life Sciences Institute, 324.
10. Hannah Allen, "Why We Should Reduce Our Meat Intake" part VI, lesson 32, course in Natural Health, Fit For Life Sciences Institute, 746.
11. George Malkmus, "Vaccines Blessings or Curses," *Back to the Garden* 34 (September–October 2005): 14.
12. Malkmus, "Vaccines Blessings," 26.
13. Michael Donaldson, "The Fine Line of Immunization," *Hallelujah Acres Health News Magazine* 56 July–August 2009): 27.
14. Chesnut, *Lying with Authority*, 125.

CHAPTER 15

Allergies

An often-heard statement is "My allergies are just acting up." Everyone seems to have an allergy of some kind. It seems to be routine these days. However, many people do not realize that the allergies they suffer from have more to do with the accumulated and overloading of toxic chemicals within their own bodies. The environmental toxins only add to the inward stress, setting the body over the edge and into a crisis mode. Outward blame does not relieve inward destruction. People tend to seek drugs, which really don't work, thus adding to this overload and only making the allergies worse.

Rose fever, hay fever, grass fever, etc., are allergies which pop up at specific times of the year, last a certain duration, and then will supposedly disappear until the following year.

Food allergies, on the other hand, are linked in turn to the environment. It all has to do with how healthy the body is. If the body is trying to combat and eliminate all the toxins that are consumed on a daily basis, then anything from the outside that is bombarding the overloaded systems makes the body just scream in agony. This condition is due to be the effects of the allergies. "No more, please," it signals.

Food allergies have increased their deadly toll in the past two–three decades There are significantly more and increasing allergic reactions to all kinds of different foods. Primarily, the biggest culprits are meats, fish and eggs, dairy products (lactose intolerant), grain flours and gluten, peanuts, soy, tree nuts, onions, garlic, and peppers. When someone looks at the above list of food items, all, with the exception of tree nuts, are unwholesome foods that the body cannot tolerate, much less try to digest. People try to consume all kinds of intolerable foods, yet the body will continue to reject them. Yet most people are woefully unaware of the hazards. According to *Living Without* magazine, people are trying to buy, eat, and consume their junk foods, cakes, cookies, muffins, and etc., as gluten-free. Tom Charla, in his article, "Diary of a Dad," is diligently trying to live in his son's food-sensitive world and to have an understanding of what the boy is living without, not being able to fit into this society of "eat whatever you want." But the problem is the family unit is not eating healthy foods to begin with. For example, the writer states that Sunday breakfast is gluten-free pancakes. First of all, the body will not tolerate any of this food type and will only accept fruit for breakfast. When only fresh whole fruits are eaten, the body is given an opportunity to cleanse and continue its elimination process of toxins. They are easy to digest, free of toxic chemicals, and well-tolerated by the human body. The writer then continues to say his lunch consists of a turkey and cheese sandwich on gluten-free bread. Whether or not the bread has gluten, meat and cheese are indigestible. The family dinner, also considered indigestible, consists of chicken cutlets and pasta. What's wrong with this picture? First and most important, where are the fruits and vegetables in these family meals? They are never mentioned throughout the entire article. The gentleman talks about bakery goods from a bakery, which sells these gluten-free items, but never about salads, fruits, vegetables, seeds, or nuts. Sandwiches, pizza, cookies, health bars, and all types of store-bought processed foodstuffs that are gluten-free are not considered healthy foods for the nourishment of the human body. It's still an excuse to continue to eat unwholesome junk foods. It's like having your cake and eating it too! There are still hazards on the body, for there are still the consequences of poor nutrition and improper digestion while still consuming unwholesome junk foods.

The biggest contributors are the food industries and companies, media, etc., that are making money off these so-called health foods. They are taking the diseases of society and turning them into money and profits. It's *big* business. There is no health in these foods. American children are suffering horribly from all the bad so-called nutrition. Years ago, food allergies were nonexistent. The human body is not designed to be eating the standard American diet with all of its chemical-laden ingredients. People will always come to alter and compromise it to fit their tastes and their way of living. Many people do not eat to live; they live to eat.

Gluten-free has become a big hype and big business to sell these types of products to the public. People are still eating improperly because they continue to consume these unwholesome junk foods. Where is the health in these so-called food products? Allergies to unwholesome foods are normal. After all, the body cannot tolerate or digest the wheat, gluten, and the ingested sugars, all of which are unhealthy.

Adults are still drinking their coffee and yogurt with their gluten-free bagels and their cupcakes. Their dinners will be the meat and potato ones, and they refuse the vegetables. No one wants to eat the fruits, vegetables, salads, and fresh whole produce.

People with food allergies react as the body is affected by the food attempting to pass through the digestive tract. The person may feel the symptoms of bloating, gassiness, constipation, or bouts of diarrhea, coughing, excessive mucous coupled with a runny or stuffy nose, or sinus congestion, and in severe cases, anaphylactic challenges. Many people with food allergies are allergic to the processed foods, preservatives, or even improper food combinations.

These improper foods also cause or contribute to depression. People are being forced to look at their diets as a contributor to their health challenges. Completely eliminating the wheat, gluten and flours, sugars, eggs, dairy and soy products from one's diet is very wise. There are allergists who promote the elimination diet, whereas all foods that have been tested as allergic are taken out of the diet then gradually added back in to verify the intolerance. This is a dangerous procedure.

I took allergy shots for years because of environmental allergies, but I had many unknown allergies to foods, especially preservatives and additives. Processed foods were killing me. Once I began to eat fresh whole produce, seeds, and nuts, it was amazing. All my health challenges cleared up. Coincidence? No, just fact.

It reminds me of the experiment of the canary in the birdcage. The birdcage was filled with gas, a little at a time. The canary in the cage didn't seem to notice, and when the toxins accumulated to a certain level, the canary died. The experiment continued, and another canary was put into the same gas-filled cage, but it died right away. The second bird's body was pure; it just wasn't used to the toxic gas as the first bird was, and it had tolerated the gas before it died.

Allergies are called into two classes:

1. There is sensitivity to foods and drugs that are ingested into the body: eggs, dairy products, meats, grains, etc.
2. There is, secondly, sensitivity to those substances that are in the environment or outside of the body: chemicals, pollens, animals, and dust, etc. These are carried through the air that is breathed into the body and can create mild reactions, which may consist of a runny nose, sneezing, or cough to more severe reactions, which would include anaphylactic shock or even sudden death.

"Allergies are sensitive reactions that happen in the body when too many antibodies are produced or when they are produced to attack harmless antigens,"[1] states John Farndon in his book, *Human Body*.

Many doctors adhere to the antibody-antigen theory and that states people with allergies have hypersensitivity to the substances that are normally harmless to others in the same sphere. They are claimed to be highly personal—what affects one person may not affect someone else. Therefore, in real life, it does affect all, just in different ways, so most people do not recognize it. It is then pointed out that for those with a life-threatening response, their bodies will trigger a massive release of histamine and other inflammatory chemicals to attack the invading antigen (a foreign protein) that stimulates the person's immune system. A shot of epinephrine will bring the system back under control. This is a body in crisis. Doctors will begin a series of vaccinations to build up the immune system. These are to supposedly strengthen the body so it can fight off any future attacks.

It is overwhelming how the scientists, doctors, and pharmaceutical companies have taken over the tail end of the aftermath of the food industry's destruction. It's too bad that people don't see what these so-called foods are doing to their bodies. It's a sad state of affairs in today's society.

Diseases are abnormal to the body because they put it in a continued cleanup mode. The effects of all the accumulated and unflushed toxins are creating so many more life-threatening allergies, especially for the younger generation. People are supposed to protect their children, but feeding them unadulterated foods is abusing them. Different forms of allergies include asthma, bronchial asthma, ear and sinus infections, eczema, hives, hyperactivity in children, and gastrointestinal allergies, among others. They are created because of all the processed foods ingested.

Food allergies, points out Dr. Herbert Shelton, are "due to the failure of the digestive system to properly prepare the food for introduction into the blood."[2] This occurs for several reasons and creates a weakness of the functioning of the digestive system, most likely due to putrefaction of decomposed proteins, which form toxins in the intestinal tract. Certain proteins are unfit for human consumption, yet people will continue to consume them anyway. Overeating puts a burden on the system. It overtaxes the capacity of the digestive enzymes. According to Susan Hazard, PhD, "All allergies result from a long-standing poisoning of the body by protein excess."[3] Meals that are eaten while under emotional, mental, or physical stress will not be digested properly; the digestive process is inhibited. It's best to wait until the next meal when the meal may be eaten when calm. Cooked proteins do not digest, so they become toxic byproducts that will create an allergic reaction in the body.

When the causes of allergies are eliminated, then the body will heal, thus the allergies can and will be eliminated also. There are simple measures to be taken for the body to heal. The first thing to do is to allow the digestive tract to rest. This is done by allowing the body to fast from all foods and drinking filtered pure water only as thirst requires. Secondly, it is important to eat proteins that are easily absorbed to the human body. These include fresh, raw fruits; vegetables; nuts; and seeds. It is necessary for proteins not to be eaten in excess, especially nuts and seeds; these should be limited to four ounces a day. If too much protein is consumed, then that will lead to protein poisoning. It is best to eat all foods in proper combinations with a calm attitude and in a calm environment so the digestion will not be hindered.

According to Dr. Robert Gross, families with a lot of allergies "violate natural laws in the same manner from generation to generation."[4] If the causes are eliminated, the allergies will cease. Health, as stated by Dr. Gross, is "the characteristic of people who live according to nature's principles and who eat good foods."[4] Good foods are those given to us by nature, not by the food manufactures. Healthy people do not suffer from allergies or diseases.

Endnotes

1. John Farndon, *The Human Body* (Miles Kelley, 2006), 39.
2. Herbert M. Shelton, "Allergy" (lesson 71, Natural Health course, Fit for Life Sciences Institute), 1499.
3. Susan Hazard, "Allergies, Hay Fever and Other Chronic Illnesses" (lesson 71, Natural Health course, Fit for Life Sciences Institute), 1499.
4. Dr. Robert Gross, "Hay Fever and Asthma" (lesson 71, Natural Health course, Fit for Life Sciences Institute), 1503.

CHAPTER 16

Migraines and Other Headaches

According to *Webster's Dictionary* a migraine headache is "a severe headache, often accompanied by nausea and disturbed vision."[1] *Mosby's Medical Dictionary* states, "Allergic reactions, excess carbohydrates, iodine-rich foods, alcohol, bright lights, or loud noises may trigger attacks, which often occur during a period of relaxation after physical or psychic stress."[2] A headache is the warning sign of a body in distress.

Mike Benton maintains, "A headache is the body's chief warning signal of the body toxicity. The toxic load in the body has increased so fast that poisons are circulating in the bloodstream and cause irritation to the brain and nerves."[3]

Swelling of the intracranial blood vessels around the scalp causes most headaches. "These blood vessels swell because of toxic matter in the bloodstream and body, and they then press against sensitive nerves." During an onset of a migraine headache, the blood vessels in the brain continue to restrict because of stress, chemicals, and improper diet, which also disrupt hormone levels within the brain and the body. The toxic flow throughout the body continues to build. Sedentary lifestyles, lack of sleep, stress, and pain medications only compound the situation.

Migraine headaches, says Pierce J. Howard, PhD, "affect roughly 28 million Americans; most are associated with vasoconstriction (tightening of the blood vessels). Vasoconstriction can be off set or prevented by limiting consumption of foodstuffs with tyramine."[3] Some of these foodstuffs are pickled, marinated, and spicy meats, fish and luncheon meats, sauerkraut, onions, breads, chocolate, dairy, caffeine, MSG, soy sauce, seasoned salts, meat tenderizer, garlic, some nuts, refined sugar, TV dinners and other packages entrees, and aspartame—in essence, most foods that have been processed with chemical additives. The human body cannot take in these things without a rebellion, whether through headaches, digestive problems, or other health challenges. It's best to avoid these foodstuffs entirely.

"Cluster headaches are more intense than migraine headaches, and typically appear with regularity, attacking the sufferer at the same time day or night. Their very predictability has earned them the moniker 'alarm-clock,'" states Pierce.[3] These cluster headaches seem to be in the region of the brain that controls the body clock, the hypothalamus, where the brain's gray matter is of more abundance. Therefore, studies have estimated those who exhibit the chronic cluster suffer more than individuals who do not.

Tension headaches are associated with unresolved stress. The person continues to be anxious and worried. "With the sympathetic nervous system," Pierce Howard said, quoting Ira Black, "stimulation of 30–90 minutes can result in enzyme and impulse activity for 12 hours to 3 days, and in some cases, for up to 3 weeks."[4]

The immune system's performance is then impaired, resulting in an even more compromised body. The chemical drugs, herbs, and foodstuffs only compound the problem by increasing the rates of toxicity. The pain halts the digestion and elimination processes. It just seems like a squirrel-cage effect on the body.

Chemicals in colognes, cosmetics, perfumes, and household cleaners affect headaches. In fact, Howard quotes a statement from Samuel Epstein, "The use of petro chemicals in perfumes is causing a rash, (yes, that's right) of adverse reactions, in addition to the positive, or seductive reaction; 95 percent of perfumes are made from petro chemicals that give off volatile organic compounds similar to the vapors of dry cleaning materials and paint strippers."[4] The symptomatic results include eye, throat and nose irritations, skin rashes, asthma attacks, headaches, central nervous system damage, cancers, kidney and liver damage, and nausea, just to name a few.

Headaches are often caused by allergies, especially to sulfites, additives, and other preservatives, wheat and other refined foods. Marti Fry quotes Dr. Alvarez of the Mayo Clinic, saying, "Breads can pass through the whole small intestine without being digested at all."[5] She adds, "Wheat also interferes with the absorption of other foods as does salt."[5] Proteinosis, which is a poisoning from excessive protein, can cause headaches and a general achy feeling. Mike Benton claims that a "high protein diet eventually destroys the entire glandular system. It places too much of a burden on the liver, kidneys and adrenal glands."[6] Allergy is defined as an abnormal sensitivity to substances that may be harmless to most people. "Migraine headaches are also classed as an allergic phenomenon," states Dr. Herbert M. Shelton.[7]

The treatments most commonly used for headaches, especially migraines, are pain medications, and nonprescription drugs—acetaminophen, aspirin, and caffeine. The doctor doesn't seek the cause of the headache; he/she just uses the symptomatic approach. He prescribes drugs, which does not make the headaches go away and stay away. Instead, the headaches always return more frequently and with more intensity because the causes haven't been eliminated, therefore, requiring more drug use. The mild headaches then develop into migraine headaches. Aspirin only adds more chemicals to the already compromised body. Aspirin does not take away the cause, only the symptoms, and these chemicals will just continue to accumulate within the body. T.C. Fry comments, "Aspirin does not cure a headache. The problems remain as before plus the toxic presence of the aspirin itself. Aspirin merely causes our body to paralyze or incapacitate the nervous system." [8]

White willow bark or peppermint teas only mask the symptoms but do nothing to take away the causes. When these herbs are taken, the body recognizes them as harmful. The circulation is intensely increased by the body and the heart speeds up. At that point, the body is just trying to eliminate these herbs as quickly as possible by increasing circulation so the elimination can continue. Mike Benton injects, "The increase in circulation due to the toxic nature of the substances has its effect on the swollen blood vessels of the head. The vessels are dilated so that the circulation can proceed rapidly and the herbs/drugs can be eliminated. As a side effect, the headache temporarily disappears."[9] The body did the all the work, not the drugs. It worked hard to eliminate the poison, and the efforts also masked the symptoms of the toxic body: the headache. The cause of the headaches, which is toxicosis, was not removed by the drug/herbs. The conditions that brought on the toxicosis—poor diet and lifestyle habits—have not been improved by the drug/herbs. The headache may have disappeared, but the original causes continue to remain. The headache will return and the body is still compromised.

Pierce claims, "One Cleveland plastic surgeon in fact had great success with Botox injections and plastic surgery to relieve the pinched nerves."[10] These are all unwise choices to an already compromised body, a body in crisis. The headaches are the body's way of trying to tell the person to stop all of the abuse to the body. But no one is listening. Many sufferers of headaches have very destructive diets and lifestyles. A friend who complained about frequent-to-daily migraines has a daily consumption of sodas and sees no correlation between the two. I suffered from headaches for years, off and on, depending upon what I ate, and I did not get it either.

The migraines and headaches disappeared when I cleared all of the preservatives, additives, and chemicals from my diet and environment. How amazing and wonderful. How simple. The few times I experienced headaches in the past four years were due to a chemical reaction of sorts.

The change of diet will be a godsend but will not come without a price. A chemical cleanup will be necessary for the body to detoxify and clear out.

"Rapid dietary change, unfortunately, often fail," claims Mike Benton. "Changing everything is extremely difficult although some have done just that.[11] The mind may be ready, but the body may not be, and that can be quite discouraging, especially when the body starts to rebel against the healthy foods. The body may revolt with nausea, vomiting, cold/flu symptoms, or headaches. The headaches may get worse at first as the sugar, caffeine, and other chemicals are purged and flushed from the body's cells. There needs to be a slower cleansing method. The withdrawals can be extremely physically challenging, and people have reverted to the old ways rather than waiting it out until the healthy balance is complete. The present state of health is the result of years of bad living, habits, and poor diet choices. Be patient with the body. Don't give up and quit; it sometimes takes a little time. The effort will gain its reward. A fast of distilled water and raw vegetable juices will be very important for the body's recovery process. To succeed, it's best to take the changes at a slower pace.

There isn't any diet for the cure of migraine headaches. Foods cannot act specifically and go directly to the affected area to produce a cure. Only the body can heal and will promptly respond when the proper conditions are provided. Take away the causes, and the healing is expedited. The change of diet to a raw produce one with fresh raw juices; clean, filtered/distilled water; and exercise will help one to sleep better and to relieve the stress in one's life so the body can relax and do what God created it to do. Be consistent, be diligent, and take it all one day at a time so you won't be overwhelmed.

Endnotes

1. *Webster's Dictionary*, Book Essentials Pub, 1990), s.v. "migraine."
2. *Mosby's Medical, Nursing and Allied Health Dictionary*, 3rd ed., s.v. "migraine."
3. Mike Benton, "Why Herbs Should Not Be Used" (lesson 42 of Harmful Practices to Avoid, a course in Natural Health, Fit for Life Sciences Institute), 482.
4. Pierce J. Howard, *The Owner's Manual to the Brain*, (Bard, 2006), 387.
5. Marti Fry, "What's Wrong with Wheat?" (lesson 7 of the Nutritional Basis of Life, a course in Natural Health, Fit for Life Sciences Institute), 190.

6.   Mike Benton, "Proteins in the Diet?" (lesson 8 of the Nutritional Basis of Life, a course in Natural Health, Fit for Life Sciences Institute), 210.

7.   Herbert M. Shelton, "Allergy" (lesson 71 of Common Illnesses and Diseases and How Hygienic Living Can Help, a course in Natural Health, Fit for Life Sciences Institute), 1504.

8.   TC Fry, "Introduction to Life Science as a Way of Life" (lesson 1 of the Foundations of Life Science, a course in Natural Health, Fit for Life Sciences Institute), 20.

9.   Mike Benton, "Why Herbs Should Not Be Used" (lesson 42 of Harmful Practices to Avoid, a course in Natural Health, Fit for Life Sciences Institute), 952.

10.   Pierce J. Howard, *The Owner's Manual to the Brain* (Bard, 2006), 390.

11.   Mike Benton, "Symptoms during Dietary Transition" (lesson 21 of Human Physiology, Anatomy, and Our Dietary Nature, a course in Natural Health, Fit for Life Sciences Institute), 484–485.

CHAPTER 17

Stress

In today's society in the prevalently fast-paced world, people expect instantaneous results on everything in life. As far as health is concerned, most people would rather take a drug of some kind and assume that surgery, or other methods, will relieve their symptoms and problems. Then they go on with life as it was, the instant cure, the fast fix. The abuse of the body continues. The disease progressively worsens and money is spent on useless items to give hope to a desperate man/woman. Desperate, yes, but not enough to change their lifestyle to rid the body of its accumulated buildup of toxins. Those chemicals are creating the diseases within the body. As a friend of mine states, "I know what you are saying is good and right, but I'm too lazy to put it into practice and live it on a day-to-day basis." That's the point and attitude of most of today's society. It takes a determined person to change the pathways that they have set in life. As Robert Frost once stated in his poem, "The Road Less Traveled":

> Two roads diverged in a wood
> And I took the one less traveled by,
> And that made all the difference.[1]
> And Jesus stated, "The broad is the way that leads to
> destruction and there are many who go by it."[2]

The pathways of life often look promising, but they do need to examine each one with strict diligence and discernment. The standard American diet of the US society is doomed to fail if it is followed every day. It isn't just the diet alone but the entire lifestyle. The stress alone will kill the body when a person is overwhelmed his/her digestion ceases. The hormone overload that engulfs the entire body creates a substantial burden on every part. The heart rate increases; blood pressure rises; blood rushes to the extremities of the body, ready to fight or flee; breathing is increased; the nervous system is tingling, ready for action with the muscular system; and the immune system weakens. If a person is stressed only occasionally and his/her body is in good health and he/she has healthy ways of dealing with stress, then the body will adjust and overcome these challenges. Unfortunately, people do live with stress daily and do not monitor their stress level in safe and healthy ways. The human body cannot take the mounting abuse that overwhelms it, and the overload of adrenaline creates an accumulation of increased toxin levels. The body will weaken and breakdown under this burden, producing a multitude of diseases. A friend who was going through cancer treatments was told by his nurse to learn to meditate and relax the body for thirty minutes daily to help it to heal from the stress levels that produce cancers. People need to slow down and learn to relax.

People continuously worry, and this produces stress on the body. People will just worry themselves to death, literally. Worry and stress cause the body to age rapidly, thus health declines severely. "Emotional stress, such as worry, causes oxidative stress within the body, which essentially increases the rate of aging,"[3] claims Rev. George Malkmus.

Fast-paced lifestyles produce too much stress with little or no way of relieving it. Lack of exercise and eating improperly are portions of a volcano waiting to explode. When disease occurs, people are shocked and wonder how all of this came about. Why me? What happened? they ask. A person cannot burn the candle at both ends because when it gets to the middle, there is nothing, I mean nothing, left. All the king's horses and all the king's men couldn't put Humpty Dumpty back together again.

Certain foods will also trigger anxiety, especially acid foods, such as animal proteins, processed foods, sugar, and caffeine. The overly acidic body cannot handle the toxic accumulations, causing body stress and weakness, which in turn will create anxiety. It's best to eat a plant-based alkaline diet to reduce this stress and restore cellular health to promote toxin removal, thus creating emotional stability.

According to Mike Benton, some forms of stress to the body that many people don't even think about can cause physiological reactions on the body, such as

1. intense heat or cold,
2. injections of any sort,
3. surgical operations,
4. trauma of any type (physical or emotional),
5. pain,
6. any debilitating body crisis,
7. emotional outbursts or anxiety attacks,[4]
8. grieving the loss of a loved one,
9. and not getting enough sleep.

In addition to relaxation and meditation, other ways to manage stress levels include exercise, walking, and monitoring the diet. Reading a good book or listening to mellow music is a good way of escaping. Prayer is the best.

Many people will just resort to their comfort foods and sit in front of the television or sleep just to hide from the world or fall back into their workaholic roles. The comfort foods add to the body's stress and anxiety levels because stress will prevent any food from digesting, halting the digestive process. It leaves the food in the stomach as partially digested particles, which, according to Nancy Appleton, PhD, "get into the blood stream which leads to allergies and most everything that ails us."[5] It's important not to eat when stressed. Eating must be done when calm, while chewing well and slowly, giving the food time and opportunity to digest.

Prevention is the key. The main key is for people to learn to say *no* more often. Take a European holiday just to relax and not be on the go constantly. The US is one of the countries in the world where vacations are not mandatory. Stop and smell the roses along the way and get off the emotional merry-go-round. Turn off the cell phones, computers, and television sets. Leave work at work and leave home at home; don't connect the two because it's very stressful. Lean to relax and learn the sleep deeply and soundly.

Endnotes

1. Robert Frost, "Two Roads Diverged Into A Yellow Wood," (1920). The Poetry of Robert Frost. Edited by: Edward Connery Lathem Pub: Holt, Rinehart and Winston Inc. NY, NY 1969. Page 105.
2. Matthew 7:13 (NKJV).
3. George Malkmus, "Stress Related Aging," *Hallelujah Acres Health News* 57 (September/October 2009): 16.
4. Mike Benton, "Stress Management, the Life Science Approach" (lesson 64, Natural Health course, Fit for Life Sciences Institute), 1354.
5. Nancy Appleton, "Don't Let Stress in Your Life Become Distress," *Hallelujah Acres Diet and Lifestyle* 49 (March/April 2008): 18.

CHAPTER 18

Stress-Related Diseases

The American Heart Association continues to present that "heart attacks are the leading cause of death in America." It continues to conduct CPR classes to save those who are having a heart attack but fail to promote prevention, which is a change of diet and lifestyle. One American dies every minute as a result of having a heart attack.

A damaged or diseased heart cannot pump sufficiently throughout the body. The body relies on the blood flow to bring oxygen, carry out wastes, and deliver nutrients to all the cells of the body. During an average lifetime, the heart pumps fifty-three million gallons of blood. The body is fearfully and wonderfully made, so it is each person's responsibility to take care of his or her own body.

A heart attack occurs when a section of the heart muscle dies because of a blood clot or stenosis due to an abundant formation of plaque within the arteries. Therefore, the clogged artery will shut off the blood-borne oxygen in the affected region of the heart. The pain and chest tightness of angina pectoris indicate that there is a portion of the heart muscle that is not receiving a sufficient supply of blood. Women may experience a pain between the shoulder blades and also unusual fatigue.

The arteries don't just happen to get clogged overnight. They are coated a layer at a time by plaque that has accumulated throughout the years as a result of a high fat diet of animal source proteins.

According to *The Atlas of the Human Body*, "In the arteriosclerotic plaque, a greasy layer of deposits of excess blood cholesterol which consist of proteins, fats, and immune system cells that have accumulated in the blood, they infiltrate scar tissue and create a bulging obstruction."[1] The cholesterol generally is the large amounts of LDL (low-density lipoprotein) that circulate through the blood and not enough HDL (high-density lipoprotein), that is, the good cholesterol that transports the cholesterol to the liver, and from there, it is moved it into the colon to be eliminated.

The slow process of arteriosclerosis begins early in one's life and progresses until it gradually takes a life as the arteries begin to harden. As the plaque begins to coat the arteries, the arterial walls lose their elasticity and the interior lumen begins to narrow as the cholesterol builds up, resulting in inflammation which will eventually result in a bulging mass. These clogged arteries can trigger not only heart attacks but strokes. In advanced arteriosclerosis, the lumen becomes too narrow for the blood flow and closes off the supply of blood. This creates an insufficient blood supply to the organs of the body; thus, the body begins an all-out emergency alert for the body to react and to try to overcome this. Cells begin to die because of lack of blood, oxygen, and nutrients. If something isn't done immediately, the organism dies.

The picture of the person who is ready for a heart attack usually depicts someone who is overweight, a possible diabetic, may smoke, drink, and whose diet absolutely defies the laws of nature. If one is to add stress to the equation, there is a bomb ticking and waiting to go off.

Even children have become victims of these adult diseases because of their poor diets. "Many overweight and obese children have arteries that are the age of a 45-year-old, and many are in the stages of arteriosclerosis. Their vascular age is at least 30 years older than their actual age."[2]

Drugs of all types are given to reduce cholesterol, thin the blood to prevent blood clots reduce blood pressure. Even so-called natural herbs and vitamin supplements won't cure the broken heart, if one is still consuming all the wrong things. Surgery won't help because the causes haven't been eliminated. Many doctors won't admit or are clueless of the causes of heart disease and arteriosclerosis, and so, many of them will die of the same diseases as their patients.

The diet of processed foods with fats, sugars, chemical additives, white flour, and animal source proteins contribute to these diseases of the heart and the arteries.

Prevention of heart disease and arteriosclerosis is to remove all saturated animal fats, other trans fatty acids and foods high in omega 6 processed fats and oils. Importantly, avoid all sugars, refined flours, and chemical additives. Too many people drink sodas with all the sugars and need to drink pure water instead. Fresh whole fruits, vegetables, seeds, and nuts all properly combined meet the nutritional needs of the human body and promote optimal health. Once the body has these severe challenges, it may be too late before a heart attack occurs that will snuff out life, so it's best to stop the body's process of disease. If you eliminate animal products from your diet, you eliminate the risk of experiencing a heart attack by 90 percent.[3]

The term stroke is in reference to the sudden death of brain tissue, which can be caused by a lack of oxygen because of the interrupted blood supply. There are two different types of strokes to be considered:

1. Ischemic stroke, a result of a blockage or reduced blood flow to an area of the brain and may be caused by a blood clot, otherwise known as thrombus. These are formed on the rough surface of the atherosclerotic plaques that develop on the artery wall. The thrombus may enlarge and block the lumen or break loose and lodge in another part of the body's vessels or organs.

2. A hemorrhagic stroke that is caused by a bleeding within the brain generally due to a burst blood vessel. The latter can be caused by hypertension, stress, or a ruptured aneurysm.

Plaque is formed by accumulated amounts of cholesterol in the blood. This sticky, gummy substance adheres to the arterial walls, forming layers that harden, thus the artery loses its elasticity and function becoming narrower until it eventually closes. Sometimes, this hardened plaque will break off in chunks, resulting in a blood clot floating off through the blood vessels. It may lodge in some organ or blood vessel, creating a dangerous situation, sometimes death to the organ, or death to the body.

A stroke or cerebrovascular accident (CVA) is an abnormal condition of the blood vessels of the brain characterized by occlusion of an embolus or cerebrovascular hemorrhage, resulting in ischemia of the brain tissues perfused by damaged cells.[4] The results of CVA depend on the location and the extent of the ischemia. The aftermath of a stroke may be paralysis, weakness, speech defect, aphasia (inability to understand or produce language), or death may occur. As swelling decreases, the symptoms will generally subside. Physical therapy and speech therapy may help to restore lost function.

The medical approach generally is an aggressive approach because of the urgency of the traumatic incident. A CAT scan is preformed to determine the location, the type of stroke, and the extent of damage. If it is an ischemic stroke, the doctors will conduct extensive tests to determine where in the body did the clot come from or if the clot can be dissolved with medication or with possible surgical removal. Some such medications would be anti-thrombin, fibrinolysin, and Heparin along with IV drugs. If it came from the heart, can it be repaired? On the other hand, if it is a hemorrhagic stroke, and then if hypertension is found to be the cause, the patient is given blood pressure drugs to quickly lower the blood pressure. Also the doctors may do different surgical procedures to remove the built-up fluid of blood on the brain. This can be done in several different ways: cauterization of the bleed, or by placing a stent in the brain to drain the fluid into the abdomen, or surgically cleaning out the blood from the brain. The objective is to reduce the swelling before it creates damage to the brain.

All of this is just the tragic aftermath and direct result of a body in crisis. The crisis was dependent on an improper diet and destructive lifestyle, destructive to one's own body. This person has depleted the number of their days prematurely. Healthy people do not experience strokes and they don't experience diseases. People need to learn from the mistakes of others. After all, no one lives long enough to make all of their own.

I have known a few people in the past year who have died tragically because of strokes and aneurysms; these people were still young, in the prime of their lives. Their bodies had been poisoned with accumulated chemicals because of their diet and lifestyle. Their deaths could have been prevented had they lived a lifestyle that practices proper nutrition and follows the laws of nature, not abusing their bodies throughout the years and days of their lives.

Rev. George Malkmus who lived eating a very nutritious diet and living a healthy lifestyle, but still experienced a stroke. He was a workaholic, continually stressing his body by his ungodly work schedule. According to George, he started to push himself beyond the body's capacity. He states, "No matter how perfect the diet, stress can cause havoc on a person's health."[5] During this exceptionally stressful period, he began to experience the repercussions of the abuse on his body and suffered a hemorrhagic stroke. His wife and son decided that George himself would refuse all medical treatments, so they informed the doctor of their decision to decline medical care. The doctor stated that George would be dead before morning without the treatments and told them to take him home. He was delivered by ambulance and placed in his bed, and his wife signed a waiver to state that he was alive when the paramedics left. His wife checked on her husband several times throughout the night, and in the morning he was still alive. She got down on her knees and praised God for his life. During the next several days, she gave him raw carrot juice alternating it with powdered barley juice, every hour for twelve hours, and on this regimen, his mind began to come back. Within a few days, he was able to carry on an almost normal conversation. After two weeks, he was back to work with his mind sharper than ever.

George states, "Approximately 50 percent of all who experience a hemorrhagic stroke die as a result of the stroke, and the other 50 percent usually are left with severe physical or mental limitations or both."[5] His life's lesson was, "We must do more than just eat the right diet. We must manage our stress level because even though the diet (Hallelujah Acres diet) is the right one, we can still get in trouble if we consistently push our bodies too hard. Managing stress and getting plenty of rest are an absolute necessity if we want to maintain our health in the long haul."[5]

Inflammatory bowel disease (IBD), Crohn's disease, and ulcerative colitis are diseases of the digestive tract, which seem to be a lot more prevalent now than ever before. This is due to several reasons created by the chemicals in today's foods and food products, animal proteins, refined sugars and flours, as well as large amounts of sodas, coffees, and other caffeine-type beverages. It is believed that one of the biggest contributors of these digestive diseases is stress-related.

Inflammatory bowel disease, Crohn's disease, and ulcerative colitis are inflammatory diseases of the intestines, which, according to the medical profession, are of unknown cause. People will continue to suffer extreme pain and inconvenience with bloody diarrhea, abdominal pain, and anemia, ulceration of the colon and small intestine, fever, fistulas, and stenosis of the bowels.

Ulcerative colitis is characterized by inflammation of the lining of the colon and small open sores in the lining of the colon. This disease usually involves only the colon and not the small intestine. The inflammatory process usually begins in the rectal and sigmoid area and then proceeds throughout the rest of the colon. Medically, drugs and surgery are standard. Complications, however, do include the disease spreading throughout the rest of the body. Many doctors claim there are genetic links and links to the environment, antibiotics, and a faulty immune system. Genetics is not a part of the same equation. It is a body that has been compromised so badly because of an enormous amount of accumulated toxins and chemicals along with a digestive system that is totally impaired.

Crohn's disease is another slow suicide attempt. Many people who have this malady would rather be dead, and they do look as if they are dead. Their attempt at living is seriously hindered. Crohn's disease is a chronic form of inflammatory bowel disease that begins as small-scattered sores on the lining of the lower end of the small intestine, the ileum. It then may continue to spread throughout the entire small intestine and may continue to damage any other part of the digestive tract from the mouth to the rectum. These small sores become inflamed, and this inflammation causes the cells in the affected area to secrete water and salt that are more than the digestive tract and colon can absorb; thus, diarrhea develops and the intestinal walls begin to swell and thicken, and then scar tissue forms. This affects the matter going through the intestinal tract, which leads to extreme pain and cramping. The feces may contain bright red blood. Sores and ulcers penetrate the walls of the intestines. These areas will be stricken with narrowing, fistulas, and stenosis. These diseases are most commonly seen in young people, twenty–forty years of age, but there is nearly no favoritism in the age of the person it attacks. Medically, diet and stress seem to be the main causes that aggravate the symptoms of Crohn's disease, but the same concept of cause attributed to inflammatory bowel disease, claims that heredity, environmental, and immune system, and otherwise unknown, causes persist in the medical community.

Inflammatory bowel disease can even be seen in children as young as a one year of age, according to L. Jodell McLemore, author of the direct reading *Radiology* magazine. In fact, the author states, "Twenty percent of IBD cases affect children."[6] Common symptoms include abdominal pain, bloody diarrhea accompanying dehydration, nutritional deficiencies, and weight loss. Instead of dealing with the cause of the disease, medically, these children continue with a lifelong drug therapy and or surgeries. At this age or any age for that matter, the physical complications can be devastating and traumatic. Dr. Paul A. Goldberg states matter-of-factly that "we do not acquire IBD due to any lack of any specific herbal or food supplement, and we are therefore not going to get well from such either."[7]

Many people whom I have questioned on their diet and lifestyle are very stressed and worried, leading a lifestyle where they are trying to burn the candle at both ends. Their diets are irregular and unhealthy. Many do not eat enough raw fruits and vegetables, but do eat a lot of improperly combined meals, ones that do not exit the stomach to enhance digestion. The stress overload inhibits digestion even further. They will continue to visit the doctors' offices and hospitals for a multitude of tests, procedures, and surgeries to remove parts of the intestinal tract or even to surgically remove a part or the entire colon. Those who have gone through these surgeries and procedures do not get any relief; they just continue to get sicker and sicker, taking more and more drugs. The cause is never addressed, and these people walk through life in the state of walking death because this is not a life to lead. I would not wish this existence on my worst enemy.

Many imitation cures are in the marketplace, such as bowel-cleansing products and a host of so-called natural food and herbal supplements of which none works.

The disease of the digestive tract and colon affects the entire body and must be addressed as such. Fasting and juicing of raw vegetable juices are important in allowing the body to heal itself. The fast allows the body to rest and cleanse, therefore, to heal itself. The determined person who fasts, rests, and starts a new life change with a diet of raw whole plant foods will achieve vibrant health, but those who are unwilling will continue to become sicker and sicker. It is a matter of making wise decisions—to choose life and therefore hope and wellbeing or choose to die slowly and agonizingly.

Endnotes

1. Beverly McMillan, *The Illustrated Atlas of the Human Body* (Argosy, 2008), 139.
2. Marilynn Marchione, "Fat Kids Found to Have Arteries of 45 Year Olds" (research paper, 2008).
3. George Malkmus, The Hallelujah Diet, Destiny Image Publishers, Inc. Shippensburg, PA (2006), 115.
4. *Mosby's Medical, Nursing, & Allied Health Dictionary* (CV Mosby., 1990), s.v. "stroke."
5. George Malkmus, "Rev. George Malkmus Experiences a Stroke—How Could This Happen?" *Hallelujah Acres Diet & Lifestyle Magazine* 49 (March/April 2008): 11– 12.

6. L. Jodell McLemore, "Inflammatory Bowel Disease," *Radiologic Technology* 78, no. 4 (2007): 294.

7. Paul Goldberg, "What is Inflammatory Bowel Disease?" (research paper, Goldberg Clinic, 1995), 2.

CHAPTER 19

Junk Food

While people will eat just about anything, not everything is healthy for the body. Humankind is the only species who cooks its foods, even the ones to be eaten as raw. All processed foods are fragmented and cooked and not really considered to be called foods. Foods are a product of nature, filled with nutrients, vitamins, and minerals. They are designed by our Creator to be easily digested and assimilated by the body. Processed, refined foods should not be eaten because they are toxic to the human body.

During the last century or so, more and more food-processing and refining companies have been established. The production of highly-refined, highly chemically oriented, and heavily processed so-called foods increasingly continues. Throughout the last four to five decades, these processed products have become much worse as far as their damage to the human organism. Most of these products that are called junk foods lack any element that began as food, and the end product is a disease-creating foodstuff. Carbohydrate type processed foods are the worst of these junk products, yet people consume them in astronomical amounts.

Chocolate is one of the most eaten sweet carbohydrate junk food. A process of fermenting, roasting, and grinding the seeds of the cacao tree makes chocolate. Andrew Smith claims that chocolate is then a complex combination of about 1,200 chemicals, none of which is dormant. The chemical theobromine is a bitter, colorless alkaloid which is found in chocolate. It is a stimulant that acts primarily on the muscles.[1] Add that to the small amounts of caffeine and the sugar that masks the bad, bitter taste of plain chocolate, and you have an extremely unhealthy product. Chocolate also contains 50 percent fat to eliminate its graininess. According to *Hallelujah Acres Newsletter*, "Chocolate contains two grains of tannin per cup (tannin is the substance that is used for tanning leather), plus oxalic acid, cannabinoids and aflatoxins, and it also contains no more than an average of 75 insect and rodent fragments per three tablespoons. The visible or solid animal excreta are not to exceed 10 mg./lb. These are the maximum level guidelines set by the US government. These insect fragments are similar to our cockroach. Sweet chocolate contains 538 calories and 35 grams of fat per 3.5 ounces."[2] What the main product becomes is a deadly poison for the body.

One hundred years ago, state the *Hallelujah Acres* authors, "the annual consumption of sugar was five pounds per year." In 2001, the average American consumed 150 pounds per year. By 2008, it was up to 170 pounds per person per year.

It is a very addictive chemical to the human body. People have been very serious about calling themselves a chocoholic and not being able to say no to these sweet confections. The sugar is high in calories and void of nutrition. It causes the blood sugar levels to fluctuate that, in turn, creates a craving for more to make you feel balanced. To break this cycle of craving, it's best to eliminate *all* sugars from the diet.

The chemical effects of cooking foods are known to be devastating, in turn adding to the destruction of the human organism. Herbert Shelton states, "Cooked foods are fiberless food. Most of the fiber has been damaged so it just coats the intestinal walls throughout the digestive process. Cooking coagulates protiens, and their amino acid molecules are broken up (deaminizes) caramelizes sugars, breaks up fats into free fatty acids, destroys vitamins and enzymes, chemically renders mineral salts unusable, leeches substances from foods, makes most foods less digestible, and alters their taste,"[3] making them unpalatable. People feel the need to use spices, artificial flavorings, sweeteners, and condiments because these products are tasteless after they have been cooked.

Doctors dealing with cancer patients have told me that their patients are not to eat any raw fruits and vegetables because, supposedly, the foods in the raw state are toxic to them; that the germs can create worse life-threatening disease, and cooking will destroy any disease-forming bacteria. They all believe that the immune system is low and impaired because of something outside of the body, but it is the improper diet of processed foods and drugs that creates chemically-induced diseases. It's sad because people can change their diets to a raw produce one, eliminating the chemicals, and the body does, at times, allow healing to take place depending on the amount of damage that has occurred throughout the years of abuse. Cancer patients have been compromised through the years by their own knives and forks along with poor choices of diet and lifestyle. According to Rev George Malkmus from Halleljah Acres and Dr. Alec Burton professor from Fit for Life Sciences Institute, their cooking of fruits and vegetables renders these toxic, void of all nutrients, and impossible to digest by the body in any proper manner.

Raw foods take only about twenty-four to thirty-six hours to digest as contrary to cooked foods, which require forty-eight to one hundred hours. Many of these improper food combinations of cooked foods may not digest at all.

The stomach will continue to excrete hydrochloric acid to digest animal flesh and also with a meat and starch meal. These foods will sit in the stomach for hours as the digestive process continues to be overburdened. The stomach will finally try and push out slowly the putrefied and fermented mess into the intestinal tract just to get rid of it. These types of meals only offer heartache, chest pains that are created by acid reflux and esophageal ulcers that come from the amount of acid backup. The foods, which have been held up in the stomach, will try to go back into the esophagus and cause GERD (gastroesophageal reflux disease). The doctors will say, "Everyone has this disease. Just take these pills (Zantac etc.)." But the cause is never addressed, and the pills reduces the stomach acid, but the stomach only produces more, and it is a vicious cycle that only gets worse. The toxins are trapped in an internal oven of 98.6°F, cooking more along the way. The foods are supposed to leave the stomach digested, but in this case, it moves very sluggishly throughout the intestinal tract. The duodenum is supposed to continue some of the digestive process, but it is also hindered in its process. The animal flesh just coats the intestinal walls, and people wonder why they are constipated and have to take poisonous laxatives to expel these deadly wastes. These foods are void of the fiber and enzymes needed for digestion.

The cooking process depletes the nutrients; therefore, the body continues to crave foods just to gain satisfaction from whole food nutrients. The person will thus continue to overeat, and the more foods that are eaten, the more of a risk of obesity. The obese body is a malnourished body seeking to be nourished.

The kidneys and the liver work overtime trying to eliminate the uric acid created from the animal flesh. The body becomes more acidic, and this uric acid creates arthritis and gout. The body seeks to neutralize these acids by pulling calcium from the bones, which contributes to osteoporosis, and the high levels of fat from the meat carry toxins and will elevate the cholesterol.

The junk food/fast food manufacturers and other food industries do not have any interest in researching and marketing raw foods. Most food advertisers promote junk foods.

Even restaurants, especially those specializing in fast foods, use their air vents to pump out their cooking smells to entice the public at large. The smells of cooked food are all the evaporating nutrients; what is left is useless to the body. These foods are void of taste, flavor, nutrients, etc., so people dump on the seasonings, spices, and condiments to make them palatable.

Proteins tend to break down when heat is applied. They begin to harden and are deemed unusable to the human body. Cooking destroys the amino acids.

When certain greens that are high in oxalic acid (Swiss chard, collard greens, and spinach) are cooked, the oxalic acid hinders the absorption of calcium and iron by the body. When these greens are eaten raw, this effect is minimal.

Cooking damages fats and changes them into fatty acids, and these cause destructive damage to the cells' absorption. It tends to coat the cells of the body with this greasy coating. According to Brigette Mars, "Excessive use of cooked oils also causes cravings for stimulants like alcohol and caffeine and also can lead one to feel unclean, depressed, and heavy."[4] The heated oils coat the lungs and affect the skin by clogging the pores, thus creating acne and eczema.

Carbohydrates are considered a large group of compounds (including starches and sugars) that contain carbon, hydrogen, and oxygen found in foods and used to give energy. Some of our primary carbohydrates are fruits, nuts, tubers, legumes, and grains. Complex carbohydrates are needed by the body for fuel to provide for the body's needs, functions, and organs.

Fruits and fruit sugars are the most important product of nature to feed our human body. These feed the body optimally and digest and assimilate quickly. They do not take from the body. The glucose from the fruits gives to and feeds the body well.

The cooking of fruits caramelize them and renders them toxic and unusable to the body. The canning process of cooking fruits and then adding sugar make these fruits highly acidic and toxic. Cooking renders them tasteless, and the sugar is needed to give back their flavor. They are horrible for the functions of the body. Fresh fruits feed the palate like a jewel, sweet and refreshing. One could not ask for a better meal.

Nuts need to be eaten raw and unsalted. Many people just gorge over cans of oiled, roasted, and salted peanuts and other types of nuts. These are so full of oil and skins. I find them unpalatable and most certainly indigestible. The peanuts are legumes, not a nut, and the body has a very difficult time trying to digest them. People come up with so many nut concoctions—honey covered, chocolate covered, and even trail mixes mixed with dried fruit for the health-minded. The body does not consider these healthy because these products pollute the body with their sugars, fruits, and nuts. The fruit eaten with the nuts is held up in the stomach and begins to ferment. The body cannot digest this burdensome combination.

The many ways and combinations that people use to cook foods are just insurmountable. One may look at these same people sometime after their meal or even the next day, see the suffering that goes on in these bodies, and not envy their lifestyles. Disease has gone rampant because of these lifestyles and diets.

Cooking at any temperature destroys all of the healthy enzymes and nutrients. This is all dead food; it has no life and gives no life. The bottom line is this: everything that a person puts into his/her mouth must be cell-building material or it will be cell-destroying material. If it is cell-building, it will be life sustaining; if not, it will be disease producing.

A diet of basic raw foods properly combined strengthens the immune system and adds vitality to the body, allowing the body to heal and maintain proper function. The aging process is slowed down. Digestion is improved, disease is nonexistent, and body odor and bad breath are not evident. The eyes are bright and clear; memory, concentration, and focus are sharp and alert. The skin and muscle tone are superb. The body has more energy; therefore, a person requires less sleep than those who continue eating the standard American diet. The natural hygiene raw foods lifestyle maintains a person's weight at a normal range, and there aren't any of those nasty cravings for all the perverted food stuffs.

Raw foods are living foods filled with enzymes, vitamins, minerals, and all the nutrients for a self-healing body. The minerals, vitamins, and hormones of the body cannot work without the presence of enzymes. Enzymes are the life of the body. They are chemical catalysts that are needed for every chemical action and reaction that happens within the body.

The human body consists of three main catagories of enzymes. The first are called metabolic enzymes. They keep the body functioning properly and are very important for every activity of the body. It depends on them and without these, the body will die. Everyone can and will run out of them. When this happens it is called death. The functions of the body cease, so life does end at this point. The more of these enzymes a person uses up, the faster the body ages, the more unhealthy a person becomes, and the shorter one's life is.

The typical, standard American diet consists of processed, refined, and cooked foods with alcohol, fluoride, chlorine, drugs, caffeine, etc. By far, cooked foods are the main cause of this depletion. These enzymes are very fragile to light and heat while pressure will deactivate them. Any temperature that is above 118°F will totally destroy them. Cooked foods are void of all enzymes, so the body must produce these enzymes to digest the food. One can use their metabolic enzymes to rebuild new and healthy cells or deplete these enzymes by trying to digest enzyme-deficient foods that rob the body of energy rather than saving and giving it energy.

One must take responsibility to make sure that nothing interferes with the body making enough metabolic enzymes to keep it healthy and disease-free. The more raw whole foods that are eaten, the more we save our body's supply of metabolic enzymes.

The second class of enzymes is called digestive enzymes. They digest the foods that are eaten. These are involved in each and every specific job of the digestive process. From the mouth to the stomach and throughout the intestinal tract, these enzymes are there to aid in the body's digestive process. There are several organs besides the stomach that excrete enzymes, such as the pancreas, the liver, and the gallbladder. These enzymes are also working overtime in the case of refined sugars, processed and fried foods so loved by the American people who are consuming the standard American diet. Raw foods help the body to function while cooked foods just add to the over-burdened stress load of disease.

When raw (live) foods are eaten, they contain their own enzymes. These enzymes are called food enzymes, the third class of enzymes. When the meals consist of fresh, raw whole fruits, vegetables, and seeds and nuts, the body can easily digest and assimilate these foods. When enzymes are heated above 118°F, they are destroyed within one-half hour. At 130°F, they are destroyed within seconds. What do you think happens to enzymes at 212°F (the boiling point of water)?

Our Creator gave this great concept to us. The human bodies are provided the proper nutrients, and by conserving the enzymes, people can remain more youthful and have great amounts of energy. The raw foods are an enzyme-conserving foods.

Breakfast is supposed to be the first important meal of the day and a time for the body to finish its internal cleansing. From 4:00 a.m. until noon each day, the body is going through the elimination process and any foods, except for fruit, will hinder this process. Unfortunately, the standard American diet only includes fruit as an afterthought. It is incredible to see what people consume for breakfast. They are abusing their bodies to the point of destruction. People are killing themselves with the aid of their forks and spoons.

Their breakfast cereals and milk sometimes are topped with fruit or they drink fruit juices. These meals are packed with sugar and are so toxic. Other sugar meals consist of pastries, donuts, and coffee. The caffeine and sugar combinations are pitiful and poisonous. The eggs, bacon, potatoes, coffee, toast, biscuits, and gravy are the items that will pack on the most food that holds one over until dinner because the food never leaves the stomach until dinner.

With all the above breakfast combinations, the recipient will not be able to have a clean body but will continue to keep it polluted with the toxins of all these indigestible ingredients. The accumulating toxins will continue to build up and contribute to the overbearing diseases as the body must eliminate and clean itself while sickness is the body's way to try and cleanse its load.

Snacking consists of eating foods in between meals. Andrew Smith states, "Until the mid-nineteenth century, snacks mainly consisted of natural foods: fruits, nuts, grain products, biscuits, and cookies with occasional cheese."[5] In this current time, the medical professionals spoke out against snacking because they believed that it promoted indigestion, and people would not be hungry for good, healthy, and nutritious meals. It was all about money because no one paid attention to these professionals, and many vendors just sold their wares to the public.

Andrew Smith declares, "At least 75 percent of Americans derive at least 20 percent of their calories from snacks."[5] Snacking in most cases has been a meal replacement that leaves out the nutrition.

There are two categories of snack foods, salty and sweet. People have cravings for both. In the 1950s, the advertisers adopted the television market to get their profits soaring. In 2004, Andrew Smith states, "Collectively these snack food markets comprise a market niche generating billions of dollars annual sales."[5] Vending machines are literally everywhere and snack goods (so-called healthy junk snacks) are even sold in health food stores.

People use spices, onions and garlic, to enhance their foods. Cooked foods in their sabotaged state are bland and tasteless. To make them palatable, people add all types of seasonings and spices for their taste and flavor. Raw food advocates believe that as long as a food is in the raw state, it's okay to eat, and in their different food combinations, they will add these spices just to be creative and be so-called healthy. In fact, not all raw foods taste good, so spices are added to make them palatable.

One can smell the nutrients being cooked. People smell the good aroma" during the cooking process. So by adding back to these foods, the smells and tastes of the spices and seasonings will excite the senses and make these foods wonderful again. All processed foods and cooked foods are augmented with something to preserve and enhance. They do not add any nutritional value to the foods. In fact, they do add to the degenerative value of these foods on the body.

These condiments and spices irritate the lining of the stomach and intestinal tract, impair digestion and absorption, and create an intense thirst for water, which cannot be quenched. One of the main contributors to high blood pressure and renal disease is salt (sodium chloride). Salt is added in large amounts to all packaged, bottled, and all processed foods as a preservative. Reading the labels on these items will shock you when you see the amounts added. No wonder people are sick with all this sodium per serving, and no one eats just one serving. Salt is also very addicting; after all, the food manufactures see to that. The Lay's Potato Chip company slogan was "Bet you can't eat just one."

If the food tastes bad, doctor it up, dump on the spices, and then they will eat all of it is the principle. Food that tastes bad is bad for the body and should not be eaten. Spices act as an irritant on the digestive tract, and some are even very stimulating and harmful to the body. They do not add any nutritional value to the body.

It is believed that spices of all kinds are healthy, and in the raw state, they are healing to the body just as they are paralleled with herbs. The body tries to rid itself of these foreign substances the same way as it tries to rid the body of drugs. The body cannot deal with any chemical substances whether they are of the health genre or drugs. A poison is a poison whether in small or large amounts. It can still kill, and timing is the only variance.

Cinnamon is toxic to the body. It contains tannin, a poisonous irritant found in teas. Tannin is a chemical used in the tanning process of leather goods. Cinnamon is now promoted as a health product for reducing blood sugar for diabetics as well as other blood sugar problems. Nutmeg is another spice that is mostly used in baked goods and desserts. The powdered outer layer of the its kernel is used for making the nutmeg spice, but the inner layer is used for making the spice mace. In large doses, nutmeg is fatal. Vanilla bean is used to make vanilla extract. The bean itself has no flavor beyond what is pulled out with the use of alcohol and other chemicals in its process to make vanilla extract and flavorings. This is a highly toxic solution that can be very harmful because of all of these toxic chemicals.

Cayenne pepper burns the intestinal tract and colon. It burns going in as well as coming out, through the skin, causing flushing, heat, and sweating. It can be corrosive to the stomach and intestinal tract. This can lead to ulcerations that people will have them removed surgically, and then continue to eat the same way without any changes.

Other types of hot peppers can be even more damaging. I have seen different television shows of how some people will consume the hottest stuff into their mouths and stomachs. The body does repel it, but this is often ignored. The shows are made into competitions of how much time it will take to eat these hot foods. Ingesting fire and destruction seems to be their goal.

People will argue that raw onions and garlic are exceptionally wonderful and healing for the body. The taste, as far as I am concerned, makes me wonder what is in their minds and mouths. The taste buds and the body reject these things, especially in the raw state. These products, raw or cooked, are an irritant and a stimulant.

They will tend to cause inflammatory issues within the body's digestive tract.

In the fast food industry, onions are used excessively. The Coney Island hot dogs, for example, are loaded with chili, onions, and excessive condiments. This combination may create a lot of digestive problems for many people. Many restaurants use raw onions in their salads; others use loads of cooked onions as a filler in their vegetable dishes. Onions are a cheap filler food, and most people will consume these with delight. Their breath and bodies smell repulsive, and even the so-called sweet onions do not taste like apples as many will say. Onions are onions, some may be hotter than others, but they still heave damage onto the human body. Toxic mustard oil, the main irritant of the onion and its family members (such as leeks, green onions, and scallions), impairs and inhibits digestion. It also causes indigestion and reflux problems. According to T.C. Fry, "Consistent eaters of members of the onion family are frequently afflicted with kidney problems."[6] Mustard oil eliminates through the bowels and skin, but mainly through the lungs (the onion breath) and the kidneys. Mustard oil passes throughout the body very fast at the body's quick effort to rid it of this toxic poison.

Garlic is the same. It is indigestible, and all of the claimed health benefits have been debunked; there aren't any. Garlic, with its toxic substance allicin, gives off a pungent odor and strong flavor. Garlic and onions both contain the toxic poison mustard oil, and I have heard that garlic and onions are from the same family. These foods need to be avoided, not praised.

Other condiments in the standard American diet include mustard, horseradish, catsup, pickle relish, pickles, and sauces sold in bottles to enhance beef and other meats. It's amazing what they can put into a bottle (read the labels and find out how ridiculous it is). The marketing on these products is ludicrous as it tries to say how great the product tastes and how many people will buy and eat these concoctions. They all contain many chemicals that are damaging to the body.

A body that is continually being bombarded with poisonous chemicals becomes a breeding ground for disease. The body in its diseased state is crying out for mercy, but no one is listening. Doctors and hospitals and food manufacturers are the only ones that are happy because they are making money from everyone else's so-called misplaced happiness turned into misery.

Refined grains are the whole grains of which the outer shell (the bran fiber) and the most inner part (germ nutrients) have been removed during the milling process. The part left is the endosperm, which is void of fiber and nutrients. Manufacturers will try to replace the nutrients with synthetic ones and call them "enriched grains." These grains are totally harmful to the body.

The body tries to digest these grains, but because there isn't any fiber, they move through the alimentary canal very slowly and sluggishly. They create excess mucus, gassiness, and bloating. When people add animal flesh to their diets, the problems are compounded even more. The animal flesh, which is also void of fiber, sluggishly moves through the digestive tract in a 100°F atmosphere, taking three–four days to exit the body. During this time, it will putrefy in the intestinal tract, thus creating mild to severe colon problems. Grains as a starch and animal flesh as a protein should never be consumed, especially together. These foods are totally indigestible and void of nutrients and will leave toxins within the body.

To be eaten, refined grains and whole grains must first be processed, cooked, or sprouted. The processing or the crushing of the outer shell is done with many different forms because of the hardness of the seed. Therefore, many cooked foods are considered dead foods because the cooking process has destroyed the living enzymes. They are no longer living and are bad for the body. Sprouted grains are created with a soaking process in which the outer shell has been softened and the roots are encouraged to sprout. These are healthy for the body to consume.

Most grains are acidic to the body when eaten. Our bodies have been designed to consume alkaline foods to maintain an alkaline environment for regeneration and health.

They must be kept alkaline to survive. The blood must be kept at 7.4 on the pH scale. If the blood becomes acidic and drops below 6.9, the body will go into a coma and die. The bone structure is kept strong in an alkaline environment. An alkaline body promotes health, an acid one, disease.

Calcium is a very alkalizing mineral, which, in its greatest abundance, resides in the bones. When the blood pH levels start to dip below 7.4 because of the overconsumption of acid-bearing foods, the body automatically steps in to correct and protect itself. The body's efforts are to sustain the alkaline levels and neutralize the acidity. It will start to draw the calcium from the bones to make the blood into its alkaline state. If the acidity in the body increases, the calcium extraction increases. Thus the bones become depleted in strength and density. They become weaker, porous, and have an increased risk to fractures.

Refined grains promote blood sugar disorders because these grains are broken down very rapidly into simple sugars that enter the bloodstream quickly. Therefore, this increased sugar taxes the pancreas as well as the adrenal glands, in turn producing hypoglycemic and diabetic reactions.

Cereals and grains, according to nutritionists and the food pyramid, need to have at least sixteen servings a day. That is astronomical. No wonder there are so many obese people; they believe this deceptive and ludicrous lie. Refined grains create obesity. These grains are void of all nutrients, therefore creating a hungry body that is seeking its vitamins, minerals, and good whole foods for nutrition. The body craves satisfaction at a cellular level to be fed. Thus a person will continue to eat. These grains *are* addictive.

When I used to eat these breads and grains, I could not stop. The stomach was full, but my mouth wanted more and couldn't get enough. That is an addiction. I have not, nor will not ever, eat any of these foods again because I do not want a repeat of that experience.

Refined grains compromise the immune system and create a variety of diseases. These grains, which convert rapidly to sugar, suppress the immune system with toxins. Refined grains build up the toxic levels within the body, and it then continues to try eliminating them. Through the accumulated poisons within the body, the disease continues as the body is attempting to clean up the mess. Refined grains are bad for the body.

Endnotes

1. Andrew F. Smith, *Encyclopedia of Junk Food and Fast Food* (Greenwood, 2006), 148–149.
2. George Malkmus, "Chocolate & Sugar," Hallelujah Acres Health Tip 105.
3. Herbert Shelton, *INHS Newsletter* (2004) (taken from "Food Cooking…Health for Millions," 1968)
4. Brigitte Mars, *Rawsome* (Basic Health, 2004), 6.
5. Smith, *Encyclopedia of Junk*, 245.
6. T.C. Fry, "All Life Conditions and Activities Affect Nutrition," in vol.1, *Fit for Life Basic Health Library*, 18.

CHAPTER 20

Junk Foods and Fast Foods

Not everything that people eat is considered to be food. Not everything that they put into their bodies will nourish them. The food industries want people to think that their food is the best, most nutritious, real food. In reality, this is an outrageous lie. According to the *Oxford Dictionary*, "food" is "any substance that people or animals eat or drink or that plants absorb to maintain life and growth." But these packaged substances do not meet these criteria. They do not sustain or maintain life and growth. They create disease and cellular death.

George Malkmus, in his article, "Are You Living to Eat or Eating to Live?" writes, "Ninety percent of the money that Americans spend on food goes toward nonfood, manufactured and processed food."[2] He also goes on to say, "Processed foods are addictive. The manufactured food industry has chemically altered their products to ensure that people never tire eating them. They are intentionally processed to be addictive."[2] The food additives are put in their nonfood products so people will not only eat these, but continue to crave them. That's why people will persist eating these products. Most of these processed, manufactured foods are loaded with all types of unnatural substances such as sugars, salt, corn syrup, MSG, and other addi-

163

tives that increase their addictive properties. Peoples' taste buds have become perverted by these manufactured products.

The standard American diet has now become the world's diet. The fast food and junk food companies now inhabit the entire planet to make a profit. From the early morning breakfasts of bagel, donuts, and coffees on the go for all of those with rushed lifestyles to the cereals with milk, with bacon, ham, eggs, toast, and hash browns. Fruit is the afterthought or what may be included with the pancakes, such as sugared strawberries or pasteurized and frozen orange juice concentrate. The lunches consist mostly of some type of sandwiches or hamburgers. Some smart, health-conscious people will take in a salad but include all the toppings of bacon bits or croutons and bottled salad dressings along with their iced teas or sodas. Dinners seem to be the biggest meal of the day and you name it and it's eaten. Pizzas, hamburgers, hotdogs, casseroles, and packaged or frozen dinners, spaghetti—mostly meat and starches—are consumed with vigor. Vegetables are a forgotten item; many won't eat vegetables unless they are cooked to mush. Children think that a french fry is their vegetable.

The deceived public believes that because the label consists of added vitamins and minerals, even stating organic, then it's considered healthy. If that were true, why are there so many sick and unhealthy people? More diseases are prevalent; new ones, unheard of even a couple of decades ago, are rearing their ugly heads because of the increased chemicals and processing of junk foods that people consume in their diets. In fact, it is known that people are consuming more chicken and beef because of the increase in fast food restaurants and the advertising that goes along with their promotion. It is now advertised that less money can buy more food. Pizza and submarine sandwich shops continue this type of promotion. Convenience stores offer big gulps, 24–32 oz. of soda for less than a dollar. These are cheap foods to fill you up but not to nourish a person. Other countries of the world are now suffering the American diseases. The fast food companies (many times subsidiaries of US fast food chains) offer cost-effective, less-expensive foods than other food establishments in these overseas nations.

In my opinion and experience, it's still cheaper to eat healthier, the natural, hygienic way. No doctors' visits, no money going toward expensive drugs to try and eliminate illnesses; you've got the idea. It's not the initial cost, but the price tag of the aftermath of what can happen to the person's body, but no one will mention that. Everyone must learn to be responsible for his or her own health.

The fast food/junk food industries are promoting their goods worldwide. As these companies know, some areas have or do ignore them, but they only push harder. These companies want profit; the bigger the areas, more people can say yes, and yes means more money. Who cares about the health of people? That is not their number one priority—profits are. People don't say no because the products are addicting and comforting. These are the true comfort foods. In excess, these products can be very harmful, especially for children when junk food and fast food compete with a balanced diet that is necessary for good health and growth. When people are snacking on junk foods, they consume less nutritious foods; therefore, they do not receive proper nutrients of a well-balanced diet. The body becomes malnourished, impaired, and a breeding ground for toxic buildup and diseases.

Another factor that inhibits people from giving up their standard American diet is that these foods are very addicting. A lot of people don't want to give up their stimulants, sugars, and refined flours, meats, grains, and dairy products, sodas, and coffees. They don't want their diseases but are unwilling to give up the items that cause these diseases. They would rather go through the surgeries, medical tests, drugs, and hospitalization.

In France, Belgium, and other European countries, the child is taught at a young age how to eat properly for good health. When taking a holiday, it is to relax, not to vacation needing to see and do everything in a small amount of time and then needing another vacation just to wind down. The Europeans go to the markets daily for fresh foods or grow their own gardens. The people grow up this way. Unfortunately, the fast food industries are seeping their way into these countries, and it is creating the American diseases for the people in these cultures as well. Obesity is becoming a big issue in many overseas countries as well.

The fast food companies and some other restaurants serve super-sized portions, and many people feel that they are getting their money's worth of food when they are buying these. In their greed, they are harming their bodies through this overeating of polluting meals. This binging abuses the body. If these meals were only an occasional occurrence, the body could deal with it, but most of these oversized meals occur several times a week, and in some cases, several times a day. The problem is that too much of the wrong foods are destructive to the body. People blame these companies and rightly so. They are to blame, but people need to also assume responsibility, to say no. They are the ones feeding these toxic foods into their bodies. So it is a double-edged sword. The best thing to do is to eliminate all the processed foods, meats and dairy products, sugars, and caffeinated beverages, or at least for the new adventurer, to cut back. It is best to eat more fresh produce and drink pure water. Yes, there will be withdrawal symptoms as the body is cleansing itself, but the body needs a chance to recuperate and regenerate.

The junk/fast foods of the standard American diet that are promoted consist of milk and dairy products, meats (especially hamburgers), steaks, pork, seafood, grains, refined sugars with the candies and desserts, and flours, fermented products, packaged processed items, condiments, and also the canned and bottled drinks with their sugars and caffeine. In fact, in the year 2006, George Malkmus stated in his *Hallelujah Acres Health News Magazine*, "On the new market, 2,800 new candies, ice cream, desserts, and snack items were introduced in comparison to 230 fruit and vegetable products. Refined carbohydrate food products are not foods at all because foods provide nutrients given by nature, and these products are void of all nutrients.

The junk food/fast food manufactures spend billions of dollars each year on advertising to sell their products and to get people to buy, buy, buy, and to make profits from their sales. They start early, targeting children who sit and watch these commercials continuously mesmerized in front of their television sets. They will be watching more than ten thousand food advertisements. Children do not have the buying power, but they do have the pestering power. Manufactures start early, knowing that these children will grow up into paying adults. These products are aggressively promoted. Without mass advertising, there wouldn't be any junk foods. People pay the advertising when they purchase these packaged processed items.

The hamburgers and french fries combinations sell in huge numbers, and children drink sugared sodas also in large numbers. These children continue to coerce their parents to eat in these establishments. It turns out to be a family affair.

These protein and starch combinations are not digested. The body digests starches in the mouth with the chewing of the foods, allowing it to mix with the saliva, enjoying the textures and flavors before swallowing it. Too many are in such a hurry to eat that they practically inhale their foods so that all of this undigested food ends up in the stomach with nowhere to go. The stomach acids will take up some of this and try to digest it, but it will just continue to churn and then be pushed through the alimentary canal. The proteins will start its digestive process in the stomach with the aid of enzymes and hydrochloric acid. When a starch and a protein are eaten together, the digestive process is neutralized, adding the condiments to the sandwich makes it even a worse mess with all the oils, vinegar, salt, pepper, and then topping it off with dressings and sodas. It makes it impossible. The stomach will continue to churn and churn, creating heartburn and reflux but no digestion. It may be held up in the stomach for up to eight hours before it gets pushed through the system, sluggishly coating and impacting the tract along the way. These proteins will putrefy and decay within the intestinal tract. I had a patient once whose breath smelled like feces. This rotting mess will continue to backlog the system. Each meal just adds to this while the organism continues to degrade. There isn't any fiber or nutrients in these foods, and the toxins and poisons are just kept within the body and will accumulate with all the leftover debris, creating more diseases. This rotting flesh and impacting grains in the intestinal tract cause flatulence, body odor, and innumerable physical problems, including IBS, colitis, ulcerative colitis, Crohn's disease, diverticulitis, and diverticulosis, and colon cancer, just to name a few.

The milk industry is another big business with all the milk and cheese products on the market. They advertised the white moustache, "Got milk? Builds strong bones and teeth." Milk, cheese, and other dairy products create excessive mucous, lactose allergies along with other types of allergies, diarrhea, intestinal distress, cramping, headaches, and immune system disorders. Milk, i.e., breast milk was designed by our Creator to feed babies, not adults or children past the weaning age. Casein, the protein in cow's milk is twenty times higher than breast milk, and its calcium is three times more than human breast milk. For the body to digest calcium, there needs to be a certain amount of magnesium, vitamin D, biotin, and manganese as well as other trace minerals. Another reason milk cannot be digested is that the human body lacks the enzyme rennin and lactase to digest the milk protein and milk sugar. This is the reason why there is so much being said about lactose intolerance. Children, as well as adults, have so many severe allergies because of all the mucous forming in their bodies as they are trying to eliminate these unwholesome foods. Cow's milk is very acidic to the body. The more these dairy products are consumed, the more acidic the body becomes and to rid the body of this acidity, calcium is pulled from the bones to neutralize this condition of the body. This reaction creates osteoporosis, a condition of a weakening of the bone density in which a person becomes very susceptible to hip, spine, and other fractures of the bones. The fat from the milk and cheeses only adds to the weight problems of this generation. Look at all the fat babies, whose overweight condition stems from the milks and formulas that they are fed, only adding to their health challenges. Children have too many experiences of allergies, ear infections, colds, respiratory infections, gassiness, diarrhea, vomiting and spitting up, also are colicky, and have excessive mucous caused by drinking milk and eating dairy products.

Homogenization and pasteurization of milk are processing techniques used to render milk safe for the public to drink. Homogenization is used to make the cream inseparable from the milk. As children growing up, we saw, in all the milk that was purchased, the cream sitting right underneath the cap. My sister opened all the milk bottles and ate the cream chunk. She was surprised when the milk began to lose its cream. At this time the word homogenized began to appear on the label, and at that time we didn't know what that meant.

Pasteurization is the heating process of raw milk to kill the bacteria. The problem is this process makes the milk even more indigestible, and it destroys any nutrients that may have existed. The vitamin/mineral elements are impaired and cooking of any proteins makes them totally indigestible.

People have been programmed since their youth by this advice: "Drink your milk it'll give you strong bones and teeth." I have two surveys that will tell otherwise.

Example 1 concerns an elderly man who still is a dairy farmer. He grew up on a farm, milking cows and drinking milk in abundant amounts as if it were water throughout his entire life. He seemed healthy enough, but he did have a couple of small health challenges and made an appointment to see his doctor. After a thorough physical exam, his doctor patiently said to the man that he had osteoporosis. The farmer retorted back, that he couldn't because he always drank a lot of milk and still does. The doctor stated that it didn't matter; he still had the disease.

Example 2 is about another elderly gentleman who grew up in a poor household wherein the only milk that was bought was one quart a week for his father's coffee. This man is now in his eighties and his bones are very strong, hence no osteoporosis. The conclusion of these two stories is that the drinking of milk is the contributing factor to getting osteoporosis.

There are other calcium-rich foods that are superior to the merits of milk, which many people falsely believe is the main nutrient of gaining calcium for the body. Some of these are broccoli, kale, dark green leafy vegetables, fresh, organic raw carrot juice, almonds, sunflower seeds, dried figs, and fresh whole figs. For the body to assimilate its calcium, it needs a balance of magnesium, vitamins D and K, boron, and other trace minerals. These all come from eating whole fresh fruits and vegetables as well as limited amounts of nuts and seeds. These vitamins and minerals are absorbed through these foods optimally and in perfect amounts.

Another major concern is that milk is acidic, and the more dairy products that are consumed, especially along with the animal flesh, the more acidic the body becomes. The only way that the body can neutralize all of this acid is to excrete calcium (an alkaline mineral) from the bones. This in turn makes the bones less dense and brittle. Eventually, the hips and spine begin to fracture. These are the first areas of the body to show osteoporosis, and then the rest of the bony skeleton will end up weakened as well.

I have a friend who drank a lot of milk daily. She just loved her milk and couldn't part with it. She ended up having bilateral hip surgeries done in a year, yet the pain in her hips seemingly worsened. I suggested again that she give up her milk and see if that helped. She had no other options, so she did eliminate her milk intake reluctantly and it worked. As I suspected, the milk was the cause of the pain. She is elated because she walks pain-free. She won't go back to her old life.

Sugar is the most addictive and common part of the standard American diet. It comes in many forms and most people are deceived in their belief that if it doesn't say "sugar" on the label, then it's okay to eat. All forms of sugar are stimulating, addicting, and destructive to the body. It shuts down the immune system; it lowers and kills the good bacteria within the body, the blood system, and digestive tract, and also adds its load of toxins. Sugar feeds cancer. It's like pouring gasoline onto a fire; after it ignites, it begins to burn out of control.

Most people on the standard American diet consume about an average of ten thousand pounds a year. Sugar is in most of the processed foods on the market in one form or another. Just reading the labels boggles one's mind: high fructose corn syrup, corn syrup, dextrose, maltodextrin, sucrose, fructose, evaporated cane juice, etc. These are staples in the diets of those consuming breakfast cereals, desserts, cookies, cakes, candies, chewing gums, ice creams, and this list will continue on and on.

When people consume their sodas, there are eleven teaspoons of sugar in each 12 oz. can. Those who have been to a sugarcane plantation have heard that it takes three feet of sugar cane to equal one teaspoon of refined sugar. Sugarcane is a living food, but after it is refined, it becomes a dead processed product, one that will take the life force from the body.

Sugar is not considered a food, but it is considered to be a poisonous, addictive, and dangerous drug, according to Hallelujah Acres author, Olin Idol in "Toxicity Refined Sugar: How Sweet Is It?"[3] Sugar is also a highly addictive substance, and it's no wonder. Just think about it. When coca leaves are refined, it becomes a drug called cocaine. When poppy extract is refined, it becomes opium (heroin), and refining sugarcane, it becomes sugar. When sugars are first eliminated from the diet, the body may go through mild to severe withdrawal symptoms. It may take the body up to thirty days to rid it of the withdrawal effects of sugar. The craving of sugar upon the body is intense.

In its processing, sugar cane has become so filled with chemicals and poisons that its end product is anything but good. It is a fragmented product with sixty-four food elements destroyed because of the processing. These fragmented food elements are the creator of the body's health challenges and nutrient imbalances. Sugar goes through several extracting and cooking processes through which different chemicals are added to, or taken, from it. Sugar's cane juice is acidic, and partway through the process, several chemicals are added to make it more alkaline. It is bleached with chlorine and ultramarine to make it white. The final residue from the sugar process is called molasses, which has all of the harmful and toxic chemicals from the process itself. It's the leftover garbage. Molasses should be dumped into the garbage, but the sugar manufactures decided that they could dump it on the gullible public as a health food for their own profits. After all, why waste anything when someone else will use it? Some of the toxic chemicals from processing, as well as some more added toxins, still remain in the molasses. Some of these are sulphur dioxide, carbonic gas, phosphoric acid, bone char, and chlorine.

Sugars of any kind are acid-forming. They decrease the body's ability to heal for up to five hours after digestion. "Sugar raises blood pressure. Sugar mixed with animal fats leads to arteriosclerosis, and by increasing the stickiness (viscosity) of the blood, increases the possibility of blood clots."[3] The main reason to avoid sugar is that it ages the arteries, also adding to the aging and destruction of the cells of the body.

It also blocks the absorption and increases the elimination of many minerals, especially calcium, from the body. The bones are the main structures for calcium content and storage. For the body to neutralize the acidity, it draws calcium from the bones to metabolize the refined sugars. Consuming sugars and animal products causes the body to excrete so much calcium that the body becomes osteoporotic and the teeth begin to decay.

Sugar is also the main cause of weight gain and diabetes, especially when it is eaten with fats, as in desserts. Many are unable to stop this dangerous practice of sugar consumption because of sugar's addictive properties. They will not stop eating their desserts, candy bars, sodas, cakes, cookies, etc. I had a friend who, after every meal, had to have her sweet confection. Even limited amounts are quite addicting. I fought long and hard to rid myself of the refined sugar addiction. It's been up to five years now, and I know that I'll be deathly ill if I take even one bite, so I do not even indulge at all. One was never enough. Look at children. If they are given one piece of candy, they will drive the parent crazy until the bag is finished. My own mother admitted a horrible sugar/candy addiction her whole life, and it brought her to a terrible end: pancreatic cancer. She died a horrible death.

Sugars can create emotional instability by interfering with the endocrine system. PMS is a common excuse for overdosing on sugars, and hypoglycemic reactions and depression are all sugar related. Children suffer from ADD (attention deficit disorder) and ADHD (hyperactivity), rampant disorders among our young. Most of them are just sugared up from morning until night without any way of slowing down. They are then put into a crisis situation when the doctors and parents put these children on another poison, a drug called Ritalin or other depressive drugs. All they have to do is to change their diets and lifestyle, and the children will become and remain calmer and better behaved.

Sugars do create a euphoric reaction, and this sugar high and instant energy keep people in its clutches. The problem comes later when the person crashes. Without any energy, hunger strikes the person because his/her blood sugar levels crash as well. A sugar crash also leads to depression and irritability. As soon as the sugars enter the stomach, they turn to glucose and pass through the stomach wall quickly and are already in the circulating bloodstream. The person who suffers from anorexic and bulimic disorders will go on sugar and processed food binges, eating compulsively, especially on sugar products and then vomit or compulsively exercise to rid of the weight gain effects, not even realizing that it has already left the stomach in a short time. To combat these maladies, fresh whole fruits are wonderful foods for the body. Their exciting sweetness digests quickly in the stomach yet offers such complimentary effects of nutrition for the body.

E. Cheraskin, MD, DMD, and W. Marshall Ringsdorf Jr., DMD, MS, spent more than two decades conducting studies based on linking diseases to the diets of the American public. They wrote a book about their research, *The New Hope for Incurable Diseases by F.K. Plous Jr.* The bottom line of their research is if people were educated on the causes of disease, would they or would they not change their diet and lifestyles to create health and prevention of any further diseases?

They stated in an article, "Twenty-Year Study Links Disease to Sugar," written by F. K. Plous Jr. to promote their book in 1972, *New Hope for Incurable Diseases,*. that all refined carbohydrates, especially sugars increase the rates of diseases. "We began collecting dietary records from two groups of people, those with a history of chronic illness and those with consistent good health. We wanted to know the answer to the question, 'What do sick people eat and what do healthy people eat?' We found out that they do not eat the same things."[4]

The people who ate less junk food, processed and refined foods were far healthier than those who consumed more. Most diseases are related to this processed, refined diet. Whole foods come packaged with their own nutrients and enzymes, so the body is capable of digesting and assimilating them.

The overwhelming statistics in 1972 were "The average American consumes 115 pounds of sugar each year—this means that each man, woman, and child eats one teaspoonful of sugar each hour 365 days a year"[4] as stated by Cheraskin. He also mentions "that the primary alteration in the average American's food intake during the past 80–100 years has been a marked reduction in starches and more than doubled increase in the consumption of simple sugars (primarily table sugar/sucrose) and syrups."[4] According to the 2008 *Hallelujah Acres Health Tip Newsletter*, the average American consumed 170 pounds per year and is still not realizing that it is doing horrible and destructive things to their bodies. They also predict that if following the same trend, people will consume ten thousand pounds of refined sugars.[5] With a rise in all that the sugar-containing foods there is an increase of chronic diseases, especially diabetes, obesity, glaucoma, arteriosclerosis, hypertension, arthritis, multiple sclerosis, and birth defects.

Even back in the late 1950s through the 1960s, when these studies were conducted, these authors, Cheraskin and Ringsdorf, concluded that vaccination and sanitation had no effect on chronic diseases because "no known communicable germ is responsible for them; they rise from the body tissue itself after something unhealthy is allowed to happen to that tissue."[6] These are the diseases that all have a relation to diet.

Although these authors promote a healthy, educated diet and elimination of all refined sugars, flours, and adding more fruits and vegetables, they both conclude that adding more animal proteins with supplementation of vitamins/minerals is promoting health. The latter also promotes disease, even if the former is worse. (The lesser of two evils philosophy.) These diseases of the 1950s–1960s were also on the rise for the younger generations to come.

I was born in the year 1950, at the start of the study, and through the years of this study, I was raised with refined sugars and white flours. The study was completed in 1971, and the years have now passed into the twenty-first century. The diseases that have wreaked havoc are tremendous. In 2006, Andrew F. Smith published his book *Encyclopedia of Junk Food and Fast Food*. With diabetes, for example, there are six hundred thousand new cases diagnosed each year and 71,372 deaths are attributed to diabetes.[7] Michael Donaldson in 2007 stated that 20.6 million people live in the "state of diabetes." That is equal to the adult population of Michigan, New Jersey, and North Carolina combined.[8]

Many people laugh when told that sugar is a poisonous drug. "Well, it's one that I'll die eating, ha ha!" The problem is that it produces a slow suicide, a walking death to some. The destruction continues, and unless the body gets a chance to eliminate these poisons, it will go through the disease process, i.e., colds, flu, sinus infections, respiratory problems, ear infections, arthritis, etc. A person may not even be aware of the internally devastating damage that is occurring.

Sugar is everywhere, in every meal that people consume, such as in the standard American diet. It is sometimes called carbohydrates. All carbohydrates are technically sugar. The body breaks down carbohydrates into glucose for the body to use as energy. What makes the difference is the rate these sugars enter the bloodstream. The fruit sugar enters it slower and is of an alkaline nature. High fructose corn syrup is a so-called natural sugar, but it is not any better than refined sugars. Both are refined, processed, and acid forming and enter the bloodstream very fast, thus the sugar high. These are both poisonous and dangerous for the body to digest and assimilate. It is best to just change the quality of the carbohydrates in the diet for optimal and quality health. People need to limit their consumption of all sugars and avoid processed food products.

Dental decay has increased to 95 percent of all Americans. Osteoporosis is now in epidemic proportions. Michael Donaldson, PhD, is in a preventive mode in his article, "The Heart Attack Helper," where he states, "Heart attacks strike down almost one out of two Americans and often come without a warning sign. If you are an American over twenty, you have a 50 percent chance that this is at work inside of you"[9] because of the standard American diet. The strong allies that create heart disease are our knives, forks, glasses, and the conventional way that people give into their utensils. But the biggest tragedy is that it is preventable. Higher cholesterol is a health marker. Only about "18–20 percent of young adults have cholesterol that is 15 mg/dl or below," claims Michael Donaldson PhD. "But as the population ages only about 2 percent of adults forty-five years and older have a cholesterol level below 150 mg/dl. The American diet, loaded with refined sugars, white flours, refined oils, meat and dairy products, and almost nonexistent of fresh fruits and vegetables, leaves no adequate protection against heart disease."[9] A radical diet change is called for.

Arthritis is just a catchall of any inflammatory disease, such as lupus, which is called an autoimmune disease. Doctors are clueless about what is causing these disorders, nor can they cure them with their drugs, so they tend to blame the patient's body. Yes, it is the patient's body, but not that the body is attacking itself. It is fearfully and wonderfully made and wasn't created to do that. The body is just in a crisis state that needs to be free of drugs, polluting foods, and cleansed. According to the Arthritis Foundation, arthritis is the leading cause of disability in the United States with "rheumatoid arthritis affecting 2.1 million Americans, osteoarthritis affecting 21 million and 300,000 dealing with juvenile arthritis." Olin Idol, author of the "Arthritis" article, also states, "By ages 55–64, nearly one out of every 10 individuals has limitations on his or her activities because of impaired function"[10] with joint and muscle pain. The Lupus Foundation of America estimated, according to Michael Donaldson, PhD, in his article, "Lupus: Disarming the Robber of Vitality," that 1.5 to 2 million Americans have lupus and more than 90 percent of them are women.[11] Lupus, fibromyalgia, multiple sclerosis, and rheumatoid arthritis are all considered to be autoimmune diseases with severe inflammation and pain. These diseases, as well as others, can be prevented and /or controlled by the diet and lifestyles of people. As the age of the person increases, the disease levels also increase because of the accumulated levels of toxic chemicals that continue to increase within the body.

Breast cancer has also remarkably risen. The National Cancer Institute estimates, states Olin Idol in his research that there are "178,480 new cases in females for the year 2007 with 40,460 female deaths and 2,030 new cases in males and 450 male deaths as a result of breast cancer. With the current trends, one in every eight women (12.7 percent) will be diagnosed with breast cancer in their lifetime."[12]

God blessed us with a body that desires to maintain optimal health, but one must be obedient to observe and live by the laws of nature that provide these conditions. One will be supporting the self-healing of the body and all of its cells. It is so much easier to live a healthy lifestyle to prevent cancer than to try and treat it after it has developed.

Quite often, if one family member develops cancer, especially husband and wife, the other family members may also develop it because both are living the same lifestyles, living in the same environment, and eating the same foods. So there is a very strong correlation between nutrition and cancer. Diets consisting of raw fruits and vegetables rather than cooked are less likely to produce cancers.

Endnotes

1. *Oxford Dictionary of Current English*, 4th ed. (Oxford University Press, 2006), s.v. "food."

2. George Malkmus, "Are You Living to Eat or Eating to Live?" *Hallelujah Acres Health News Magazine* 58 (November/December 2009): 6.

3. Olin Idol, "Toxicity Refined Sugar: How Sweet Is It?" *Hallelujah Acres Health News Magazine* 55 (May/June 2009): 24.

4. E. Cheraskin and W. M. Ringsdorf Jr., *New Hope for Incurable Diseases* (Exposition Press Inc., 1971), 21.

5. George Malkmus, "Alcohol Does the Body Bad," Hallelujah Acres Health Tip, *Hallelujah Acres Health News Magazine* 558 (2008).

6. *Cheraskin* et al., *New Hope*.

7. Andrew F. Smith, *Encyclopedia of Junk Food and Fast Food* (Greenwood, 2006), 71.

8. Michael Donaldson, "The State of Diabetes," *Back to the Garden Health News* 45 (2007): 18.

9. Michael Donaldson, "The State of Diabetes," *Back to the Garden Health News* 45 (2007): 19.

10. Olin Idol, "Arthritis," *Back to the Garden Health News* 47 (2007): 20.

11. Michael Donaldson, "Lupus: Disarming the Robber of Vitality," *Hallelujah Acres Diet and Lifestyle Magazine* 48 (2008) 22.

12. Olin Idol, "Breast Cancer," *Hallelujah Acres Diet and Lifestyle Magazine* 49 (2008): 20.

CHAPTER 21

Artificial Sweeteners and Additives

There are many artificial sweeteners on the market to keep people out of the sugar bowl. These are designed to feed the sweet tooth but not gain weight in the process. All of these have their dangers, and some of them happen to be worse than others. All are digested and metabolized by the human body as chemicals, and these toxic chemicals will create disastrous effects.

All of these artificial sweeteners are approved by the FDA (United States Food and Drug Administration): acesulfame-K, aspartame, neotame, saccharin, and Splenda. According to Scripps Wellness (Scripps Hospital System in San Diego, California), Daniella Blau and Alisa Scherba, MPH, RD, CDN, claim that all of these sweeteners are probably safe to use with the exception of saccharin and acesulfame-K.[1] Most people think if the FDA approves it, then it must be okay to use. Unfortunately, it's a wrong assumption to make.

The *Artificially Sweetened Times* newsletter used twenty-five pages to show factual evidence of how dangerous aspartame, Splenda, and neotame are from its beginnings (December 1965) to its present research (July 4, 2005), citing examples of deaths, diseases, experiments done on the aspartame contents on cans of Diet Coke by an eleven-year-old girl and her impressive and shocking results.[2]

It was too bad that she couldn't open the eyes of the government and the blind public to the neurological damage, muscular sclerosis, and Parkinson's disease symptoms, to name a few, and the dangerous chemicals that are in these products. A few examples include formaldehyde that accumulates in the brain and damages the central nervous system and the immune system, aspartame that converts to wood alcohol, as well as aspartic acid, an excitotoxin.

Excitotoxins are a chemical protein food additive that are in processed foods and drinks and create neurological damage to the brain and central nervous system. The most commonly consumed food source of excitotoxins are aspartame (e.g., NutraSweet); MSG (monosodium glutamate), a taste enhancer; and hydrolyzed vegetable protein (which is on the labels of processed foods containing "natural" flavors, spices, yeast extract, and soy protein extract). The non-food source excitotoxins are pesticides and insecticides that are put in our food supplies and poison the foods, consequently the body.

These chemicals cause many neurological diseases such as MS (muscular sclerosis), Parkinson's, or ALS (amyotrophic lateral sclerosis), commonly called Lou Gehrig's disease. When the body breaks these chemicals down they are changed into compounds that are thought to cause damage to the nerve receptors of the brain.

In fact, Dr. Dan E. Chesnut states that aspartame (NutraSweet brand)) "breaks down within twenty minutes at room temperature into several primary toxic and dangerous ingredients:

1. DKP (diketopiperazine) when injected, converts to a near duplicate of a powerful brain tumor-causing agent,
2. Formic acid (ant venom),
3. Formaldehyde (embalming fluid),
4. Methanol (cause blindness: extremely dangerous substance)."

Aspartame is now in more than six thousand products, claims Chesnut.[3] Even a little of these poisons is not okay; it will still kill a person, just a little bit slower. Yet people are still drinking and eating too much of these laced products. In place of sugar, many people use aspartame as an artificial sweetener for dieters desiring to lose weight and who are trying to have their cake and eat it at the same time. Aspartame causes neurological problems. It causes abnormal dopamine levels in the brain that mimic mental illness and seizures. The increased use of this chemical as an artificial sweetener is creating a significant increase in too many once unknown neurological disorders.

Splenda isn't any better of a substitute for aspartame. It is just refined sugar that has chlorine as an added ingredient. Aspartame is considered to be an excitotoxin along with MSG (monosodium glutamate) and hydrolyzed vegetable protein (listed on the labels as natural flavors, natural flavorings, yeast extract, textured protein, and soy protein extract).

Aspartame is placed on all types of products on the market, more than six thousand food items (in addition to soda drinks), many processed foods, dietary supplements, medications, and the worse culprit, chewing gums. I read all the labels on the packages of chewing gum in the drug store aisle while waiting for a friend's prescription. I was appalled. Every package, including the ones with sugars, all contained aspartame. The mouth is the best and fastest way to absorb anything into the body because of the amount of blood vessels. The people who chew gum, from youngsters to the elderly, buy and chew astronomical numbers of packages of chewing gum and this, with all the other aspartame-based products, are helping to kill the ignorant public. It's a dangerous product, yet it is promoted and is advertised as safe. Artificial sweeteners are chemicals *not* food. These are dangerous even in small amounts approved by the FDA, so they are to be avoided. How does one know what or how much the body can or cannot handle? These sweeteners confuse the body and the brain. When they are consumed, the cells wait for an insulin surge that doesn't come, and then the brain feels deprived. The caffeine that comes from the sodas then gives a stimulant's effect. The body waits for the energy, which does not occur, so the body starts a craving for carbohydrates. People tend to eat more because of the mass confusion and will still gain weight, and then people will wonder why. The confused body eats more to get what it wants and needs. One can keep his/her blood sugar levels balanced and maintained by the eating of healthy whole foods, not processed products. All human beings desire sweetness. God created these in the taste buds but designed the bodies for sweetness to come from fresh, whole, sweet fruits, not chemicals.

Sorbitol is an artificial sweetener that is used by diabetics. It does have a laxative effect on the body, therefore causing bouts of diarrhea, bloating, gassiness, and irritable bowel syndrome. This chemical sweetener should be avoided. It is used in sugarless candies for diabetics.

Stevia is better alternative sugar substitute, and long-term studies indicate it is free of side effects. This does not stimulate sugar cravings, nor spike insulin levels. It does contain about one-half the calories of sugar and is about twenty times sweeter than sugar and is not digestible by the small intestine. It is produced from the leaves of a South American plant (stevia plant) with leaves naturally sweet to the taste.

Xylitol is another alternative sweetener that is made from birch tree pulp. It looks like sugar and can be used just like sugar without the spiking of insulin levels and other hormone levels. It is used in chewing gums and toothpaste, and some dentists claim that xylitol is a deterrent to tooth decay. It can help to prevent osteoporosis when taken as a supplement, according to Dr. David Williams, who has conducted studies on the product xylitol. He states that this product can increase bone density, but "exactly how xylitol helps to increase bone density isn't fully understood. It appears to increase the intestinal absorption of calcium. It also makes the vitamin D receptors more sensitive and enhances the beneficial effects of vitamin D." He also claims that the human "body makes as much as 11 grams of xylitol per day."[4] Williams promotes this as a great sugar substitute, especially for diabetics and those with hypoglycemia.

In other studies, Williams claims that xylitol has shown "to re-mineralize tooth enamel, reduce cavities, dental plaque, and the plaque acids that erode the teeth."[4] I assume that this is an alkaline-based product because all the things that he stated are acid-based body health challenges. I personally have and do use stevia and xylitol occasionally, but I mostly eat fresh sweet fruits to fulfill the sweet needs.

One of the most-used sugar substitutes, placed in almost all processed and packaged foods, is high fructose corn syrup. When one reads the labels on different products, it is horrifying. High fructose corn syrup, corn syrup, fructose dextrose are many ways that sugars are added, allowing people to believe there isn't any sugar because the word "sugar" isn't written on the label. The corn syrups are the cheap sweeteners. I recall as a child my mother would add Karo syrup (corn syrup) in the baby's water bottle to entice the infant to drink it. It was also used as pancake/waffle syrup until pancake syrups became more popular and not as expensive. No wonder children are so wired up, considering the numerous items they eat and drink that include some type of sugar.

It's best to eat unadulterated, unprocessed, fresh whole foods. Most of these processed foods that society at large consumes are the cause of America and the world's (at large) diseases. The sweet tooth starts at birth with the parents who feed their babies and children junk foods that they will continue to crave into their adult years.

People need to eliminate all the chemicals of any kind from their diets and homes in general. They need to eat the freshest, raw whole fruits and vegetables and drink the purest, cleanest water. Our brains need glucose to live on and to continue to function properly. Glucose is the primary fuel that feeds energy to the brain. The needs of glucose for the brain and nervous system are great. The brain, that runs the entire body, consumes 25 percent of the body's glucose. Excitotoxins and food additives are in every processed food product, and a lifetime of eating these food additives and excitotoxins creates even more havoc and destruction of the brain, an extremely sensitive organ. These excitotoxins continue to accumulate in the brain and spinal cord, creating a powerful and enormous breakdown.

The adult body and brain have a very difficult time dealing with these poisons, but a child's developing brain and body is even more burdened. A child is at least four times more sensitive. Their bodies are smaller, and the junk foods and drinks they consume are the same amount as an adult, so they are fatally damaging to the child's cellular and genetic structures and contribute to the brain's cellular destruction. Diseases are running rampant. Genetics? Runs in families? People in these families who live the same lifestyles and eat the same foods with the same toxins will inherit and die of the same diseases. The curses are passed down.

When MSG is consumed, it will create damage and deterioration of the memory portion of the brain cells, thus Alzheimer's disease will come about. The energy-starved cells will shrivel up and die.[5] There has been a significant increase of this dementia-type disease in the past three decades. The elderly usually does not consume a healing diet, nor live a healthy lifestyle. Many have so many health challenges because of this, using too many prescription drugs, only compounding the situation even more. These bad combinations add to the destruction of the body. I have heard from some physically-challenged elderly people that the reason for not changing their lifestyle is "I'm such and such age, and I'm not going to do anything different now." MSG of any form, consumed in large amounts tends to be selective on its neuron damage.[5] In the case of Alzheimer's, it seeks the hippocampus area of the brain. The areas of memory seem to be attacked and killed. It is sad to see these people degenerate so badly that they are walking dead.

When more than one excitotoxin is consumed, it only intensifies and multiplies the damage these additives create. "Glutamate and aspartame are even more toxic than either one used alone,"[5] states Russell L. Blaylock, MD. He goes on to say that "many foods contain glutamate, aspartate, cysteine, and hydrolyzed vegetable protein. Many diet colas contain aspartame, of which the primary ingredient is aspartate."[5]

The more a person consumes excitotoxin food additives along with the duration indicates the extent of damage. Young children, of course, are much more sensitive based on their height, weight, and purity of their bodies. If a young person only consumes a small amount but daily or weekly, the extent of damage may or may not be as bad as the one who continuously eats and drinks daily, seven days a week. These repetitive abusers may not live into their elder years.

Excitotoxins have only been on the extensive market since the 1950s, but they double each succeeding decade. Those who may have started with small amounts as a youngster, now are in their middle years and contracting the diseases of those who are elderly. Blaylock asks a question, but answers it in the following: "Is Alzheimer's disease causing energy failure of the brain? There is growing evidence that it plays at least a major part of the story."[5]

The glucose adequately received by the brain on a continual basis includes three conditions.

- First, the glucose must be properly digested and assimilated before it can enter the blood.
- Secondly, the glucose in the blood must be transported across the blood-brain barrier into the cells of the brain.
- And lastly, the brain cells must be able to convert the glucose into useable energy.

Many elderly people do not consume enough raw, wholesome, fresh fruits and vegetables. They do tend to eat a lot of canned produce; soft foods; and cheap, processed, additive-saturated foods. Because of their poor diets and lifestyles, many of these people have poor digestive powers, especially with their lack of teeth and use of dentures. The years of poor eating have weakened their digestion and assimilation, and because of the drugs they have consumed, there will also be a lack of elimination. These drugs, with the continued use of MSG, glutamate, and aspartate, have all but destroyed their taste buds and they no longer can taste "real foods" because the foods they do eat have so many additives and taste-enhancers, that the real thing doesn't taste good any more. These foods also deplete the vitamin/mineral levels of the body and the brain thus reduces the adequate functioning of the organism. The excitotoxins in the blood can inhibit glucose from entering the brain, thus the brain is starved for energy. This is another reason to rid these poisonous chemicals from ever entering the body. It is so important for the brain to receive adequate amounts of glucose in the diet. Regular exercise is also necessary for the body to keep its blood sugar levels maintained and stabilized.

Other serious disorders and neurological diseases caused by excitotoxin food additives and sweeteners are seizures, headaches, strokes, ischemia-anoxia, hypoglycemia, and dementia. Aspartame can cause and increase the risk of brain tumors as well as other brain-related diseases of Alzheimer's and Parkinson's disease, multiple sclerosis and Huntington's disease as well as ALS (Lou Gerhig's disease).

The companies that manufacture NutraSweet, which contains aspartame, and the Ajinomoto company, the main manufacturer of MSG and hydrolyzed vegetable protein, as well as the Food and Drug Administration have their reasons (money) to make sure that their products are continued to be in high demand. It doesn't matter how dangerous these products are to the body; these companies have protected their commodities and will not let anyone take it off the market for any reason. The public as well demands these products for their own taste-enhancing properties.

The most unprotected are the unborn babies. Their mothers are consuming these products in ignorance, and the unborn will suffer the most. The toxins cross the placenta and invade their little underdeveloped bodies many times to the point of destruction. People need to be educated and stop this horrible abuse to future generations.

The US public has and is eating the wrong things, and their bodies are suffering because of it. One of the worst parts of the standard American diet is all of the chemical additives and preservatives that most people consume in their so-called foods. Pick up a can, box, and package of any kind then try to read the label. Most of these ingredients are not even understandable and do not come anywhere near what a food is. More problematic is not just what is in these products but what is not written on the label.

How safe are these additives? How do they affect the human body, and what do they do to the body's health in the long term? The human body does not tolerate foods that are chemically altered in any form. Most are claimed to be harmless, and what the FDA calls GRAS (generally recognized as safe) are assumed not harmful because there weren't any negative effects recorded during the testing of these products, or those were possibly ignored. Dr. Dan Chesnut states, "Labeling is a sneaky, rotten business. Cleverly, deceptive. A label screams out, 'No trans fat' or 'Organic,' but contains other bad additives and may have been gassed or irradiated."[7] He goes on to say that there aren't any completely safe processed canned and packaged foods, very few are anyway. Some, such as vitamins and minerals, are even claimed to be beneficial and nutritious. But these are synthetically-added and also just as damaging to the organism. Many of the chemicals are added to enhance these foods and to gain the consumer's eye appeal and to feed a perverted pallet.

A number and variety of these chemicals accumulate and alter the body's hormone, chemistry, and cell function. A continual daily and yearly overload of these un-eliminated toxins will mutate the cells and their reproductive functioning. The body's cells will age at an accelerated rate, employing destruction to the whole organism.

In his book, *Lying with Authority*, Chesnut states, "There are at least 4,000 different additives plus thousands more from foreign sources and from chemical changes through processing and cooking, including cooking at home."[7]

Most of the standards set by these chemicals have been at the expense of animal studies, but these animals have a shorter lifespan and different chemical makeup from humans, so it is still difficult to judge long-term usage of these additives. Once a drug and/or chemical enter the body, there is not any control over what happens.

I really wish people would realize that. Because if they did, they would change and take control over what they consume and would be burdened with fewer diseases. The FDA is not there to protect our nation and its people. These chemicals are, in small and large amounts, carcinogenic. The chemical hazards that we as people are living with are real and dangerous, no matter how those who choose to minimize it.

The FDA okays small amounts as safe, but there are *no* safe amounts. The consumption of all these chemicals throughout one's lifetime will cause severe health challenges, diseases, and cancers. The danger of the chemical additives is accumulation to the point of saturation. They will continue to amass and add to toxicity levels, creating sensitivities, serious impairments and diseases, cancers, and death to the organism. What we eat does affect the health of the body. People need to be accepting and responsible for their own health.

The body is wonderfully and fearfully made. The body is a beautifully created, functioning mechanism that can render small amounts of these chemicals almost harmless if digested and eliminated, but many people continue to consume overwhelming amounts, of which many are so addicting that most people refuse to give them up. People will not even look and accept the truth behind the lie; people think that the government and the food manufactures won't allow these so-called poisons to be put in our foods. In fact, a person may consume approximately 150 different food additives with each day's meals, eaten on the basis of the standard American diet. All processed foods, including the ingredients in the salt and peppershakers, contain the poisons that obstruct and hinder physical healing and the body's recovery mechanisms. People need to remove their rose-colored glasses and put on the spectacles of truth. The government (FDA) has indeed approved of the preservatives, coloring agents. There are about 140 different kinds of coloring ingredients that are considered to be unsafe, and yet, the FDA has not taken them off the market. There are also flavorings, and the most dangerous of these is MSG (monosodium glutamate). It damages the brain and the nervous system. People continue to consume these chemicals in products because it boosts the flavors of their foods. Public demands keep a lot of these chemicals from becoming obsolete. Ruth Winter states that processors "embalm their products to keep them feeling fresh." One example that she gave was balloon-type bread that underwent rigor mortis thanks to its additive, plaster of Paris.[8] The bleaching agents used in flours and sugars are used just for appearance sake.

To sell their products to those who are health conscious, manufacturers will enhance their items with nutritional supplements because the natural nutrients were removed during the processing and will need to be replaced, so the public will think these products are healthier than the others on the market. Ironically, when foods are free of chemical additives, the price is much higher. The cost though may be higher, which is a crime, but at least a person will not be paying double for it later with a sick and diseased body and a multitude of doctors and hospital bills.

We as the public, consumers, need to be informed and responsible about our health with the overuse of chemicals. People need to request and buy only clean, fresh whole foods. This is how people can strike back at the greed and ignorance by these manufacturers in the food industries.

Food additives include artificial sweeteners, such as aspartame, artificial colors, artificial flavors, flavor enhancers such as monosodium glutamate (MSG), and preservatives such as nitrites. Aluminum-based additives (found in antacids and double-action baking powder) seem to have catastrophic on the nervous system. These can include nervous system disorders such as Parkinson's disease and multiple sclerosis. Some brain/nervous reactions may include insomnia, poor concentration, short attention span, aggressiveness, and irritability. It is best to avoid all food additives or chemicals of any kind. These all do the body bad.

How does the body really react to these chemical poisons? One fact stands alone in its truth: the body cannot and does not remove all of these chemicals as long as they are consumed and ingested in excess. The enzymes and acids of the stomach and intestines, in their work to destroy them, may alter their chemical makeup, which can actually be worse than it was before they were taken into the body. Pesticides especially love an acid environment. The body does have a tendency to take in all these chemicals and absorb them into the cells all in good faith. Then the reactions start to occur, chemicals start to bond with the cells, and then the cells start with the process of inflammation and destruction, producing free radicals. Some chemicals will store in the fat cells, liver cells, and the blood.

The liver is an amazing organ, yet people in their thoughtlessness dump all kinds of crud into the body, and then the liver becomes overwhelmed and begins to deteriorate and break down. The liver will begin to enlarge and swell, creating new cells to replace the damaged ones, and the body will become distended and bloated. Energy sources will be drained and the body will malfunction thus starving for nutrients. Chemicals take their toll on the nutrient reserve.

People need to decrease these chemicals for the normal body defenses to work and function properly and optimally.

The body, as well as the brain, needs nourishment, and that nourishment comes from fresh whole foods with no processed ingredients, additives, or chemicals of any kind. The brain keeps the whole body in check. If it isn't fed well, its function will become impaired and will be lost, especially during the golden years of life, according to Peter Howard, author of *The Owner's Manual to the Brain*.[9] A diet that is important to consume is one of fresh whole foods for a lifetime of health and optimal brain function.

The proper foods to consume for brain-functioning are proteins, complex carbohydrates, and fats. Many people though will consume too many simple carbohydrates, which are sugars. These only add to a sluggish brain and body. The refined sugars provide a quick rise in blood sugar, which might give a false sense of instant energy, but then there comes the letdown. At lunch, many people will eat some type of sandwich combination followed by a soda or coffee and then wonder why they are falling asleep. Lunch should give energy to carry one throughout the rest of the day. Eating a meal of fresh fruits, vegetables or a salad with a few nuts will sustain a person and help the body to maintain the blood sugar while keeping the brain alert and functional. The nuts, especially flaxseed and walnuts, and avocadoes feed the brain functionally with omega-3 fatty acids. When the brain is optimally functioning, so is the nervous system; therefore, the entire body responds to the kindness of a healthy lifestyle.

When there was a shift in the omega 3 to omega 6, which is in all processed foods and oils, there has been an increased rate in many or all diseases because of free radicals created by these rancid oils and the cooked and processed foods.

Furthermore, concerning the brain and nutrition, there is a strong correlation to high sugar diets and violent behavior. With a high sugar diet, the body is left depleted and malnourished. The blood sugar is lowered when the sugars wear off because the insulin is released to turn off the body's production of glucose. According to Pierce J. Howard, "The limbic part of the brain then gobbles up the available glucose, starving the cerebral cortex and thereby making emotional behavior dominant (the limbic system is in control) and pushing rational behavior into the background."[9] There are many people in prison systems because of their lifestyle and diets, and the prison systems don't help at all.

Processed foods, preservatives, and additives continue to rise, and the health of the world at large decreases in value. They are addictive and further the body's health on a downward spiral. For example, there is more dieting at this time, yet there are more and more people who are obese. According to Michael Donaldson, "Fourteen percent of Caucasian children ages 6–11 are overweight, 21 percent of African American, and 23 percent of Hispanic children are overweight; also 65 percent of adults are overweight with 31 percent of these being obese. Diabetes is an epidemic with 8 percent of all adults with full diabetes and another 40 percent prediabetic."[10]

The grocery stores are continuously selling more of these artificial fat-free and low-fat foods. There are no fat-free, low-fat, diet, fake foods, sugar-free foods to feed the perverted palates of desperate people who want to continue to binge on their favorite foods, but not suffer the consequences of increased calories, weight gain, and the like, when they eat the real thing.

Dr. David G. Williams states in his *Alternative Newsletter*, "It has been reported that there are 5,000 low-fat and fat-free food products on the market in the United States." Yet with all of these products, people are all gaining weight. Dr. Williams goes on to say, "These artificial products have been created to trick the body into thinking it's consuming fat or concentrated carbohydrate (sugar) when in fact the substitute is really some chemically-altered protein."[11]

The food industry gets involved and continues to create more ways to make the public think they are getting a healthy low-fat and fat-free product. However, taking the fat out doesn't necessarily make it a healthy food. The dieter is still suffering malnutrition because their bodies are just starved for good healthy nutrients, not processed concoctions. Many will feel that they can feed their bodies with a supplement pill that, according to the advertising, helps to supplement their diet. Never is this happening more than right now. Unfortunately, these pills create even more harm than the intended good.

These altered fat-free and low-fat products have more additives, chemicals, sugars, and flavoring to make them taste good, but they are worse than the real thing. For example, they sell all types of low-fat margarine (a butter substitute), but this is one molecule less than plastic. Butter (unsalted and organic) would be a wiser choice.

The American Heart Association had claimed that all of these fat-free and low-fat products are the major contributor in the rise of obesity and diabetes as well as other diseases. These are not healthy but a waste of money and a poison to the body.

People will change their ways of eating to where what is called a healthier approach, i.e., low-fat and fat-free products, because the health challenges they are facing at the time. Many obese people will even resort to surgeries, such as gastric band laparoscopy surgery, gastric bypass surgery, and stomach stapling just to be thin and healthy. Most of these types of surgeries will kill a person because of even more malnutrition problems than the person had before because of the damaging effects of malabsorption of nutrients and poor, if any, digestion.

Many of the foods that are bought in grocery stores are grown conventionally in depleted soils and the biggest factor, according to Jackie Graff, is "what affects the calorie-to-nutrient ratio is cooking. When a food is exposed to temperatures over 110°F, many nutrients are damaged, becoming unusable by the body." Cooking is the process of destroying the enzymes, vitamins, and minerals of the foods, creating a new challenge: overeating. The overeating and food cravings are due to the effect of the body, in all of its intelligence, having desires to have nutrients at any cost. One will continue to eat even to the point of stuffing oneself just to get those nutrients, which will never occur until they come from nutrient-filled, whole raw fresh foods. This overeating creates weight gain. A cooked-food diet is not a long-term diet to lose weight. In fact, it helps one to gain weight because all the processed foods are considered cooked foods and are unhealthy.

Many people have been led to believe that fats are the main reason for obesity, high cholesterol, and heart disease problems. So deceived consumers will buy and eat these fat-free snacks, thinking they can eat as much as they want after all as there isn't any fat. In the meantime, the manufacturers have added more artificial sweeteners and flavorings, thus these products need to be higher in calories and chemicals than the regular products with normal fat. This all has resulted in a doubled increase in obesity in the past twenty years, and also in a significant increase in type 2 diabetes in the last ten years.[12] People may be insulted, but the United States has the fattest people of any nation at this point. Thin people are the minority and many of the thin ones are fat people in thin bodies with all of the same diseases.

With all of that obesity, there is a huge market of dieting shows on television, diet books in the marketplace, diet pills, and surgeries to help people lose some weight, but the problem is that the diets do not work because they are only temporary, not designed for long-term use. People will lose weight, but they cannot keep it off, so they do what's called yo-yo dieting. The weight goes up and down continuously, always ending up heavier than before. People must realize that they need to find a healthier lifestyle that they can live with; one that doesn't include all of the processed, addictive foods that got them fat to begin with.

Everyone agrees that sugars and refined, processed foods are the main contributors to the declining health in this society. The human body was not created to consume these substances and yet maintain health. The body cannot keep up these huge sugar levels any more than it can keep high stress levels. It will just break down and crash.

Endnotes

1.   Daniella Blau, "The Facts on Sugar Substitutes," ScrippsWellness. com (2010), 1–3.

2.   *Artificially Sweetened Times*, "How Diet Soda Becomes Poison," *Artificially Sweetened Times* (Winter 2005): 6.

3. Dan E. Chesnut, *Lying with Authority* (Restoration Health, 2008), 192.

4. David G. Williams, "A Sweet Solution to Brittle Bones," *Alternatives Newsletter* 10, no. 3 (2003): 18.

5. Russell L. Blaylock, *Excitotoxins: The Taste That Kills* (Health Press, 1997), 153.

6. Ruth Winter, *Consumer's Guide of Food Additives* (Crown, 1984), 1.

7. Chesnut, *Lying with Authority*, 147.

8. Winter, *Consumer's Guide*, 2.

9. Pierce J. Howard, *The Owner's Manual to the Brain*, 3rd ed. (Bard, 2006), 121.

10. Michael Donaldson, "Why Are We So Sick?" *Back to the Garden Health News* 34 (September/October 2005): 8.

11. David G. Williams, "When It Comes to Instinct: Trust Not Verify," *Alternatives Magazine* 19, no. 14 (August 2002): 10.

12. Jackie Graff, "How I Got Fat Eating No Fat," *Back to the Garden Health News* 36 (January/February 2006): 24.

Beverages

Water is the fountain of life. The human body is composed of water, which makes up about 65 percent of total body weight. All of the cells and tissues of the body cannot function without pure water. Its main purpose is to be a transport system for all of the organic compounds and electrolytes inside each cell. Water flushes and cleanses the body of its toxins and all impurities. Water also maintains the temperature of the body and aids the proper functioning of its glandular system. Humans can live for some time without food but can only live for three days without water.

Pure water is an odorless, colorless, and tasteless liquid made of two hydrogen atoms and one carbon atom. It refreshes the body as nothing else will. Every living thing is made up of water. Our Creator in His blueprint called life designed this.

Water is one of the main nutrients needed and used by the body. Without it, death occurs. The water that is to be consumed by the body needs to be the cleanest and purest possible to keep the body free of toxicity and disease. The best water for the human body is from fresh, raw fruits and vegetables. Fruits are the perfect form of pure water and they contain typically 80–90 percent water. Vegetables contain water also but maybe not in such abundance as fruits. The raw, organic produce has its own water source, which is free of all inorganic minerals that would be harmful to the body. The secondary source of water should be distilled water. It is water that is in its purest form and assists proper functioning of the body. Tap water or bottled water is poison to the body because they both contain so many pollutants and chemicals.

While I was going through my adult years of dieting, it was always told to me to drink a lot of water to help curb the appetite. Drink a lot of water before meals to fill the stomach, so I wouldn't be as hungry and would consume less food. Drink at least two–three liters of water a day for optimal health. Well, I found out that these were all wrong and dangerous practices for the body.

The body does need a lot of water, but pure water, and at the time of thirst only, not just a continuous flow dumped in all day, and never with the meals. There are specific rules for drinking water to have optimal digestion. Drink water at least thirty minutes before meals, although it can be had fifteen minutes before a meal if only a small amount is taken. Other liquids move through the stomach a lot slower. It is wise not to drink water until least two hours after a meal, for it will dilute the digestive process. It dilutes the action of the stomach acid and the pH balance.

When one feels exceptionally thirsty and continues to consume water after a meal, the meal must have been cooked, also containing an abnormal amount of salt (sodium chloride). This is the case of all processed and preservative-laden foods. These types of meals are quite common in the standard American diet. I had this occur a few years back, and it was a horrible and unbearable experience. Never again will that happen.

Water must be consumed at room temperature for optimal digestion. Drinking it either hot or cold contributes to indigestion. Hot beverages may then damage the sensitive nerve endings of the mouth, sometimes to the point that the taste buds will not function properly. These hot beverages will also burn all the way down. The body temperature is 98.6°F and hot beverages are well over 110°F. These beverages will alter the body temperature.

Cold beverages will also interfere with the body temperature. Did you ever notice how cold the body feels after consuming an icy drink? The cold drinks will also halt the digestive process.

People will consume milk with their meals, and milk, which is considered a food, should be consumed alone. Milk is improperly combined if it is consumed with any other foods. Soups are another food, not a drink. Fruit and vegetable juices are also food, not beverages. If one drinks these as beverages throughout the day, the body will be consuming too much food. People will drink fruit juices assuming that these are a healthy beverage. These all have been cooked (pasteurized) and are fermented, preserved, refined, and oxidized foods. The best juices are from the fresh fruit itself. Worst of all are the coffees, teas, hot cocoa, and soft drinks. These are not foods or drinks but toxic poisons to the body. These all stimulate the body rather than adding any nourishment or nutritive value.

Alcohol is a legal drug consumed by millions of people in this country. We live in an alcoholic society with alcoholic problems, and most of these are continually ignored. The troublemakers are the only ones who are addressed. This drug does not have any place in a healthy lifestyle.

Alcohol is a dangerous legal drug. It is American's public enemy number one and has caused at least one hundred thousand lives each year. Alcohol takes away the quality of life from those who are unfortunate to have become addicted to this drug and to the family and friends who will suffer even more because of the effects of alcoholism in their lives.

Alcohol kills. According to reports, alcohol is the main factor in 50 percent of traffic fatalities, 30 percent of all traffic injuries, 83 percent of all fire and burns fatalities, 86 percent of all homicides, and 64 percent of all attempted suicides. "There are 160,000,000 Americans who drink alcoholic beverages," reports Rev. George Malkmus, "which is approximately 60 percent of the population and of those, 12 million are alcoholics, of the remaining 148 million, at least 10 percent will become alcoholics."[1]

The manufacturers of these alcoholic beverages think that they are not in any way responsible for any of these problems because they state warnings on all their labels, "Please drink responsibly." They feel this takes them off the hook. The problem is this is an alcoholic society and these companies in their greed help contribute to this problem. Society itself has a massive repair bill because of the alcoholic. People drink alcohol not necessarily because of the taste of it; the alcohol itself is distinguishably disgusting. It is the mixing of other ingredients that may give it its flavors, the sugars, grains, fruit, etc., all fermented together to make a unique potent drug that supposedly tastes good. In the end, it's the effect that people crave. The first drink tastes terrible, the second maybe a little better as the taste buds, mouth, brain, and the body in general start to blur. A person will no longer taste anything. The body's craving just takes over, especially for the alcoholic.

There are social drinkers; those who can have one drink, taking the entire night to sip it, or leave it, all for the sake of being social. It's amazing what people will do in a social setting. Everything revolves around food and drink, especially alcohol. These just pollute and destroy the body. Alcohol makes drinkers feel good while they are drinking it and bad when they stop. This is all part of the addictive process.

Alcohol poisons the cells and leads to many physiological malfunctions. It also leads to many disorders of the central nervous system, especially the brain, the liver, cardiovascular system, and gastrointestinal tract. Literally, every cell of the body is harmed with the consumption of alcohol. Alcohol, when consumed by the alcoholic with the intentions of getting drunk, destroys more than one hundred thousand brain cells. For those alcoholics who black out (alcoholic amnesia), even more brain cells are irreversibly damaged, especially in the memory portion of the brain. As we go through life, many cells of the brain may regenerate, but not the ones lost during a blackout. They are gone forever, and never will these memories be retrieved. It's called liquid fire for a reason; it consumes everything in its path of destruction as a forest fire does. As I said before, alcohol kills everything and everyone in its pathway. Do not be deceived.

Soft drinks do serious hard damage to the human body. Phosphorus in sodas fights with the hydrochloric acid (used to digest proteins) in the human stomach and renders it ineffective, therefore halting digestion. This promotes indigestion, bloating, and gassiness in many individuals. The sugars in these sodas are approximately eleven teaspoonful per 12 oz. can. The number of sodas consumed daily by the average adult can be anywhere from six to twelve, and the average child may consume one to three per day. These products are damaging to the young's growing and developing body, but the added caffeine makes it unbearable for the child's body. The human organism cannot tolerate these poisons. The body needs only pure, distilled water and only as thirst requires. People seem to drink out of habit, not out of need. People will say, "I'm getting my water out of these drinks." I doubt they will ever realize the extent of damage that continues to harbor within their bodies.

To sell more sodas, soft drink manufacturers increased the size of the soda containers. It went from a 6½ oz. bottle to 20 oz. At the convenience stores, movies, and at many restaurants, they sell no-limit refills, and fast food restaurants now sell 64 oz. containers. They are selling cheap poison. These companies are gearing their advertising efforts to sell to children and teens. In 1998, the Center for Science in the Public Interests Study called it liquid candy. According to Andrew Smith, they reported that the soft drinks "provided more than one-third of all the refined sugars in the diet."[2] These products contribute to tooth decay, delayed bone development, diabetes, and obesity. Diet sodas have many more dangerous ingredients that contribute to chronic diseases. Aspartame for example, is an excitotoxin and contributes to central nervous system's disorders. Other toxic, poisonous ingredients include high fructose corn syrup (cheap sweetness), carbon dioxide, sweeteners, colorings, and artificial sweeteners. All of these are poisonous to the human organism and its parts.

Gatorade is a product that was initially invented to hydrate football players at the University of Florida. This is a non-carbonated drink containing water, carbohydrates, and the bragged-about electrolytes. The claim in advertising is that athletes will lose many electrolytes during exercise. These sports drinks are high in sugar and calories. Distilled water is safer and healthier than these toxic beverages.

Endnotes

1. George Malkmus, "Alcohol Does the Body Bad," Hallelujah Acres Health Tip, *Hallelujah Acres Health* (2008).
2. Andrew F. Smith, *Encyclopedia of Junk Food and Fast Food* (Greenwood, 2006), 250.

CHAPTER 23

Caffeine

Caffeine is one of the most used and abused drugs on the market. It is an addictive and stimulating toxic substance obtained from the cacao bean that is used in different drugs, coffees, teas, some sodas, and chocolate. (Chocolate's form is called theobromine). This drug is used by all ages of human beings, from babies to adults.

Approximately 80 percent of Americans consume some kind of caffeinated beverages daily. According to Rev. George Malkmus, "Fifty tons of caffeine is consumed by Americans each day. The dosage of 75 cups of coffee placed in a body at one time would kill a person,"[1] yet very few realize its addictive properties.

The one or two cups tends to lead to more and more to receive the same stimulating perk up effect, thus the addiction has taken over. Also stated in Hallelujah Acres Health Tip, "Injected into human muscles, caffeine can cause paralysis while 10 grams of caffeine accumulated suddenly in a human body would result in death. One cup of coffee is not considered fatal, but the kidneys do have to work overtime to rid the body of this poison to prevent accumulation."[1]

The first thought of most people when caffeine is mentioned is their morning and daily coffees to get them going and keep them alert. These same people would never give their children coffee but do allow them to drink all sorts of sugar-filled caffeinated sodas, also consuming chocolate candy bars, chocolate milk, and hot cocoa. These are all filled with sugar and caffeine. A cup of brewed coffee, a cup of green tea, a 12 oz. can of caffeinated soft drink, and an 8 oz. milk chocolate bar contain 50 mg. of caffeine each.[2] These youngsters are weighing half the size of an adult, so their bodies are much more sensitive to the effects of caffeine. One can of cola to a child is equal to three cups of coffee to an adult. The caffeine and the sugar make an unmanageable child and create much physical damage.

Many college students, truck drivers, and people needing to stay awake will not hesitate to buy an over-the-counter stimulating drug called NoDoz. Now, there are other products on the market. For example, Red Bull has four times the amount of caffeine and sugar to put a person into an extra stimulating mode for the duration of the day. It does overstimulate to the point of destroying the body, a complaint from some of its users. Their physical symptoms were at dangerous levels.

Some stimulating effects of caffeine include irregular heartbeat and increased heartrate, high blood pressure, frequent urination (because of its diuretic properties), increased stomach acid, irritability, nervousness, insomnia, loss of appetite, (there are diet pills that are manufactured that contain significant amounts of caffeine), nausea, and diarrhea. Caffeine also contributes to osteoporosis due to the effect of the body trying to neutralize itself of the acidic effect of caffeine by taking calcium from the bones.

The withdrawal symptoms can be very severe: migraine headaches, anxiety, drowsiness, tension, and depression that can last for as long as a week or more. I experienced a four-day weekend going through extremely debilitating caffeine withdrawals. After it was over, I never touched anything with caffeine again, so I would not have to relive that experience. It was a horrible nightmare except I was awake through it all.

According to Dr. Russell Blaylock, "The worldwide consumption from various sources now approaches 80,000 metric tons a year."[3] Most of this is in the United States and is through coffee consumption, which is now up to 75 percent, and in Canada, it is up to 60 percent from coffee drinking. Teens the world over consume substantial amounts of caffeine from drinking sodas. The average 9-ounce cola contains about 30 mg of caffeine, which is higher than a cup of coffee, and these teens and children alike tend to drink at least three–four sodas per day."[3]

Hot chocolate contains even more caffeine (40 mg.), and a chocolate candy bar has about 30 mg. per bar. Caffeine stimulates the brain, and used with these excitotoxins, these stimulate it too much in combination, adding to the destruction of the brain neurons, compounding the risk of neurological disorders.[3]

Hallelujah Acres Health Tips gave a partial list of some commonly consumed caffeinated products. "The amount of caffeine is in milligrams per 7 oz. cup of coffee or 12 oz. can of soda;

- drip coffee, 115–117;
- brewed coffee, 80–135;
- instant coffee, 65–100;
- decaffeinated coffee, 2–4;
- iced tea, 70;
- Mountain Dew, 55;
- Coca-Cola, 45;
- Dr. Pepper, 39;
- Pepsi Cola, 37;
- chocolate bar, 30;
- NoDoz (stay-awake pill), 100;
- cold tablet, 30–200;
- diet pill, 100;
- Excedrin, 65;
- Midol, 32."[4]

The effects of caffeine on the brain and nervous systems are more destructive than the use of morphine. Yet people would think that is ludicrous, but they continue their caffeine addictions.

The body is trying to tell us something if it is fatigued. People need to pay attention to their bodies and give it what it needs—sleep and rest and proper food to replenish it. People need to learn to accept the laws of nature. One can't beat a tired horse to run a race;

eventually, it will collapse. It's the same with the human body; it will just give out and stop.

Endnotes

1. George Malkmus, "Caffeine—A Dangerous Drug," Hallelujah Acres Health Tip, *Hallelujah Acres Health Magazine* 170 (Archives 2001).
2. George Malkmus, "Caffeine Does the Body Bad," Hallelujah Acres Health Tip, *Hallelujah Acres Health* 555 (2008).
3. Russell L. Blaylock, *Excitotoxins: The Taste That Kills* (Health Press, 1997), 190.
4. Malkmus, "Caffeine—."

CHAPTER 24

Fermented Food Products

Fermented foods and beverages have become the common place in the diets of the standard American. Most are being promoted as health foods, great for the digestive system, helps the bacterial flora of the large intestine, etc. According to Mike Benton, who puts it well, "A fermented food is basically a food that has been carefully spoiled."[1] So it is basically rotten food with a lot of processing and chemicals added to create the good flavor to disguise its rottenness.

Yogurt is one of the primary dairy products to hit the junk food market as a health food. This is promoted as a perfect diet food, the dieter's delight since cottage cheese was so fattening. It is a milk product that has been soured and altered to the point of making an indigestible product. It is also promoted for the increase of flora in the digestive tract, mostly in the large intestine. The bacterium that is put into the yogurt isn't a part of the healthy body, so it is just excreted out with the bowel movements. Most of these yogurts are prepacked with fruit and sugar, which is even more toxic on the body and totally suspends the digestive process even further, adding even more toxins. It is still a milk product, and with all of the stuff added to the yogurt, it is completely indigestible. Dairy products are bad for the body.

There is now another dessert based on the yogurt manufacturers' need for more profits. They add even more harmful ingredients into the yogurt to entice all the other people who don't eat yogurt because of its ugly taste. These manufacturers have gone into the dessert market for a better flavor, using more sugar and flavorings. It's still just like regular ice cream, so-called healthy with all of the pollutant ingredients, which are not even listed on the label.

Another fermented dairy product is cheese. Cheese is marketed for the young and old alike and is another dairy product that is indigestible to the human body. Cheeses contain and are made of mold. For example, blue cheese is made from a process of blue molds, thus the name. These products are in a continuing molding process even in the refrigerator. These cheeses are wrapped in plastics, which add to the toxic levels of the body.

Other cheeses sold are not cheeses at all. Velveeta cheese or American cheese slices are not cheese. They have a list of whatever ingredients, but none is food-related. They promote string cheese and all these products that are sold and bought for the youngsters in mind as snacks, using slogans like "Got your cheese?" and "Get your milk with cheese in mind." People will have wine and cheese parties, and it's no wonder people become ill after eating these improper and toxic combinations together.

Sour creams, cream cheeses, and buttermilk are more fermented dairy products that are bad for the body. They are all full of preservatives and additives to keep them from becoming totally putrid. These products are made from soured milk to feed the perverted palates of the American public. For example, some ill-combined combinations are: baked potatoes with sour cream, buttermilk pancakes with syrup and fruit, cream cheese and bagels. These are all horribly indigestible, toxic and polluted substances for the body.

Pickles, sauerkraut, and other fermented vegetables are totally indigestible. The stomach's digestive juices bounce off of these chewed-up items like an object bounces off rubber. These vegetables are eliminated through the digestive tract just as they were in the stomach.

It's amazing when I watch some of the cooking channels on television. These people will make and sell fried pickles. How horrible and disgusting for the body. The vinegars and salts that have been added to these products add to the already accumulated overload of chemical poisons.

Sauerkraut is also indigestible. Raw cabbage will digest from the stomach in about two hours. If cooked, it will take about eight hours to digest, but if fermented with all the vinegar and salts it won't be digested at all. The foods that accompany it in the same meal also will not be digested. It's no wonder that most people have digestion problems every time sauerkraut is eaten. Many people will have GERD, diarrhea, gassiness, and bloating. Sauerkraut can be continually rinsed, but the toxin, vinegar, and salts will still remain because of the processing.

Soy and soy products have properties that interfere with the functioning of the thyroid gland. They also add estrogen-like chemicals in the body, and these types of products interfere with the functioning of the endocrine system.

Soy contains lectins and this causes the clumping of red blood cells, causing the immune system to react abnormally. According to Lorette C. Luzajic, "Soy contains oligosaccharides, sugars that cause gas and bloating and oxalates, which prevent calcium absorption, cause painful kidney stones, and vulvodynia which is a vaginal disorder."[2]

Soymilk is filled with sugars and rancid fats, and soy cheeses contain hydrogenated oils. (The government claims that a small amount of hydrogenated oils is safe in products, but the safety level of these oils is zero.) Health advocates claim the wonders and miraculous claims of health attributed to soy products when, in fact, there are far more dangers involved because of soy.

Manufacturers of soy products continue to defend hydrogenation, not because they have the public's health interest in mind but because of the money and the profits it turns up. Soy ingredients are hidden in all types of processed foods by the food manufacturers. Most of the labeled "vegetable oil" in the United States is actually soy oil, which is also in margarine. It is even hidden in chocolates and meats.

Soy is one of the main contributors of deadly allergies and chronic diseases, weight gain, and abnormal endocrine function. Soy fats and oils are carcinogens.

Products that use soy include items such as tofu, soymilks, and soy formulas (for babies who are allergic to regular formulas and milk products.) Also in the vegetarian marketplace, they have incorporated meat replacement meals made of soy. Soy sauces and tamari contain at least 18 percent salt and quite a bit of added alcohol has been added to these products.

Beer and wine are fermented drinks made with sugars, hops, and barley, producing an alcohol-based drink. These are very poisonous to the human body and should not be consumed.

The body will warn of all of these items by trying to expel them rapidly. These fermented products can be habit-forming and addictive because of some of the substances in them. These are not good, wholesome foods for the body; they do not have *any* nutritional value.

Endnotes

1. Mike Benton, "Fermented and Putrefied Foods in the Diet" (lesson 37, Natural Health course, Fit for Life Sciences Institute), 865.
2. Lorette C. Luzajic, "Spilling the Beans: The Trouble with Soy," *Hallelujah Acres Health Magazine* 56 (July/August 2009): 12.

C H A P T E R   2 5

Excessive Protein

Protein is essential for the building and repair of muscles and body tissues. What the body needs in moderation for optimal health is probably 25–30 grams daily. The best way to get this is in the fresh raw foods in the diet each day: fresh fruits and vegetables with moderate amounts of sprouts, seeds, and nuts, which are concentrated proteins. Protein needs to be eaten sparingly.

Wholesome proteins are nontoxic, nutritious, easily assimilated, and meet all the needs of the body. Proteins from sources other than fresh, raw foods can be hazardous to the health of the body. They can create an overload and, by their excessiveness, can poison the body. Protein poisoning causes general aches and pains, including headaches and joint pain. Allergies are considered part of the protein-poisoning process, an accumulation of toxins that the hypersensitive body is attempting to unload.

Bodybuilders and various other athletes believe that they must supplement their bodies to achieve their supreme health status. It is a very dangerous practice and many are just completely ignorant of what they are doing to their bodies in their attempt to compete in their sport.

For example, to gain weight, Lou Ferrigno ate anything he wanted so he could gain and weigh 300 pounds.[1] Hungry or not, he'd force feed himself. He went overboard on the tuna and fish protein. All he wanted to do was be huge and be a famous bodybuilder. He went on a strict diet, meat, tuna and water. He only ate one piece of fruit per day. This was his competition diet. Fortunately, he did and does not believe in taking drugs (steroids) as many athletes do, but he did and does believe in consuming a lot of supplements, especially protein supplements and powders. Nutritionally, he and others feel that animal proteins are an important part of the balanced diet. Fortunately, when not in competition, he consumes fresh whole fruits and vegetables but believes that whole grain products are for creating energy.

It became a grueling obsession with him. He worked out and trained every available moment, wanting to be huge, gigantic, and strong. It became a full-time job, a full-time career. He had an intense fierceness as well as determination to look the greatest and look the best.

At twenty-one years of age, he stood six feet five at nearly 300 pounds, with 22½-inch biceps. He realized that the continuous eating was thickening his waist. Although he eliminated the sugar, the protein he ate was still a tremendous amount. It was for the sake of bulking up. According to him, it was too much because he needed to build muscle, not more mass. This lifestyle takes its toll on the human body, and obsession becomes ignorance. The one thing that bodybuilders do after a competition is to eat and eat. The straight high-protein diet that leads up to the competition makes the body terribly hungry for good, healthy food. The body says, "Give me nutrients now!" Ralph C. Cinque does not object to weight-training or bodybuilding, but only to the excessive bulking that many weightlifters develop. This can be detrimental to their health.[2]

Many athletes who follow this unhealthy regimen will develop acute and chronic diseases, sometimes serious, such as liver and kidney malfunctions or failures. Many people feel that if they exercise, they are healthy, but they do very little about feeding their bodies correctly. "A high alkalinizing diet composed largely of fresh fruits and vegetables enhances one's oxidative powers and one's ability to sustain muscular effort,"[2] says Cinque.

Taking any supplements is dangerous. The body reacts to these pills and concoctions just as if they are drugs or poisons. "Protein supplements," says Hannah Allan, "should never be used. Dried and crystallized tablets, protein powders, or various protein concoctions are even more dangerous than other food supplements because the consequences of protein overconsumption, especially as an isolated food element, may be disastrous."[3] Food is the only thing that is proper and healthy, for the body needs nutrients with their complex mixture of food elements. The body cannot and does not take nutrients in isolation; it is for the overall good of the body. All the vitamins/minerals in a properly-combined plant food diets combine together for the whole of the organism.

There is a stimulating effect to supplements and protein powders. While it is in the process of eliminating them, the body will work overtime to protect itself. These toxins are an overload and will place a burden on the kidneys as will any other animal protein, but in synthetic protein supplement form, they are even more dangerous to the body. Protein drinks are a burden on the heart and the mineral balance of the body. Many athletes end up with gout, arthritis, and other serious challenges, including cancers. Arnold Schwarzenegger had a couple of coronary bypass surgeries made necessary because of his abusive past of bodybuilding, steroid consumption, and intense protein overdosing. It's part of the lifestyle. I do hope he has a better diet and lifestyle today. "The average American," claims, Ralph Cinque, "consumes two to four times as much protein as he needs, and cancer (which is characterized by runaway protein synthesis) is killing one person in four. Cutting down on total protein, in general, and animal protein, in particular, is a desperate need."[4]

Michael Dye states, "Protein requires more energy to digest than any other type of food. Protein is a negative energy food and is credited with being an energy producer. However, energy is used to digest it, and energy is needed to neutralize the excess ash it leaves. Protein uses more energy than it generates."[4]

Athletes need the same amount of protein that nonathletes need. Protein does not give a person extra strength. All of these supplement hypes are outlandish and deceiving. Dye claims that there are star athletes who are vegetarians, including Andreas Cahling, Mr. International bodybuilding champion, and Roy Hilligan, Mr. America bodybuilding champion.[5] One of the most famous vegetarian athletes of all time was Walter "Killer" Kowalski. He was a giant of a man, standing 6'7" tall and weighing 275 pounds. Kowalski became a vegetarian at age twenty-two. He has been given credit for changing the sport from a sedate entity to one that became high-flying. He attributed his style to the extra energy he had from consuming only vegetables.[5]

We need our protein from raw plant foods. The building blocks for the living cells of the body need to be living, not dead. Cooked proteins and supplements contain mutants that are hazardous to the health of the body. It is very difficult, if not impossible, for the body to digest them.

"Glucose is the starting molecule for glycolysis, an energy producing process common to almost every life form on Earth,"[6] states Janet Shagan, PhD.

It is glucose that makes the body run. It, not protein, is the energy-producing component for the body to absolute health. Glucose from fruits is for the health of the body. A person needs to achieve health and life that is in a balanced state. A fresh, raw produce diet, exercise, sunshine, pure water, a peaceful, calm attitude and disposition are the keys to health and wellness. Moderation, not obsession, is the goal of a productive life.

Endnotes

1. Lou Ferrigno and Douglas Kent Hall, *The Incredible Lou Ferrigno* (Simon & Schuster, 1982), 52.
2. Ralph C. Cinque, "Exercise: A Hygiene Perspective" (lesson 97, Natural Health course, Fit for Life Sciences Institute, 2032.
3. Hannah Allen, "Protein Supplements" (lesson 85, Natural Health course, Fit for Life Sciences Institute), 1794.
4. Ralph Cinque, "Protein," part II, lesson 8, course in Natural Health, Fit for Life Sciences Institute, 219.

5. Michael Dye, "Protein and Propaganda," in *God's Way to Ultimate Health* (1995), 135–136.
6. Janet Yagoda Shagan, "Unlocking the Secrets of Parkinson's Disease," *Radiologic Technology* 79, no. 3, January/February 2008): 231.

CHAPTER 26

What the Media Sells

The media does a job of promoting truth as well as exaggerated lies and deception. The year 2015, claim several news media anchors on television, is going to be a healthy year. The commercials are popping in more and more "healthy lifestyle" changes.

One example is the sales of a particular bag of salad that is said to be "so fresh and good-tasting that you don't even need dressing." That's good, trying to promote these raw vegetables even if they are in a bag, especially to eat plain. This is so much better than the stuff people are eating on the standard American diet.

On the downside of the media is the Food Channel's cooking shows. These are promoting the comfort foods. Many of these shows are cooking competitions that highlight taste, flavor, and presentation, not the health issue. Another show is called *Man vs. Food*, a competition to promote gluttony, a pig-out show. It is all about how much food one can eat in a certain amount of time; the quantity of food, not the quality, is paramount. Most of the food is perverted and unacceptable for the human body. For example, a 15 lb. ice cream sundae or a 20 lb. hamburger with fries and the works or the hottest, spiciest foods to be eaten in ten minutes.

Another show promotes restaurants that sell deep-fried bacon, deep-fried pickles, or deep-fried Twinkies. These are promoted as a "heart attack waiting to happen." They tell people that they cannot come into this place to eat all of the time, and most of the people who are the clientele are obese. But, it is still promoted as a fun, good-tasting place to be. It is downright disgusting.

People are addicted to the flavor, texture, and the comfort that these foods give them. These foods just make people feel good when they are consumed. It makes them experience euphoria, stimulation, and regressive emotions of the past. But their bodies end up taking a beating, and they continue on the road to destruction.

This downward spiral to destruction has to stop. The world around us has gone mad: lost in gluttony, lust, and despair. When people decide to give up their comfort foods, it's a small price to pay to halt the growth and spread of diseases, especially cancer. That is what the media promote, disease and insanity. Let's get off the merry-go-round and get a life.

On the other hand, there are folks who sell movies based on truth that needs to be told. These people put up their own money to help the public to become wiser and make better food choices.

Health is a commodity that is sought, desired, and coveted, but most people do not want to take the time or the effort and be disciplined to live on the pathway to health each day. Health is not found in the standard American diet.

CHAPTER 27

Cures

Only healthful living produces health. The *Oxford Dictionary* states, "a cure is the healing of an ill person; an end of a disease, condition, or problem by treatment or appropriate action."[1] That seems to be the problem with most people; they feel that they have to take or do something to get well. They feel that the symptoms that are making them miserable are there because someone or something made them sick. The cures are sought by external aid. People are sick because they just eat and live horribly. People need to look to where the fault actually lies within themselves. The best of all cures is to do nothing. Allow the body to rest, and it will heal itself. There are not any so-called cures.

The healthy state of the body is the equilibrium and homeostasis of the body. It functions well, the organ systems are in balance, and the cells are properly eliminating toxins. The body is not burdened or overwhelmed with toxic garbage; it is clean. There are no cures, only faulty thinking and living.

Disease is the body's effort to heal, so *disease* is the *cure*. The cure is in the corrective action of the body. Remove the cause, and the body goes back to its balanced state of health.

Many people, especially in medical science, resort to drugs to attempt to heal or cure the human body. Its true action must be taken to be healthy, but it's in the way we live, not by the world's standards, but in being obedient to the laws of nature. Therefore, this does take an amount of determination and diligence. The attitude of a person who seeks health must be one of "I will do whatever it takes, no matter what." It takes a person who will live stubbornly set apart from the world's standard diet and lifestyle. That is the only cure.

People need to know what is going into their mouths and bodies. They need to educate themselves. There is a true cost to buying and eating cheap foods. In recent times, the fats, sugars, and high-calorie foods have declined in price while the low-calorie healthy foods have soared. "The cost of fruits and vegetables have increased 40 percent since 1985,"[2] state the Malkmus authors. Eating these cheap foods has detrimental effects on the body. The cost of one's health will be an even more expensive decision. Most studies have concluded that several medical and health conditions, especially cancer, high blood pressure, and type 2 diabetes are caused and aggravated by the high-calorie and low-nutrient foodstuffs.

Complementing the disease aspect of doctors and hospitals, drugs, and ill health can cost more in out-of-pocket healthcare expenses than buying the good foods to begin with. The grocery bill will actually be less than buying the processed packaged goods because there will not be worries of poor health and disease. People don't want to go through their lives becoming bankrupt, not just in the pocketbook but with the health expenses as well.

When living foods are consumed, the body will have the nourishment; it needs to produce health and continued healing. The general public must learn to take responsibility for their physical health, and by doing that, they will also learn to make wise choices to promote that health. These choices are not only dietary, but lifestyle choices as well. People need to keep informed and guarded with that information to stay on the pathways of health. This includes information about product labels, not just what is eaten, but also the products that are used in the home, and personal body needs (see appendix). People also need to keep informed about needless tests and useless drugs prescribed by so-called well-intentioned doctors.

Successful cures, according to medical doctors, come from the outside of the person's body. They supposedly come from the drugs, surgeries, and procedures. But according to Patch Adams MD, "If success really depended on cure rates, primary care physicians would suffer great agony over all the patients they cannot cure."[3] Doctors are given all the benefits of a so-called cure, and the patient is just a passive beneficiary of the so-called cures. If it doesn't work, the doctor puts the blame onto the patient, or the patient will charge the doctor with malpractice. The patient needs to take full responsibility of his/her body and of disease or health, not just believing the doctor is the panacea. People need to investigate, study and research, and come alive with passion to achieve a healthy, happy lifestyle and live it abundantly.

Many people are so miserable with their lives, jobs, etc., that this stress just eats away at their bodies and attitudes. Stress kills and eats the person alive. That is why Jesus said, "Do not worry, and do not be anxious!" [4] He is just trying to protect everyone from the harm that people create for themselves. Stress begets poor health. People need to learn to relax, not take life so seriously, and learn to laugh again, even at their own mistakes. Adding a little bit of humor will tear down the mountain, turning it back into a molehill. Learn to love life, find and focus on at least one good thing in every situation, and allow one to bend before the break comes. People will need to keep the stress levels low in their daily lives, finding ways to manage the stress within the body when their world feels overwhelmed.

A soft touch, a kind word, and a caring and compassionate heart move people's souls. We need to learn to look outside of ourselves to help and serve others. When we are just looking inward with contempt and self-pity, the world looks dark instead of bright. When we help a stranger in need, it does our spirit good and brings a smile to our hearts. We must choose to be happy and to commit to living a joyful life. We can choose to be happy or to be miserable. We need to make the wise choice to maintain a good, healthy attitude and body. The world is too stressed. Let's change our priorities and have a great life.

Endnotes

1.   *Oxford Dictionary of Current English*, 4th ed., s.v. "cure."
2.   Paul Malkmus and Ann Malkmus, "Yes, You Can Afford To Be Healthy," *Hallelujah Acres Health News* 56 (July/August 2008): 8.
3.   Patch Adams with Maureen Mylander, *Gesundheit!* (Healing Arts, 1998), 53.
4.   Matthew 6:25 (NKJV).

CHAPTER 28

Holistic Medicine

The field of holistic medicine emerged to offer an alternative from the overuse of toxic medication. Doctors continue to prescribe drugs long past the time people should have discontinued their use, creating even more dangers than the malady originally produced. Prevention is the key elements that people and doctors fail to look at. Prevention versus drugs. Even in the holistic applications, the main purpose can still be about what will cure, not how to prevent disease.

When listening to the advertising that goes on about different drugs, it is astounding to hear about the huge list of side effects; the list goes on and on. A smart person would be better off not ever beginning to take these drugs because the side effects are generally worse than the person's present problem or disease. Some people are smart enough to want to avoid these hazards, but not smart enough to get off all drugs and change their lifestyles. The holistic approach is better, but still has its challenges, i.e., these holistic medicines are still drugs, only in a different form and are still taken in the context to avoid symptoms; thereby, the accumulated toxins still exist in the body.

Proper nutrition and a healthy lifestyle are still the most optimal approaches to regeneration and healing of the body to have good health. It's too bad that the doctors are just as ignorant as their patients. It's the case of the blind leading the blind until they both end up in the pit, the pit of despair, disappointment, and disease.

Other holistic applications will now be discussed. The first is called chiropractic medicine, which does not use drugs. The chiropractic doctor will use spinal manipulations as well as muscle pressure procedures to release endorphins as well as to relax the tension within the muscles, producing a healing for the body. The doctor will also use what is called a TENS unit machine as well as ultrasound equipment and electrical stim treatment for relaxation and pain management. These doctors may also suggest supplements and herbs. Sometimes, they may speak of nutrition, but do they preach it, teach it, and live it? Many of their patients come to them for help to eliminate their pain, but most would be pain-free, or at least minimally free of pain, if their diets and lifestyles were changed as well. A lot of these people instead are dependent on the doctor for temporary relief that comes in the form of bi-weekly/weekly adjustments and manipulations. Those due to injuries do get some relief if given a chance to heal in between visits instead of having to come in every day; but the others with noninjury pain will be coming in continually and do not seem to get permanent healing because there hasn't been any change. The toxic accumulations are still creating the pain, which creates more stress, thus more pain, and so on and on. "At least I don't have to do any drugs" is their attitude.

There have been some entirely injurious situations caused by chiropractors who have provided faulty treatments. Fortunately, I have been lucky enough through investigative efforts to have competent and qualified doctors. Doctors need to be checked out by many reliable sources, especially if they are going to do procedures, manipulations, or anything to the body.

Most of the chiropractors, whom I have utilized in the past as well as the present, are just as nutritionally unhealthy as their patients. They agree with the nutritional aspect but claim they have their vices, and they are healthy enough and don't get sick. Most are severely overweight, and some have type A personalities, are workaholics, and possess very commanding personalities. Stress levels can be high in these types. These doctors have a passion for their field along with a strong desire to help other people, especially their patients. Some to the extent that all else falls apart around them in their personal lives. Most do not believe in surgery. "Just let me adjust you, and you will be healed," they boast. If it fails, they maintain, "A person was just born that way." It's never the doctor's fault.

As far as my own personal experience, I have had several chiropractic doctors adjusting my spine because of the injury in which my disk was herniated. The only good thing that came from all of these adjustments wasn't a cure, but that I was able to have a surgeon repair my back eleven years past the injury, which is generally unheard of. Most surgeries must be done right after the injury, to be successful because, generally, without adjustments, the spine would have fused around the nerve and healed in a deformed manner. The surgery I had was successful and free of any complications. I went against all of my chiropractors' wishes and had the surgery because I was losing nerve functions. My gait was becoming complicated, and I lived in continual pain, no matter what I did, and I could not live the rest of my life that way, eventually becoming confined to a wheelchair. This happened to a friend of mine. He had the same type of injury, no adjustments, just pain and truckloads of drugs only. His back became fused, impinging on the nerve to the point that he lives on pain medications. He can barely walk and now is developing Alzheimer's disease and muscular dystrophy because of the stress on his body, the toxic use of drugs, etc.

I believe everything has its place in the area of healing due to an injury. There just need to be investigative efforts and discernment to what can and will happen in the area of repair to the body; investigating every avenue with a fine-toothed comb; and judging all approaches, not just leaving everything in the hands of the doctor. I have seen some real horror stories, so even the doctors need to be checked out through careful scrutiny. Of course, a person has to be very in-tune and informed of his/her body and all of its ways. I had a better advantage than the general public because I work in the medical field of radiology and in a hospital setting. I have worked in the operating room with surgeons and had investigated every back procedure, including surgery, along with every option, including the risks involved with each procedure. Once I had my surgery, I obeyed all the laws of recovery to never go through a repeat surgery. I learned more than my own surgeons, getting information from many other doctors, including a special chiropractic doctor whom I highly respected as a friend. I learned all about the anatomy/physiology as well as the functioning, maintenance, and care of the spine itself for my own personal situation. We must always keep ourselves with an open mind for learning. The healing always starts after the repair and the willingness to treat the body well. There will always be changes to be made, and we must be willing and determined to complete that part of the recovery as well.

I have seen others go through continual surgeries and repair because of ignorance and stupidity. Many people do not take care of or respect their bodies. The human body does have its limitations, and when it is abused, the body will fail. Chiropractic is not the end-all result but can be used with some benefits in the context of health. People need to be responsible for their own health, healing, and recovery. It's important to learn all we can about living with the one and only body given to us by our Creator.

Acupuncture is from the Chinese culture and medicine. The Chinese are very health-oriented, thus structuring their diets and lifestyles with vitality and longevity in mind. Their diets and medicine incorporate herbs in addition to standard medicine. Today, the Chinese normally don't use acupuncture, but there are still some clinics. In the US, acupuncture is offered by quite a few naturopathic practitioners. Those who choose to incorporate acupuncture and herbs in fact are practicing traditional Chinese medicine (TCM), a term used to differentiate between traditional and modern medicine in China.

Along with the herbs used in TCM, acupuncture is used as a way of keeping the flow of energy moving to achieve harmony and balance. This is achieved by the use of hair-thin needles placed in precise locations of the body to correct the malfunctioning channels of energy, thus allowing an energy flow for healing and health, creating a so-called cure. Along with the acupuncture procedure, in the US version of TCM, the person is also persuaded to consume different types of healing herbs. There are herbs that can reduce pain and inflammation. Some of these herbs are to be taken daily for general health and regeneration, and some are used as antibiotics for diseases that are already present.

These herbs, however, can have toxic effects on the body in the same way as the drugs, but most people who take these different herbs consider them safe. Some will say the herbs are the lesser of two evils, better than the pharmaceutical derivatives. Acupuncture can, in most cases, be less dangerous than the Western procedures and surgeries, but sometimes, these TCM approaches used with modern techniques can be painful and may create a worse situation.

I had a friend who had ankle pain due to an injury, so she made an appointment for an acupuncture treatment. After her first visit, it was perfect, no pain. After her second treatment, she had so much pain that she could barely walk. The acupuncturist stated that this was a normal occurrence and encouraged her to continue the treatments because it may get better. That was her cue, no guarantees, just might get better. She discontinued any further treatments. Eventually, her ankle did heal. Many studies have indicated that those who claim almost instant success using acupuncture are, in fact, experiencing a placebo effect.

I had two treatments that were done to my lower back a couple of years before my surgery. The Chinese doctor promised that I would never have to have surgery if I continued the treatment protocol. Both were just excruciating. This man used the needle procedure, but he also used light electrical currents to go through the needles to stimulate healing. It only stimulated the pain, and I never went back again. I have heard anecdotal statements from people who used TCM methods, indicating that they felt better. But I'm not going to be a candidate for them because I do not believe that herbs can be a cure-all any more than drugs for healing. The body will heal itself if the cause of illness is taken away.

Hypnosis is supposedly a way of curing someone from addictions, i.e., smoking, excessive drinking, or overeating. It is a practice of causing a person to be in a very relaxed, suggestive state of semi-consciousness whereby the mind ready to receive suggestions or commands from another person or self-induced to bring about a change in behavior.

The person may be cured of one addiction, but the problem lies in the fact that the person may resort to another one. Addictive people must eliminate the cause of the addictions, allowing the mind and the body to accept that they have an addiction and the desire to stop and change these behaviors. People keep running to addiction to fill the voids in their lives.

Some addictions are physical in nature, in relation to the hypothalamus of the brain. This part of the brain regulates water-balance and thirst, food intake, feelings of hunger and satiety. Some people will eat or drink themselves to death because of a malfunctioning hypothalamus. I believe an alcoholic starts off with a psychological fixation, but because of the damaging effects of alcohol on the body, the brain and the liver cannot eliminate the large amounts, and the body and brain will begin to degenerate at a very fast rate. Thus, the damaged brain cells cease to produce adequately, and the hormone levels of the brain also malfunction, creating the vicious cycle of addiction. In cases of recovering alcoholics using only hypnosis, it's always been a failure, at least from the physical sense. The body is so very malnourished and damaged, sometimes to the point of no return, that the psychological state does not get addressed for the alcoholic, who has an addictive nature, and he/she will just seek another addiction to fill the void.

The food addict shares the same symptoms. The body and the mind (attitude) desire to be brought back into homeostasis with proper amounts of nutrition along with fasting to promote the body to heal and regenerate. If the food addict seeks only hypnosis, it will also be a failure. These people may then tend to seek smoking, drinking, gambling, shopping, or some other addiction, to fill the gaps in their lives.

Therefore, hypnosis can be a very dangerous avenue for people to seek for cures. They need to address the reason for these addictions, admit to them, and revamp their whole destructive and abusive lifestyles, seeking to live a healthy lifestyle and to be free of the chains and bondages of addictions.

Vitamin supplementation is a huge business. Manufacturers of supplements will make their profits based on the fact that other junk food/fast food manufacturers are supplying low-key wannabe foods, and the biggest factor is that people will continue to buy and eat all of the processed foods. Because of poor diets and lifestyles, the public will buy many vitamin/mineral/herbal supplements but will never change their eating styles. People believe when they are consuming the supplements that they are getting a healthy body, so taking daily supplements is promoted for health. They will think that they are getting all of the good nutrition based on the supplementation because it has been made known that the body needs more than the foods will provide. That's true because they are eating "dead foods." There is a particular manufacturer that takes the fruits and vegetables and processes them into a concentrated pill form for people who do not eat produce. But, no one seems to realize that all of these concentrated fruits and vegetables are just another processed junk food. They have been chopped, pulverized, cooked and jammed into a capsule that is absolutely useless to the healing of the body. Many will say that their health is much better because they take these vitamin pills, but much of this is due to the placebo effect.

A placebo is an imitation medicine that convinces people that they are taking a drug of a "pill of health;" vitamin/mineral/herb supplement and they are miraculously cured. The fact is that the body is a self-healing organism and if people think they are on the pathway to recovery, then their attitude may trigger some of the healing on its own, but it's not the pills.

The problem with all of these supplements is that they will leave a trail of toxins within the body that will disrupt the healing process. Nutrition is the right idea for the recovery and regeneration of the body, but it must be with fresh and properly-combined whole foods.

Fresh whole foods contain more than essential nutrients. They contain enzymes, fiber, and dietary components, substances required for a healthy digestive tract and colon. No vitamin pill will ever substitute for all the good anticancer, anti-disease agents of nature's treasure of delicious and perfect, unprocessed foods. What God made, we can eat; what man made, we must never eat. Like the nutritionists have often said, "You are what you eat." People don't want to see it, but closing their eyes to something doesn't make it untrue.

A doctor friend of mine is an advocate for popping all sorts of vitamin/mineral/herbal supplements, sixty-five pills per meal. He continues to be very diligent about his lifestyle and thinks that everyone who gets cancer, or any other type of disease, needs to consume more of his supplement products. Yes, he does eat somewhat healthy foods, at least better than the general public, but those are definitely not wholesome. He just boasts that because of the supplements, he takes daily, his eyes (retinal detachment) are much improved, he has great bone density, etc., although he recently had some skin cancers (melanoma) removed. I have made my point. His own father died of esophageal cancer, and all he commented on was that his dad quit taking the supplements and that is why he contracted cancer. He said the same thing about my husband. "While you were taking the supplements, you were doing very well (my husband has had chronic lymphocytic leukemia since 1997), but that is why your cancer has progressed." In other words, he persisted in getting him to continue taking all of these pills again. We were duped into believing this and spent approximately $500 a month for all the vitamin/mineral/ herbal supplements. Sad but true. We still continued to develop diseases because they didn't keep us healthy. Many others are just as deceived.

The body needs to be free of toxins but mostly by not consuming these in our foods and diets. Less food is best. Many people have a tendency to consume too much food. Even good foods taken in excess are toxic. Pills do not take away the toxins or add anything in the form of health to the body. Nutrients are in the form of fresh whole foods, not in a bottle of pills.

Endnotes

1. Earl Mindell and Hester Mundis, *Earl Mindell's Vitamin Bible* (Warner Books, 1991), 190.

CHAPTER 29

Are Herbs and Vitamin Supplements the Fountain of Youth?

People have become excited about the vitamin supplementation/ exercise regimen to remain ageless but fail to change their diets or stressful lifestyles. They will go from one so-called healthy lifestyle and diet to another but continue to consume an abundant amount of unwholesome foods. This is done not just in ignorance but also because of laziness and lack of discipline. This in turn only creates a more disastrous physical situation. The body's health only spirals downward, leading to more impaired health. People need to remove the burden to the body's health by eliminating the processed, addictive, and unwholesome foods. These substances will only enhance the perverted palate. "Do not be deceived, God is not mocked, for whatever a man sows that he will also reap."[1] Diligence and persistence are the only ways to move forward. People need to cease looking back; after all, look what happened to Lot's wife (Genesis 19:26). No one wants to die before his/her time. When people continue living by the standards of the world, their days are definitely destined to be shorter and fewer than our Creator meant them to be. The bridges to the past must be burned, thus new windows will open up to a new, better future for optimal health. People must become realists and give up their stubbornness, which will only lead to continued cravings along with food and lifestyle addictions. Mankind needs to start making healthy choices or will it continue to suffer a horrifying existence. The human body can only take so much abuse before it just gives up and gives out.

Herbs are another form of supplementation. Consuming and eating these natural plants daily to promote health and healing has become a part of some people's nutritional practice. It's an alternative to drugs, only in a different form. It's considered food by some sources, but the body reacts to them as a drug, a stimulant, as it tries to eliminate the chemicals quickly from the body.

There is a particular herb company that manufactures and sells herbs as a food product to prevent illness and to regenerate the body. While I look at the distributors who sell these products, I can't say that they all look like they have vibrant health. In fact, if they get sick, they just overload on certain herbal products to get well. It's a bit backward for me. I want to stay healthy by eating raw, fresh whole fruits and vegetables, not by popping herbal pills or drinking these herbal beverages which do not keep me well. These people spend thousands of dollars each month on so-called foods. I spend my hard-earned money at the farmer's market, and when I eat the fresh, raw produce, my body stays well, not poisoned like theirs. They take their herbal products and still have weight gain issues and struggle with the flu and colds. People use these herbs rather than change their diets and lifestyle. It's all about money; it's a big business. The herbs in this case are used as food supplements and concentrated foods. But these concentrated foods are very strong and, in some cases, toxic. Even small amounts of some of these herbs have created diarrhea, showing that they are a burden on a healthy body. The herbs are indigestible by the body because the body cannot assimilate these plants and herbs. Some will even create a stimulating effect. The herbal supplements, as well as other supplements, imbalance the body, disrupting the body's functions, impairing the body's metabolism and forcing the body to eliminate these products, sometimes in disruptive ways.

I have lived the natural hygiene lifestyle since 2007 and have maintained my weight and all of my health challenges are gone. My body does feel like I have found the fountain of youth. As a life scientist, I continue to experiment and the raw, fresh whole produce diet is the one for optimal health and disease-free life.

Vitamin and mineral supplementation has become normal in our society; everyone just wants a quick fix without changing anything else in their lives. It has become a monster business. Because of it; one can buy a supplement to cure anything. Everyone has his/her views, but everyone does agree that health is important and all are trying to buy it. No one seems willing to change and take away the cause of disease so the body will be free of disease. Most will just take the supplements believing that these will give them health and energy.

Yes, the body does need vitamins and minerals, from raw, fresh, and properly-combined whole fruits and vegetables, not from bottles of pills, liquids, and rancid oils. The amounts of pollutants in these alternative drugs are still enough to do the body great harm.

Earl Mindell's book is written very simply, for the unknowledgeable, health-minded novice. I became involved with his books years ago to try and gain health, but not changing any of my diet and lifestyle because of lack of knowledge and ignorance. There is a vitamin for everything that we do, according to Mindell's book, and there are many cautions he has written, but unfortunately, there are more than he even realizes. It has to do with, "You are what you eat," including these supplements. They are just false security, like putting a Band-Aid on a broken leg. These supplements just overload the body with a continued flow of toxins that will accumulate until the person acquires more sicknesses and diseases.

All of this vitamin/mineral/herbal supplementation throws the body off-balance. For example, taking too much of a zinc supplement can deplete the copper in the body. Fat-soluble vitamins A, D, E, and K need other vitamins, fats, and/or minerals to be absorbed into the body. They cannot be taken in isolated forms as people will do to supposedly heal specific diseases. People will continue this practice and wonder why they still have health challenges, sometimes very severe ones at that. Much mega dosing is done, and this damages the liver, kidneys, and other vital organs of the body.

Earl Mindell is a pharmacist who realized that all the people he was selling prescription drugs were taking many drugs, not for illnesses alone, but to just get through the day. People take an amazing amount of drugs just to take away the side effects of other drugs. No one even questions why they take the drugs and use the excuse of just because the doctor told them to. Mindell states, "I had one regular patron who had prescriptions for pills to supplant virtually all his bodily functions, and he wasn't even sick."[2] Earl began to learn more about nutrition and vitamins in general, but these synthetic vitamins have their cautions. One has to be a scientist just to get through the lists of what each vitamin and mineral does, what they are for, how they work for the body, and how much must be used in conjunction with other vitamins, dosages, the enemies of the vitamins, where these vitamins come from, and most important, the toxicity of these supplements.

The public is disillusioned with all of the hype of what they are told that they need. What they really do need is to stop eating all of the junk foods/fast foods, refined sugars and white flours, and pill popping. There are no cures. If there were, we would have made history by now. Human beings have become quite creative by now in attempting to find ways to make up for their shortcomings as to their diet and lifestyle.

Nowadays, there is a big hype about getting enough of a good omega 3 fatty acid supplement. The processed, additive-filled foods found in the standard American diet have been found to consume too much of the omega 6 oils, the trans-fat type oils that bombard the body with free radicals. These trans fats are cooked oils. Cooked oils of any kind added to the diet slow the digestive process, sometimes by as much as half, as well as add toxic poisons to the body.

At the turn of the twentieth century, the human body had more of a balance of omega 3 and omega 6 fats. It wasn't until the oil salesmen started peddling different vegetable seed oils, also boasting how one could cook with these oils to make different food products taste wonderful that the balance of omega 3 fats became out of whack.

Then the problem with the increase of omega 6 fats in the body began. These fats began to increase the disease rates, and the ratio of omega 6 fats far exceeded the omega 3 fatty acids.

Rev. George Malkmus claims, "It has been established that the omega 3 fats prevent cancer and stop its spread by reducing inflammation. Conversely, an overload of omega 6 fats speeds the growth and spread of cancer."[3] That may be true, depending on what type will be used for the body. Fish and fish oils are definitely out because of the mercury in the fish. Also, it is not digestible animal protein, and fish oil capsules contain fragmented and rancid oils and are poor substitutes for healthy fatty acids that the body can use. The body needs fats for sure, for the proper functioning of the brain, skin, joints, kidneys, and prostate; prevention of gallstones; and hair loss. Fatty acids also help the endocrine system function as well as help defeat depression and keep the nervous system properly functioning.

The body can get adequate amounts of fatty acids from avocadoes, nuts, and seeds. A person can also add to this raw, fresh, wholesome fruits and vegetables, and the body will be well-supplied and healthy without an excess of the unhealthy fats.

Let us not get caught up in all of the dangerous claims brought on by the manufactures of supplements. They are just their ways of using their scientific background to try and cure diseases with their products, making profits at the cost of the public's health.

Fasting, not herbs or food supplements pill-popping is the way for the body to heal from its toxicity. For the body to experience optimal health, one must have a proper diet, healthy lifestyle, and fasting as needed. There isn't any healing that comes from any substance outside the body. The body is a self-healing organism when it is taken care of properly.

Endnotes

1. Galatians 6:7 (NKJV).
2. Earl Mindell and Hester Mundis, *Earl Mindell's Vitamin Bible* (Warner Books, 1991), 2.

3. George Malkmus, "Is There a Place for Fish Oil in the Hallelujah Diet," The Hallelujah Health Tip, *Hallelujah Acres Health* 624 (November 2009).

CHAPTER 30

Natural Body Cleansers

Many people like the effect of a clean body; it's sad that people will go through a fasting and cleansing process and then return to their former ways. What have they gained? Their desire was to get a clean body so they could be healthier, but they have failed to realize that it isn't just a diet, which is something temporary. It has to be a healthy lifestyle to be lived daily for a lifetime. These cleanses are parallel to yo-yo dieting; the body only gets worse with each of these bouts.

There is a popular cleanse that people use to cleanse their body of mucus and so-called debris. It consists of pure maple syrup, lemon juice, and distilled water. Some will add apple cider vinegar to this concoction. I have heard others will add Epsom salt. This is a catastrophe, a misery for the body. Pure distilled water, as needed for thirst, is the only healthy fast to cleanse the body.

A work associate generally does a juice fast along with maple syrup, lemon juice, and water to remove excess mucus. Apparently there is a lot removed as well as other cleansing effects within the body. She and her husband do this regimen for one week to ten days at least twice a year. She does her regular work schedule during this time, so rest is not applied. She did attempt the distilled water-only fast and barely made it to twenty-four hours. She claimed it was too intense, and she didn't feel very well. Her body was overloaded with toxins, and yet she claims that she eats healthy. The gallstones and kidney stones that were eliminated from her body were of a great number. People *think* they are living healthy, but this is not health. All of this debris shouldn't be in the body of a healthy individual. Then returning to one's so-called normal lifestyle instead of introducing a change is ludicrous. According to Hannah Allen, "The relationship between fasting and nutrition must be recognized. Recovery from pathology can often be accomplished through fasting, but permanence of the recovery is dependent on the continued diet and lifestyle."[1]

People want instant cures and feel that pills and potions will be their answers. They just want to feel good again but do not want to eliminate the cause of their body's distress. Bad habits must be converted to new and healthy ones to bring freedom from diseases.

One of the most frequent bowel problems today is constipation. Constipation is a slow transition time of the elimination of toxic wastes through the digestive system caused by animal proteins, cooked foods, improper food combinations, grains, and drugs. The longer the transit time, the longer the toxic wastes sit in the bowel. The longer the body is exposed to this decaying matter, with a chance of these toxins becoming reabsorbed, the greater the risk of developing disease, especially cancer. One needs a good transit time to expel the three meals that are eaten during the day. The natural, hygienic lifestyle with fresh, raw whole fruits, vegetables, seeds and nuts, will give the body a twenty-four–thirty-six hour motility rate (three bowel movements a day). Thus, eating the standard American diet will give a motility rate of forty-eight to seventy-two hours, sometimes up to one hundred hours, and many people who are on excessive medications may not have bowel movements, if lucky, once a week or more, without the help of stool softeners or laxatives. Oftentimes, the peristalsis of the digestive system becomes severely challenged and weakened with all these chemicals. Disease usually begins with a toxic colon. A healthy colon usually weighs about four pounds. Once that is filled and coated with impacted mucoid plaque, it could weigh as much as forty–fifty pounds.

I had a patient receiving a barium enema in my X-ray who had problems with diverticulitis and constipation (these two go hand in hand). He stated that he only had two to four bowel movements a month, but his wife had two per day. The difference makes a big difference in the state of health.

A fast of pure distilled water has a way of allowing the digestive system to rest and have time to eliminate these toxins. The colon, through improper lifestyle and diet, develops layer upon layer of mucoid plaque that weakens the colon. This plaque will harden and continuously add more layers. Through a fast, this will eventually become softer and slough off. While the plaque is there, the body is unable to absorb the nutrients from the digestive system. Cleansing the colon may take time. Some of the other types of cleanses that people use do not work, the chemicals and toxins in them just add to the toxic and poisonous burden of the already challenged body. It's not surprising that the body will continue to eliminate during the fast, especially of the impacted stools. People have remarked that they continued to have bowel movements even though they were not eating any foods.

It's best to eat raw fruits and vegetables that consist of significant amounts of pure water, just what the body needs to keep the organs of elimination clean, especially the colon and the kidneys. For optimal health, eliminate cooked and processed foods after the fast to keep the digestive system free of the mucoid plaque. The raw produce is nature's fiber. One must never use the synthetic fibers, enemas, or other cleanses. When the body can be properly eliminating, including the cells as well as all the parts of the body, the body will not have a buildup of toxins. The body can then accomplish optimal health, remain pure, and have freedom from disease.

The kidneys can remain clear and free of kidney stones and disease by eating a raw whole produce/plant diet and eliminating processed, cooked, and perverted (chemical-based) foods. Fresh raw foods provide an abundant amount of pure water that flushes the kidneys and purifies the blood, producing radiant health. Kidney stones are formed by excess calcium intake, inorganic mineral supplements, milk products, and animal flesh.

God created the body for a perfect purpose in mind. We have two kidneys to keep the blood of the entire body filtered and cleansed.

When the kidneys fail to function, a person can be put on dialysis to filter the blood or death occurs. We must take care of these as well as the whole body; it is wonderfully and fearfully made. Our kidneys do an overload of work unless we live a healthy lifestyle and eat correctly for the optimal health of the body.

Juicing is the process of extracting the liquid portions of produce: enzymes, vitamins, minerals, and micronutrient portions of the produce and eliminating much of the fiber for quick and easy absorption through the digestive system and into the body. Another benefit to juicing is that it will digest quicker and can be godsend for those who are unable to eat raw vegetables or fruits, for example, those persons who have trouble with chewing and mastication. Also included are those who refuse to fast with distilled water only. Alternating juices and water would be beneficial for recovery, and it also helps the body to detoxify. Some I have worked with who have had esophageal ulcers and have accomplished a healing by alternating juicing and water until they were able to chew and swallow masticated fresh produce again. Juices are to be sipped very slowly and mixed with the saliva, not to be gulped, as it can be very challenging for the stomach to incorporate that much food at one time.

Some people believe that, with years of abusive eating and compromised intestines, juicing is a wise choice. The poor choices made in the past have limited the ability of the body to absorb the nutrients from the foods, especially raw fresh produce, while juicing tends to keep this absorption ability.

Juicing is also a very good way to start children who have been raised on a conventional diet to transition to the natural raw produce diet and lifestyle. This helps them to get excited about their health and trying to improve their body's functioning if they have been in poor health. These juices must be made from raw, fresh whole produce, not commercialized, pasteurized, bottled, canned, or frozen, which are a toxic blend of juices. These types of juices are damaging to the human body because they are fragmented and cooked although no one seems to be aware of all the poisons that reside in them. People just want the simplest method—to eat the fruit from its wholly raw state. Fresh juice from the fruits and vegetables is the best, freshest and most wholesome, the natural source. People have been deceived in their thinking that they can buy their juice in the store and that will contribute to better health. They bought the lie.

The brain and the body have been created to eat the fresh, raw whole fruits and vegetables, not drink them. When only juices are consumed for meals, the mouth, tongue, and stomach are totally unsatisfied. The act of smelling, seeing, biting, chewing, masticating, and swallowing the foods make these pleasurable experiences and also satisfy the body's needs. The foods must be consumed slowly to grant satiety to the body so one will desire to not overeat.

People need to consume raw, fresh produce daily for the best possible health, but it is best to eat the produce fresh and still filled with whole nutrients, not fragmented. Fragmented foods are oxidized and rendered useless to the body. Freshly juiced vegetables can become acidic even though they came from alkaline vegetables.[2] Vegetable and fruit juices must be consumed promptly after juicing because they become oxidized and lose their nutrients.

George Malkmus, in his proven Hallelujah diet, claims that no one can eat enough raw vegetables to restore optimum health and afterward to maintain it, so the answer to the problem is juicing. The juicing of fresh raw produce feeds the cells yet saves the energy that the body uses to separate the juices from the solids, not overburdening the digestive system. He advocates the eating of raw fresh whole produce with the juicing during the day to receive the needed fiber. George Malkmus stated, "Juices are the key to the Hallelujah diet and provide most of the power for internal cleansing and restoration of optimal health."[3] There isn't any nutrition in fiber; the nutrients are in the liquid part of the produce.

It is best to drink the juice immediately following the juicing to eliminate drinking oxidized juice. "Oxygen accelerates the enzymatic digestion of live foods,"[4] and it's best to happen internally inside of the body not on the kitchen counter or in the refrigerator. Juice must be sipped very slowly, allowing each sip to mingle with the saliva in the mouth before swallowing.

Because juice is a liquid, it doesn't remain in the stomach for long. It exits quickly, continuing through the digestive tract while the nutrients continue into the blood stream, feeding the cells of the body. Many people will consume nothing but diluted juices and distilled water for detoxifying and cleansing the body. Different sources will claim admirably the marvels of the juice and distilled water fast, singing praises for its safety and the healthfulness of juicing.

Fasting is a total abstinence of all foods. Drinking pure water as thirst dictates, allows the body to rest and cleanse. Some people will drink juices during a fast, but juices are still considered as food because of the raw materials of nutrients in their makeup. People will consider a fast as just liquid, but anything other than water still forces the body to go through its digestive processes to digest these liquid foods.

George Malkmus claims that the distilled water fast can be more intense, resulting in more sickness and less energy than fasting with fresh vegetable and fruit juices. George advocates juicing continuously every day as part of his healthcare program. He states that he worked at the Shangri La Health Resort in Bonita, Florida, a natural hygienic fasting resort retreat in the 1970s. While he was there, he watched the effects of the distilled-water-only fasting anywhere from three days to forty days. He feels that they had too rapid a detoxification and had to go to bed. The idea is to rest the body, including bedrest, if needed. He feels that they lost weight too quickly and many seemed to be excessively challenged in a physical sense. He feels that water-only fasting is too dangerous. He also believes that a person needs to allow the body to heal by extracting the juice from fresh whole fruits and vegetables, therefore allowing these nutrients, vitamins, and minerals to flood the body at a cellular level in its attempt to restore it to health. Subsequently, all the cells will be fed, and because of the limited fiber intake, a person "will save most of the energy that the body uses to separate the juices from the solids. The body uses less energy with this method, and the cells are fed much more quickly with less loss of energy."[5]

"There isn't any nutritional value in the fiber," state the authors of the Hallelujah diet. "The nutrition is in the liquid parts of the fruits and vegetables that we eat."[6] According to these authors, it is advocated to "drink eight ounces of vegetable juices at least two to three times a day or up to six to seven times if you are fighting an illness rather than a large amount all at once."[6] Large amounts of vitamins, minerals, and nutrients are ingested.

The water fast, according to natural hygiene principles is far superior to a juicing diet. According to doctors Immerman and Burton, "The elimination of salt from the body which occurs so rapidly while fasting and results in health improvement will not occur at all while on juices."[7]

A fast of pure water only has its advantages as well as disadvantages. During the fast of pure water, the accumulated toxins are removed and eliminated from the body's cells and tissues. As the body rests and regenerates, the aging of the body slows down and youthfulness and vitality are restored. The body will begin to function as it was created to. The mind will become more focused, clear, and alert. A fast is the best way to detoxify and cleanse the body's organs and systems.

During the water fast, the body will continue to function, cleanse, and heal itself. The causes of disease have been removed along with the drugs and food chemicals; therefore, the body can inevitably eliminate the accumulated toxic waste products, maintain a blood acid/alkaline level, excellent blood pressure level, proper body temperature, steady heart rate, and normal functioning of the kidneys and lungs. Instead of the body going through its digestive processes, it will be resting and devoting all its time to the function of waste elimination. The nutrients that the body uses during a fast are from the reserve stored up within the body, therefore protecting itself.

Some of the disadvantages of the water-only fast can include too intense detoxification and rapid weight loss. The cold and flu-like symptoms can be alleviated in this manner, but the body may experience weakness, headaches, and loss of energy, to the point of bed rest. I have done a thirty-six–forty-eight hour water fast to clean up the body of toxins that are trying to release, but it can be challenging, especially for the novice who is unaware of what the body is experiencing. If the fast is too prolonged, one may risk kidney damage. Then people may tend to gorge instead of starting light and small amounts of food, mostly light vegetable/fruit juices. All fasting must be done with discretion. Some bodies may tend to detoxify too fast on the all-raw diet and raw vegetable juices while others may recover easier from all the cleansing effects.

People will try and use a fast for the curing of all of their diseases. A fast does nothing to cure; it just provides the basis of a condition that the body will use to clean out its environment and then it will effectively build its health. The body is doing the work, not the fast. The fast just provides the opportunity for the work of the body to do what it was created to do. We need to get out of the way and watch what it can do.

Endnotes

1. Hannah Allen, "Fasting Does Not Make the Body Disease Proof" (lesson 48, a course in Natural Health, Fit for Life Sciences Institute), 1070.

2. Robert O. Young and Shelley Redford Young, *The pH Miracle* (Warner Books, 2002), 96.

3. George Malkmus, "Stress Related Aging," *Hallelujah Acres Health News* 57 (September/October 2009), 16.

4. George Malkmus with Peter and Stowe Shockey, *The Hallelujah Diet* (Destiny Image, 2006), 164.

5. George Malkmus, "Why Not All Raw?" Hallelujah Acres Health Tip, *Health Acres Health Magazine* 404 (August 2005).

6. George Malkmus et al., 164.

7. Alan Immerman and Alec Burton, "Introduction to Fasting" (lesson 45, a course in Natural Health, Fit for Life Sciences Institute), 1020.

CHAPTER 31

Healing Therapies

The body will begin to heal and restore itself if the causes of the diseases are removed and completely eliminated. The second part of this process is taking a course of action for health and healing of the body. The damage created by years of chemical abuse may in some cases be healed, depending on the extent of damage. It is through a three-fold process: mental, physical, and spiritual.

Mental aspects work to heal the body. If a person has a good, healthy, proper diet and is dealing with any type of emotional upheaval, a stressful burden that will be destructive to all the cells and organ systems will be placed on the body.

Attitude can change the healing aspects of the cancer patient. In fact, I had a friend whose oncology nurse who prescribed to him a period of one-half hour per day of meditation—to just to lie in a recliner, listen to a relaxing meditation tape, and to allow each muscle in the body to relax, especially the brain. He was to focus on his breathing, which will help the state of relaxation of his body to slowly occur. This, she said, would help him in his recovery from his cancer.

While I was going to college, raising a family, and working full time, I definitely needed to do the relaxation therapy because I was so overwhelmed with stress. Relaxation therapy, as well as going to the gym, allowed me to alleviate the damaging stressful hormones that I knew would destroy my body. I listened to the sounds of nature tapes and allowed my body to meditate and relax until I felt suspended. This is a state of relaxing without going to sleep but remaining semi-conscience; the brain was aware but was relaxed as well as the body. I reclined in the chair, but I did not feel it beneath my body. It was a very peaceful time. (It took a lot of practice for me to learn this because I'm either falling asleep or hyper.) The best part of all is just to let the brain, the thinking and emotions, slow down as well to let the hormones balance and heal.

I'm sorry that I didn't retain this practice throughout the years because now, when the world is getting in my face and the stress begins to mount, I definitely need a break. I am trying to incorporate it back into my life. When I do, I definitely sleep better, feel like I can focus and deal better with life, and feel more relaxed. Stress slows digestion, and I need that to be corrected.

Along with relaxation therapy is what I call an attitude adjustment. Most of this takes practice, practice and more practice. Developing a servant's heart can relieve a person of his/her rut of selfishness, and eliminate the plague of "me-ism." If I'm able to look at other people and their problems first, I'm not as focused on my own quandaries anymore, and my problems won't seem as significant and important. If we were asked to take the other person's load, we would rather grab our own back, because it's a smaller load. The grass always looks greener on the other side until we get over there. Then we find out that it still looks greener on the other side (our own this time). This is called human depravity.

Another attitude that needs practicing is learning to live in the present, in the here and now. Many people tend to focus on their past guilt, sins, or they are off on a tangent of what their future could be. Thereby, the present is totally forgotten, only adding more stress into one's life when the body needs peacefulness and serenity. This can be very difficult, but by continuously focusing on the present situation and circumstance, a person will learn to become calmer and more serene. Alcoholics Anonymous has a standard that is a good philosophy: Living for Today One Day at a Time. I call it "One moment at a time." The Alcoholics Anonymous's Serenity Prayer, "God grant me the serenity to accept the things I cannot change, courage to change the things I can, and the wisdom to know the difference," is a lifesaver if it is practiced and lived continually in a person's life.

Another form of relaxation comes by the way of music. Music soothes the soul as well as the body. It tends to take the mind off the anxieties and just focus on the sound itself. It involves more than just the sense of hearing; it will include the inner being, especially the brain, emotions, and hormonal changes. Soft music seems to calm while a fast pace tends to put the body into a frenzy and a state of hyperactivity. While patients are in the waiting rooms of doctors' offices, the types of music played can have an important impact of the anxiety levels of their patients.

Many doctors, anesthesiologists, surgeons, dentists, and chiropractors have used music as a way of helping to relax their patients. They also have used earphones plugged into their patients' favorite music before performing the procedures. The patient, who is relaxed beforehand, may have much fewer anesthetics used, and the patient associates these experiences as pleasurable rather than painful and without the anxiety.

Generally, the softer the music that is played, the lower the stress levels. The person remains calmer, especially if it is kept as background music. The louder the music, the more agitated the body becomes. Experiments have been conducted on human babies and animals using different types of music while viewing and recording their physical reactions.

Music introduced before the birth of babies, especially soft music played while the baby was still in the womb, helped these babies to remain calm after birth. Music has been shown to reduce infantile colic and excessive crying in infants. Breast-fed babies had soft music playing while being fed, and this calm experience reduced the anxiety on both the baby and the mother. These babies experienced less, if any, colic. The babies and their mothers were more relaxed and bonded more closely. Soothing music reduces anxiety and tension on the baby.

I do remember one particular scene in the movie *The Shawshank Redemption* in which the main character, who was in prison, broke into the warden's office and put a record onto the loudspeakers that broadcasted throughout the prison. The music was opera music of some kind performed by a woman who sounded like an angel singing. All the prisoners in the entire prison and courtyard stopped what they were doing and stood mesmerized, just listening to the beauty of the song and the singing. The narrator spoke, "No one understood the words, but it didn't matter anyway; she was beautiful." I think about that scene quite often and do wish that they could do that in real life, using music therapy to calm the hostile and angry.

There are too many angry people, and most don't even know why they are. I believe that the foods (improperly combined), additives, sugars, and processed foodstuffs contribute to this anger. All these disrupt the hormones, which in turn affect the angry ones adversely.

I had to practice to not be angry. There were so many triggers to the inner rage, but as I became in touch with other emotions, relaxed, prayed to God, and ate properly, the anger began to defuse and melt away. It does take willingness, at least in my case, along with a determination to get well emotionally and mentally.

Psychotherapy can help in some cases but there also needs to be a healing of the body involved, a regeneration. When the body begins to regenerate, many people get a false sense of security and begin to substitute something else for what the body really needs, nutrition. Many physicians give drugs to relieve depression and psychological problems, including children and teenagers who have been diagnosed with attention deficit disorder (ADD) and attention deficit hyperactivity disorder (ADHD). It's sad that these drugs are replacing what the human body truly needs, good and healthy nutrition. The problem is the destructive diet with all its colorings, additives, processed foods along with the drinks which contain sugars and chemicals that are highly poisonous to the growing body. Even earthly environments are filled with contaminations and things that affect the body's chemistry. Replacing all of these so-called manmade foods with God-made fresh whole foods can give adequate nutrition to the starved body. The body and the brain need fresh whole fruits and vegetables, nuts, seeds, and pure clean water. The rule of thumb is if one feeds the body and the brain, they will function and behave normally and optimally. If not, they will act abnormally.

The standard American diet is a poor substitute for the real thing, and everyone who eats this as standard fare suffers tragically because there are not any vitamins or minerals to feed the body properly. The children and adults who eat this way have a brain chemistry imbalance thus becoming irritable and wired, ready to go off at the drop of a hat.

I remember reading an article many years ago about Kelly Lebrock, an actress whose children suffered too many childhood diseases and also ADD-type behaviors. She was very disillusioned with what the medical system wanted to do with her children, with the prescribing of drugs that were useless and dangerous. She decided to move out of the city, buy a farm, and raise their own foods, and coincidentally, her children lost all of their antisocial behaviors and became very healthy and happy people.

It's the same important element for all growing bodies; correctly feed these young people well, and they will stay healthy and grow up to be healthy, functioning adults. So it isn't all just in the mind, it's the whole body that's affected as well.

What also helps to heal the body is laughter. A good belly laugh ten minutes a day is called internal jogging, "which is massaging the internal organs," says Norman Cousins.[1] Laughter can ease the pain of a broken spirit and aching body. It can bring one back to life again. Laughter can release the person from a prison of despair. Laugh and the world laughs with you; cry and you cry alone, or so they say. Laughter is contagious, and one must learn to laugh at ourselves and our own mistakes. "If I wasn't laughing then I'd be crying," has often been said. The problem was that through the years, I found very little to laugh at. Many people also share a lack of a sense of humor, which is unfortunate because it creates a burden on the body, soul, and attitude.

Life can begin again as one can laugh. Dr. Patch Adams and Norman Cousins, both by their own personal experiences, know about laughter therapy and its beneficial effects. Both used different approaches to the subject of health and healing the body, but the common bond of both is humor therapy.

History speaks of laughter medicine. In the Bible, the book of Proverbs 17:22 states, "A merry heart does good like medicine."[2] I've even heard in the thirteenth century some patients, before and during surgery, were distracted by their doctors through the use of laughter. It's an interesting concept, much better than the whiskey that was used by other doctors before amputation and the removing of bullets.

Patch Adams was one of the first to use laughter and humor in his medical practice. He was at one point in his life so depressed that he checked himself into a medical hospital because he was thinking of committing suicide. According to Patch, his two-week stay was the pivotal point in his life. Through his roommate, he learned to get out of himself and really listen to another human being with his heart not just his ears. He said, "For the first time in my adult life, I empathized with another person."[3] He learned about loving someone else, not only how to give love but to receive it. Loneliness was the chain broken by love.

He wanted to be a doctor, but not just an ordinary medical doctor; he wanted to have fun at his work and with those around him. He learned to come out of his inner lonely existence with love and humor. This helped his confidence levels, and he spent the next years experimenting on how to get to know and interact with people. He carried on learning how to be silly and help others to have fun with him. He continued to learn about people, especially his patients, and to be comfortable being himself.

It was difficult going through medical school with a silly, nonchalant, happy attitude. He was so despised by doctors and their interns, but his patients were happier because of the humor, silliness, and fun. Many patients became happier, healthier, and recovered faster than those in other wards. It is an interesting concept to turn one's attitude from sorrow to joy, even in sickness. The disease will tend to go away with other recuperative measures.

This is the way of life for him now in his personal life and medical practice. It is a different approach. He bases health first as prevention and teaches this philosophy in the general care of living a wellness lifestyle. People need to work together for a common good, the health of humanity.

A few years later, Norman Cousins took laughter and humor in a different direction. Norman proved in his life that laughter and humor stimulate the endorphins of the body. This adds a feeling of health throughout all of the body processes, in turn relieving nervous tension and stress. The quality of one's life is in how it's lived, and when one is happy, life can be joyous and meaningful. Many elderly people complain about the misery of getting old. "The golden years, bah," they say. Misery is a choice as well as poor health is by the chosen lifestyle. Someone once said to me, "Happiness is peacefulness and contentedness. You can sometimes be content and not be peaceful or the other way around. Then there will be times of sheer happiness with peacefulness and contentedness. It's not something you will have all the time, so don't continue to *look* for it." What a freedom to have the burden removed. I quit looking for happiness. I was happy sometimes and other times ok—it's just a matter of perspective.

Positive emotions are life-giving experiences. They add years to life, a sweet spirit to the soul, and peace to the heart. Positive emotions though can be lost in the spiral of negativity that the world can throw in your face. These positive emotions must be continued to be stimulated to overcome the negative influences. Negative emotions produce negative chemical changes within the body, so with positive influences and positive chemical changes, the body will restore and maintain balance and health. Norman Cousins says, "Laughter and humor can make one forget about their problems and life for a little while. It not only adds a smile to your face and a sparkle to your eyes, but it will let joy and hope fill your soul and spirit."[4] In the meantime, laughter stimulates your hormones, including your production of endorphins, which heal and release tension, pain, and balance the body.

Norman Cousins worked to improve the quality of his life. He contracted ankylosing spondylitis, a terminal disease in which the connective tissue of the spine disintegrates. He was hospitalized, given many forms of tests, drugs, and procedures, which nothing helped and only made everything worse. He began to investigate how to strengthen his endocrine system, especially his adrenal glands.

He was administered so many different drugs and felt like they were giving him a toxic load to his already compromised body. He needed to be free of these for his adrenal glands to function normally again. Drugs do more harm than any good preached by the medical profession. He was in severe pain because of the deteriorating joints of his body. He studied medical journals and also investigated about the effects of vitamin C (ascorbic acid). Then, he began to administer vitamin C through an IV. His attitude, he maintains, was an important factor, and he did have the will to live. How could he keep this attitude? It would come through laughter therapy. He checked out of the hospital, rented a hotel room, rested, continued the vitamin C, and watched reels of funny movies, anything he could get his hands on. He was finally able to sleep. Cousins reported, "Ten minutes of genuine belly laughter had an anesthetic effect and would give me at least two hours of pain-free sleep."[4] As stress decreased, the pain levels also lessened, giving him a better quality of life. His body continued to heal because of this therapy and regimen.

Laughter enhances the respiratory system, opening up the lungs for more oxygen. Laughter also increases the immune cells and lowers blood pressure, thus there are fewer repeated heart attacks. Norman Cousins calls laughter "internal jogging for the internal organs of the body."[4]

Laughter takes away the fear in the lives of people, so they are able to deal with life's circumstances and situations that seem to overwhelm them. It's best to learn to laugh in a tense situation, find something humorous about it to laugh at, for humor will relieve the stress. It helps to keep things into perspective, to keep the molehills from becoming mountains. It also helps to stimulate the brain's creative resources and assists people to just cope with the world around them. It helps fight depression. The will to live becomes stronger, and courage can help to overcome adversities. Each hormone of the human body is unique, and all of the hormones need to work together in accurate balance for the body to function optimally. Hormone balance is extremely important if one wants to end the addictive craving cycle. The chemicals that have been consumed tend to imbalance the body's hormones.

One of the hormones of the endocrine system that seems to go awry is the thyroid hormone. The thyroid hormone affects all of the adult cells of the body— brain, spleen, uterus, and testes—with the exception of the thyroid gland itself.[5] This hormone is regulated and controlled by the pituitary gland. When the T3 and T4 hormones secreted by the thyroid gland are low, that stimulates the pituitary gland to excrete thyroid's stimulating hormone, i.e., the negative feedback system.

"Estrogen," according to Dr. John Lee, "also tends to suppress thyroid gland function. Estrogen causes food calories to be stored as fat."[6] Many different chemicals tend to turn on the hormone estrogen switch, for example, environmental chemicals as well as the chemicals that are consumed in the foods of a person's diet. Meats that have been fed grains with pesticides, drugs, as well as estrogen itself will play havoc with the body's endocrine system. Plastic and Styrofoam containers used for hot foods emit gasses that are hazardous to the body and affect the hormone levels, especially the estrogen hormone. Dr. John Lee's hypothesis is that "estrogen inhibits thyroid action in the cells…estrogen may compete with the thyroid hormone at the site of its receptor."[6] Many people are prescribed the synthetic hormone drug, Synthroid. I have been prescribed thyroid medication for the past twenty-five plus years. I have been investigating ways to reduce or discontinue this drug but to no avail. At this time in my life, the thyroid is crippled and can no longer function on its own since I have been on the drugs for so long. Fortunately, it is the only drug that I consume daily. The sad part about it is that I am stuck taking this for the rest of my life. Many others have fallen into the same medical handicap of ignorance.

Today's standard American diet disrupts the thyroid function, especially when drinking milk or eating milk products, such as cheeses and yogurt. Meats especially tend to interfere with the hormone functions of the body, but continually adding all the other junk foods, processed, and fast foods along with sodas, desserts, and the like also adds to the imbalance of these hormone levels. This imbalance also produces more food cravings and adds fat to the body's tissues. Estrogen attaches to these fat receptors. The fat cells will also hold in the chemicals consumed from the diet. Therefore, anything that is consumed into the body that imitates estrogen also attaches to these cells and creates more of an imbalance.

Dr. John Lee states that when he "became aware of estrogen dominance syndrome, I noticed that the taking of thyroid supplements was especially common in women with this condition." He explained why he believes in adding natural progesterone cream. "When I attempted to correct their estrogen dominance by adding progesterone, it was common to see that their need for thyroid supplements decreased and could often be eliminated. Thus, I became aware that estrogen, progesterone, and thyroid hormones are interrelated."[6]

The endocrine system works in perfect harmony throughout the human body. If one is off, this will affect the other hormones because these chemical messengers rely on each other to properly help the body to maintain and function optimally. The endocrine system also works with the nervous system, and the hormones also affect the body's metabolism. They work with the body as a unit. It is utterly amazing that each hormone cooperates with each other. The body is wonderfully and fearfully made.

The body in its created genius works its wonders because of the programmed efforts of its Supreme Designer and Creator. The body has its own healing powers if given the correct ingredients and people are obedient to these laws. The spiritual attitude of relying on a Supreme Power outside of the self, whom I choose to call God, will instill an inner peace and calmness within the body. When stress strikes, prayer and Bible reading can be extremely important to focus on, and you realize how unimportant these external issues may be in respect to keeping the body calm. After all, stress will slow down and, in some cases (with agitation), halts the digestive process. Is it any wonder that during a time of stress, while eating, the stomach and bowels can feel horribly distressed and uncomfortable? The foods just sit as the acid continues to build, attempts to digest but cannot. If one wants to have a body that is tuned in and balanced to whole-hearted health, it is significant to remain calm. Stress can also immobilize a life as well as the body. It accelerates the squirrel-cage process of stress, begetting even more tension.

It is amazing how the mind with a positive outlook helps the body to heal. I know of some people who will themselves to health and healing while others experience depression, illness, and even death. Given the proper resources, the body can do a remarkable recovery.

One of the best ways to relieve tension is to focus on something or someone else, and its best to focus on someone bigger than us, whom we know can take care of us, especially in our time of need. This can help us relax as we put our trust, faith, and burdens on God.

As they read the Word of God (Bible) and His promises, many people become exceedingly calm, especially when that is followed by prayer. Prayer helps to relieve pain and anxiety in some.

People also need to learn to say no, for even Jesus, when He and His disciples ministered all day, said, "Come with me by yourselves to a quiet place and get some rest."[8] People also need to get more sleep, restful sleep. With all of the rushed lifestyles that consume the lives in today's fast-paced environment, there is hardly any time for relaxing, and when people get to bed, the body is still running, thus it's difficult to unwind and sleep. Insomnia seems to be normal; the insomniac tossing and turning half the night. When morning comes, these people will resort to drugs of some kind, such as caffeine and uppers, to stay awake and try to be alert. At night, they will also opt for drugs, which, in fact, do not promote restful sleep. The race is on. These sleepless nights create a lack of energy that takes its toll on the body. Naps are a short rest and a break, but unfortunately, they are not always possible. People need to change and alter their priorities, learning to say no to the many unimportant, trivial things of each of the days of our lives.

It's good to take time off and just relax. The Lord said that He worked six days and rested on the seventh (Genesis 2:3). God expects the same from us. We need to be obedient so that we won't burn ourselves out. Relaxing is so important for the entire body to work, stay balanced, and function properly.

Getting proper sleep is so important for the healing, function, and energy of the organism. To perform, the brain must be free of anything processed. Only fresh whole foods feed the brain its correct nutrients. Sleep and rest along with correct combinations of whole fresh foods give the body its energy, energy to work and to play. Proper sleep seems to take the burdens off life. A person will be able to go with the flow of things rather than becoming irritated at every little mishap.

Endnotes

1. Norman Cousins, *Anatomy of an Illness as Perceived by the Patient*, (W. W. Norton, 1979), 39.
2. Patch Adams with Maureen Mylander, *Gesundheit!* (Healing Arts, 1998), 35.
3. Cousins, *Anatomy of an Illness*, 1.
4. Elaine N. Marieb, *Human Anatomy & Physiology*, 5th ed. (Benjamin Cummings, 2001), 624.
5. John R. Lee with Virginia Hopkins, *What Your Doctor May Not Tell You about Menopause*, (Warner Books, 1996), 98.
6. Anonymous, *The Prayer Prescription* (Rodale, 2002), 4–5.
7. Mark 6:31 (NKJV).

CHAPTER 32

Drugs

Do US lifestyles proclaim health care or disease care? In Western medicine, doctors and drugs are specialized. That means there is a drug for every symptom imaginable and a doctor who is specialized in dealing with different diseases, so-called prevention and treatment, including surgeons who will perform different tests, procedures all for the care of the patients. Many doctors will not do anything for the good of humanity. They do it for payment.

The current medical practice has very little to do with the promotion of healthful living. There are too many sick people, more than the system can handle. They continue to get sicker, and no one can understand why. People just don't want to take responsibility for their own illnesses. They don't want to believe it because then they would have to change what they are doing—their diets and lifestyles.

The drug companies are in the medical field for money. It's a *big* business. In fact, the advertising and promotion of their drugs to the doctors and the general public is so astronomical. It is in the hundreds of millions. The drug companies pay for luncheons, big dinners, vacations, conventions, schooling, anything to promote their drugs to the doctors, including the future doctors, the whole medical field, and the population at large from birth to death. More space (by law) is allotted for the side effects rather than the benefits because, in reality, there aren't any benefits to these drugs. Drug companies depend on the diseases of the public and the continuation of these diseases for their income. Drugs don't cure. If they could, then every news media on the planet would report that news in headlines.

According to an unnamed source in one particular pharmaceutical company, there is less research going into the drugs at this time, and there are many layoffs in the big pharmaceutical industry at large. The money that has gone into research for all of these years hasn't gotten anyone cured. The body is the only thing that will heal if all the causes are taken away. People keep going to the doctors and drugs for their healing and cures. The blind are leading the blind at this point, and both will fall into the same pit together.

Drugs are so much a part of this worldly generation. This is a drugged society. Street drugs are prevalent, but even more common are the legal drugs, namely prescription drugs and the over-the-counter drugs. Also, for those who want to get away from the dangers of medicines, the herb and supplement companies have jumped onto the profit bandwagon. All are used to take away the symptoms of disease, which only creates more disease.

Greed is the biggest part of all this. According to Patch Adams, MD, greed "is one of society's worst malignancies, and it appears to have metastasized to every corner of the earth. The sense that greed is incurable may well account for its escalation. Unless greed and its symptoms are excised, society will perish."[1]

Olin Idol, ND, CNC, states empathetically that more than $200,000,000 has been spent on cancer research over the last thirty-eight years, and after spending all of this money, there are more people dying of cancer than ever before. People are dying because of *bad* nutrition. People are dying because of the way they eat more than by smoking, alcohol consumption, or any other lifestyle or environmental factor. There are too many chemicals being consumed in today's diets.

Modern medicine is becoming increasingly dangerous, and drugs are extremely dangerous to the human body. Drugs kill, not heal. All drugs, no matter what type, have some kind of side effects. Some can be very mild while others are life-threatening. Many will require another drug to counteract the previous drug's side effects, and this can create a monster inside the body because it keeps compounding as each one needs another drug. It becomes a squirrel-cage effect that no one can escape except to be bold by saying no to all drugs. This society is programmed to reach for a pill, a miraculous cure for all symptoms. No one realizes that they are the cause of the symptoms of their diseases. The drug companies don't want anyone to know, and they keep coming up with more advertisements for their "wonder" drugs: "Check with your doctor if XXX drug is right for you," "Take more! Take more," "What are your pain levels? We can help you," "We have a drug for XXX or whatever your ailment is." It's pathetic. Drug attitudes consume our nation and world. It's an endless cycle that isn't going to cease unless people take responsibility for themselves.

Drugs only worsen the situation. They can alter or rearrange the balances in the bloodstream, causing it to clot slower or faster. When an emergency situation or surgery is to take place, it puts that drug-taking person into a critical and life-threatening situation.

Hippocrates insisted that it is natural for the body to heal itself and that this healing process can generally take place without the intervention of a physician and to avoid any treatment that would interfere with that process because that would do more harm.

Vitamin/mineral deficiencies are very real today, especially with the large dependence on processed foods. This nation is too overfed yet extremely undernourished. Fifty percent of all patients admitted to the hospital are undernourished (improperly nourished), and the leading cause of death in the United States has been linked to diet. *Knowledge* is the key that unlocks the prison of ignorance. Even God said, "My people are destroyed for lack of knowledge, because you have rejected my knowledge."[3] God did not design the body for any pills.

The trouble with science is there are those who are making conclusions that are not consistent with the facts. They will continue to do the massive research, using the public's charity monies, but the health of this nation hasn't gotten any better only worse. We are *being poisoned* to death. Testing of these drugs only has proven their threat to humanity. Drugs are chemical poisons that are destroying the human body, not bringing health. Life science is proven by the body's ability to live within the realm of health and wellness and freedom from disease. There are many people who represent this truth, who understand it, live it and continue to be an affirmation of the truth.

Pain pills are at, or near, the top of the pharmaceutical sales list. These include not only prescription drugs for pain but over-the-counter drugs as well. Aspirin and ibuprofen are the most common ones used. People have died taking these OTC medicines and yet they are still on the market, and people will continue to consume them. Everyone seems to be suffering from pain. In fact, what many people do not realize is that the more drugs one takes to mask the pain, the more pain one will experience. Now if someone has an injury, surgical procedure, or the like, there will be drugs prescribed for the pain. While many can take these drugs for a short duration in their recovery and not have a problem, others may experience its addictive properties, thus continuing to have serious multiple problems.

But the majority of people who take these drugs are just experiencing pain from an unknown cause or phantom source. These are the people who may not be aware of it, but their pain is created by their diet and lifestyle. Their bodies are screaming out to be fed properly and for proper nutrition and elimination. Of course, one thing leads to another. The digestive system begins to shut down when there is pain. At that time the digestion ceases; therefore, people will continue to eat then everything backs up and constipation occurs. More drugs are taken for pain as well as the constipation, and they create more back up and continued accumulation of toxic wastes. It is a vicious cycle that doesn't end unless one decides to stop the drugs and fast, resting the digestive system to allow the body to clean house, which will release the toxins. Thus, the pain will reduce and eventually disappear. The body will now have a chance to be free, free of pain and inflammation. Drugs are trial-and-error antidotes. It's a guessing game to see which ones will reduce the patients' symptoms. Drugs produce side effects, and people may spend the rest of their lives just monitoring these side effects. Once a drug enters the body, the body and person are no longer in control. The drug has control over the body, and anything goes.

There are many diseases, painful diseases, that just continue to become worse, not better, because of the effects of drugs. These are fibromyalgia, arthritis, lupus, Crohn's, just to name a few. Today, there are more people getting around with walkers, canes, and scooters because of too much pain. It's debilitating to say the least and their sedentary lifestyles and poor diets have contributed to this pain.

In 1987, Dennis Slamon, an UCLA chief of the division of oncology and hematology, became obsessed with the traumatic and gruesome treatments many women were receiving for breast cancer. The cancers were becoming more aggressive and treatments were failing. Surgeries were doing more harm than good. Women were dying more from the treatments than the disease itself. Dennis was the scientist chosen to lead the research project to create a drug to cure breast cancer: Herceptin or HER2. He had a compassionate heart and dove in head first to the project in spite of many obstacles from drug companies and the research grants. He was continually opposed and ridiculed by his colleagues. This man not only had a goal, a dream, and a project, he had an emotional interest in the welfare of the women who were dying of an aggressive form of breast cancer. He knew that the breast cancers would reoccur, but he believed that the drug he was working on to be tested on humans was not as harmful as the chemo drugs were and would be a success. Too bad he couldn't have researched more into the areas of nutrition based on the laws of nature along with his study. HER2 was eventually approved and marketed in 1998.

Other drugs that are given in great force are statin drugs for high cholesterol and high blood pressure medications. These drugs are extremely dangerous and should be outlawed. People will obediently consume these drugs in spite of the dangers because they do not want to give up their poor, addictive diet and sedentary, lazy lifestyle.

The side effects of these drugs are killers. The muscle and joint aches then the muscles begin to atrophy until they just give out and quit working because of the poisons in these drugs. There are two serious potential side effects:

1. Liver damage occurs by increasing liver enzymes, which can lead to irreversible liver damage.
2. There are muscle problems, muscle pain, and tenderness. In severe cases, the muscle cells can breakdown and release a protein into the bloodstream, which will damage the kidneys. Unfortunately, doctors will have their patients on these drugs for life. Their life and health will deteriorate more.

There are better methods of decreasing one's blood pressure and cholesterol, thus enhancing one's health, and it's not with drugs. Protect the body at all costs and do not use drugs. Dietary lifestyle changes should be the first factor for any disease reduction.

Antibiotics came on the scene as a miracle drug, able to destroy bacteria and microorganisms beyond the reach of other drugs. Unfortunately, because of the overuse of these drugs, the bacteria became resistant to them. The antibiotics kill the good bacteria in the colon and body, thus the body can develop yeast infections as well as other diseases. At this time, other drugs are prescribed then the cycle begins again until the body is in such a weakened state that it will continue to develop other diseases just by trying to clean itself out. People are just ignoring the blatant warning signs.

Incidents of obesity and diabetes are overwhelming, now in epidemic proportions. More than 60 percent of this nation is obese. Which of these diseases came first? They both are linked together in a pathological body. They are not looked at together but as separate entities. The medical profession will give insulin medication for diabetes. Unfortunately, once on insulin, the person may be condemned to a lifetime of this medical nightmare because the pancreas may atrophy and cease to function on its own with these drugs.

Diabetes can be prevented, and the body may heal itself of diabetes before one succumbs to the insulin drugs. Weight loss, exercise, and a raw produce diet will help to control type2 diabetes so the body may come back to somewhat normal. Prevention is always the best avenue as not to get on the pathway to destruction. Other drugs that are damaging to the body are taken for gastrointestinal reflux disease (GERD), acid reflux. Reflux is a disease that is caused by improper food combinations that most of the general public eat, which is the standard American diet. The food isn't emptying from the stomach. It keeps churning in the stomach acids, trying to exit the stomach, and these acids will try and back up into the esophagus. The sphincters of the stomach are weakened by the state of acid in the stomach, which can also contribute to a hiatus hernia (the top portion of the stomach which out pouches into the esophagus above the diaphragm.) Zantac and other reflux medicines are given to reduce the acid. The problem is that the stomach needs acid to digest the foods, so it creates more. It becomes an endless cycle, more drugs, decreased acid, and then the stomach makes more. When the acid continues to rise up the esophagus, it creates ulcers, sores, and it weakens the tissue itself. It can even create diverticula in the esophagus. The diet needs to be changed, stress-levels need to be dealt with, and all medications need to be stopped for the body to allow itself to heal and regain health.

Antidepressant drugs are given for depression, bipolar (manic depression) disorder, and schizophrenia. There are many different types and strengths. The dangers are extreme with these types of drugs as they alter the hormone levels of the body and interfere with the serotonin levels of the brain. These drugs are found to be ineffective for nonclinical depression. Alternative drugs (herbs) such as St. John's wort are given, but this also proved to be toxic and ineffective. The major side effects are suicidal tendencies, aggression, and lashing out. Look at the children and young people who took guns into their schools, killing some of their classmates and injuring others. These psychotic drugs, Ritalin, for example, are used for behavioral changes but have only produced the opposite effects. What is happening to our children is tragic. All they need to do is to get rid of the additives, chemicals, sugars, and processed foods and start to eat fresh whole produce.

Vaccines have in many cases become mandatory for children for them to attend school. Many of these vaccines contain dangerous chemicals that have been known to cause brain inflammation and autism in children. Thimerosal causes neurological brain disorders. "Flu vaccines," according to Dr. Dan Chesnut, "given during pregnancy can dramatically increase the risk for autism and schizophrenia. Most flu vaccines," he continues, "contain mercury (thimerosal) and aluminum and could contain viral fragments."[4] They overstimulate the immune system, especially the brain, and can decrease the immune function of the body for weeks following the injection.

There are currently many vaccines that are given, all of which are dangerous to the human body. The only way for the body to avoid disease is through good proper nutrition. Of course, in the nature of drugs, included are the drugs of caffeine, alcohol, and nicotine, which are consumed daily worldwide. Of these, alcohol is the only one that is a mind-altering drug although they all can be body-altering drugs. These drugs, as well as all other drugs, are damaging to the human organism. They do not nourish the body as foods but are extremely addictive and poisonous. They are promoted, accepted, commercially-advertised, medically prescribed, and even the US government protects them. These drugs create disease, especially cancer, and should never be consumed in any form. The body needs to be cherished, nourished, and protected.

People are deceived into believing that vaccinations are the way to prevent diseases. Babies begin receiving these toxic injections from birth. In fact, Michael Donaldson, in his *Hallelujah Acres Health News* article, states that currently before the age of six, a child will receive eighty-eight antigenic exposures, while in 1985, they only received thirty-three.[5] These drugs decrease the immune system and, according to Dr. Dan Chesnut, who quotes Russell Blaylock, MD, "A large number of studies have shown that when you vaccinate an animal, inflammatory chemicals increase dramatically in its brain. After a vaccination, these animals become activated and move around rapidly as if signaled to fight an invading enemy."[6] There are many contaminants in these vaccines that kill the cells of the body as well as induce shrinkage of the brain.

Pharmaceutical companies invest their resources into advertising and selling doctors, hospitals, and the public their products, especially vaccines. They are trying to make it mandatory to be inoculated for the swine flu and the H1N1 vaccines as well as the shingles vaccine. Shingles is a disease of a completely depleted and compromised body, and no vaccine will ever prevent it but will only add to the nightmare of it. Most people who get shingles are stressed, malnourished, and many are taking too many drugs. These companies have, and will continue, to use scare tactics on the public, using diseases, germs, and viruses as excuses to fill their pockets with the profits of the diseased nation. People are so frightened of being a part of an epidemic that they will do anything. The hospitals in the state of New York have made it mandatory that their health care personal get the H1N1 vaccination or they will not be able to work. In other words, they will be fired. Drug companies are trying to make it mandatory for young girls to receive the vaccination drug Gardasil that is to supposedly prevent cervical cancer. Dr. Dan Chesnut claims. "Gardasil contains sodium borate (a common roach poison) and polysorbate 80, linked to infertility in mice studies."[7]

Flu vaccines are another profit drug for the big pharmaceutical companies. Every year, these vaccines include three strains of the most prevalent flu virus that they think will strike the public, but it is never the correct ones because everyone gets sick anyway, especially the people who have received the flu vaccines. It's always a guessing game at the public's expense. Flu vaccines overstimulate the immune system and the brain, according to Dan Chesnut MD. "The mercury and the other contaminants are the cause of hearing loss, memory loss, decreased immunity, vertigo, and even death. It's just not worth it. Ever since I myself stopped receiving the flu vaccinations, I stopped getting the flu. How ironic. Protection from the influenza comes from good nutrition."[7]

"A compelling amount of research shows that our resistance to infectious diseases is highly dependent on our nutrition. Even a single nutrient deficiency can suppress immunity and raise one's mortality from infections,"[8] states Russell Blaylock, MD.

The flu season comes at the same time of the year when most people are starting to be confined indoors because of cold weather and rainy seasons. They stuff themselves with all types of junk foods (comfort foods). The holiday parties begin at this time, and most people live this unhealthy way, overeating on the wrong foods, mostly sugary foods, and the body continues to weaken. Therefore, all of these people tend to get sick around the same time, and they blame it on each other, saying, "I caught the flu from so and so." They place the blame outside of themselves. It starts at Halloween with all the fall parties and continues through Thanksgiving, Christmas, and New Year's with the overeating of all the wrong foods, no exercise, not getting enough sleep, and just going until they crash and get sick. People are lazy. They just want to get a shot or a pill and continue to live the same lifestyle and not get sick. They literally want their cake and eat it too.

Vaccines aren't safe and don't last a lifetime like natural immune diseases do. More people will get sick and die from the vaccines than from infectious diseases themselves. Prevention of the flu includes a properly combined fresh, raw fruits; vegetables; limited amount of seeds and nuts; pure water; sunshine; exercise and fresh air; and dealing with the stressful situations in a healthy way as not to let the body deplete. A good, positive attitude will do wonders for the health of the body.

Health is a valued commodity, but it definitely has to be chosen and acquired. It needs to be taught from childhood on. It needs to be practiced, lived, and taught to the next generation. What seems to be taught instead of health is sickness. It is sad, and what is even sadder is that there aren't any victims.

Endnotes

1. Patch Adams with Maureen Mylander, *Gesundheit!* (Healing Arts, 1998), 53.
2. Olin Idol, "Cause of Most Cancers Revealed," Hallelujah Acres Diet and Lifestyle Health Tip, May 2009.
3. Hosea 4:6 (NKJV).
4. Dan E. Chesnut, *Lying with Authority* (Restoration Health, 2008), 125.
5. Michael Donaldson, "The Fine Line of Immunization: Johnny and His 88 Vaccines," *Hallelujah Acres Health News* 54 (July/ August 2009): 27.

6. Chesnut, *Lying with Authority*, 122. (Restoration Health 2008), 124

7. Russell Blaylock, "Vaccines: What You Should Know," *Hallelujah Acres Health News* 59 (January/February 2010): 6.

CHAPTER 33

Pain

Pain is not the ultimate enemy. According to Norman Cousins, "Americans are probably the most pain conscious people on the face of the earth."[1] For years, people have been bombarded in print, over the television, on the radio, in everyday conversation that any hint of pain is to be banned as though it were the ultimate evil. As a result, "this nation has become a nation of pill-grabbers and hypochondriacs, escalating the slightest ache into a searing ordeal. We know very little about pain and what we don't know about pain makes it hurt worse."[1]

The most ignored fact of all pain is that the best way to eliminate it is to eliminate its abuse. People are very intolerant of any type of pain and just reach for a pill. Harvey Diamond states, "Pain is the number one treated health concern. It's a silent epidemic with 89 percent of Americans, that's 9 out of 10, experiencing pain on a monthly and 43 percent, which is 93 million Americans, have pain on a daily basis."[2] The purpose of these drugs is to kill the pain, but it cannot cure or take it away. Most of the pain is of unknown cause, and people have to learn to cope and to live with this pain through pain management techniques. Unfortunately, this doesn't work well at all, and people are caught into a web of deceit and despair, continually taking more drugs.

Hospitals have signs all over that say, "Please tell us if you are in pain we can help" and "What are your pain levels on a scale of 1–10?" At the same time, they are willing to dish out any medicines that the public asks for. Many painkilling drugs actually make the pain worse. They just add more toxins to the already inflamed areas, which just intensifies the pain while the person will continue to need more of the over-abused drug to receive the same effect. It thus creates an addictive process within the body. I have seen many people on narcotic pain medication, suffering from the addiction of these drugs, unable to be set free from them because they cannot deal with the intense pain and the withdrawals. Some of these drugs (especially aspirin) seriously interfere with the ability of the body to metabolize food properly, resulting in malnutrition. The pain itself does slow down the digestive processes, thus adding these drugs just halts everything. People will cease to have any bowel movements on their own. They will take other drugs, suppositories, laxatives, and stool softeners without avail, not understanding why they are even more miserable for now while the entire body is backed up and seriously affected with poisonous toxins. It is a vicious cycle that has to stop, but many won't. People are caught up in this until the body gives up, breaking down with severe diseases.

Over-the-counter painkillers, such as aspirin and ibuprofen, are the most commonly used pain suppressants. Doctors will even give heart patients daily doses of aspirin to be used as a blood thinner, and these drugs are combined with all types of other drugs. The drug lists of some people rank in the line with a pharmaceutical drug company. Ignorance and their doctors are killing them, and they wonder why they continue to experience so much pain and disease in their lives.

People ought to know that nothing is more remarkable than the regenerative and recuperative process of the human body if it is treated correctly. People are more afraid of pain and disease than of death itself, and they continue to take the avenue that leads them there. Pain is the warning system of the body that something is wrong, out of kilter, and needs to be checked and adjusted. It's like a car—one cannot ignore the dashboard warning lights that continue to blink and the sensors that are flashing a warning, telling you the car needs to be taken care of before the car ceases to function and break down. If oil isn't replaced, the engine will seize up and melt down, just as the human body, a delicate piece of machinery, will similarly cease functioning and stop. One can't continue to ignore the warning signs by using drugs to cover up improper diets and lifestyles.

Pain is a result of the body trying to get attention and tell a person something is wrong and warning him/her to do something now. Drugs don't fix the body. They just deaden the pain.

Steroids are another type of drug that is severely abused by doctors and their patients. They're the cure-all for anything—pain, infections, and inflammations. They are even given to cancer patients and organ recipients to make sure that their bodies will accept and not reject the blood transfusions and organ transplants. The body rejects all outside interference, and anything brought into it will be rejected, including drugs.

I have seen cancer patients given continuous rounds of steroid drugs to hold in the numerous amounts of red blood cells and blood platelets. Without question, the body that continues to reject it is a healthier body. Steroid drugs interfere with the endocrine system, creating dramatic disturbances. Some caretakers of those who take these drugs reported aggression, severe mood swings, and violent behaviors. It can be very disturbing, especially because no one questions, "Can it be the medicine?" These drugs cannot be stopped midway without serious danger to the patient. A natural health advisor can take the person through the process, but they need to be very closely monitored.

The Food and Drug Administration needs to be more interested in acquainting the public of the dangers of drugs, pain relievers, etc., and the harm that will be produced instead of so actively trying to close down and reduce the vitamin supplement corporations. Yes, these would and are considered by the body to be drugs also, but the FDA doesn't want to educate anyone on anything but their own agenda—drugs. They just continue to advertise, not educate, and keep the public ignorant.

Endnotes

1. Norman Cousins, *Anatomy of an Illness as Perceived by the Patient* (W.W. Norton, 1979), 89.
2. Harvey Diamond, *Living without Pain* (VP Nutrition, 2005), 9–10.

CHAPTER 34

Gesundheit!

In the US, we have a health care system that is in deep trouble. It is crying out in pain. First of all, people are not treated in a humane way. They are just a number, a disease and a dollar sign. The doctor is the knight in shining armor, the god who is there to save the people, but these doctors have failed at their job. In the present system, each patient is given a small amount of allotted time. History and current reports aren't read or looked over before the patient is seen. The patients aren't given time for questions, much less well-explained answers. The doctor will just rush through the exam to get to the next group of patients.

Doctors' offices and hospital staff are not designed to work together as a team to help alleviate the patients' suffering. They do not even have a clue of how to help their patients in the area of prevention and nutrition, so they won't develop diseases in the first place. The doctor is ignorant about how to prevent disease, much less how to cure or heal people. It's a guessing game, one of elimination. That's why it's called a medical "practice." It's the blind leading the blind, and they both fall into the same hole of despair.

Many tests and procedures that prove to be futile and hopeless are performed for the sake of diagnosis. They can lead to a medical nightmare. All of these senseless tests and procedures are hopeless, and they can be painful and often traumatic, especially in the case of children and the elderly. Most of the time, a good doctor could spend an extra amount of time with the patients, getting to know them. The doctors could find out more about their patients as people, the stresses, their diets and lifestyles and how to approach their stress in this direct way instead of pushing pills and ignoring them. Just learning how to be a friend, a person, and have some compassion. According to Dr. Patch Adams, "Friendship is great medicine. It overcomes many of the inadequacies of the medical profession."[1] It puts the doctor into a human level instead of just a god. The doctor will never be a savior.

Health is a valued commodity, but it definitely has to be chosen and acquired. It needs to be taught from early on, from childhood to be continued and taught as an adult to the next generation. Doctors should be teaching it to their patients. But you can't teach what you haven't learned. So each generation's health is becoming nonexistent. Their idea of nutrition is eating vegetables (french fries) or as their fruit, sugared strawberries on top of their pancakes. Even small children are becoming obese.

According to Dr. Adams, "Greed is one of society's worst malignancies, and it appears to have metastasized to every corner of the earth. The sense that greed is incurable may well account for its escalation. Unless greed and its symptoms are excised, society will perish."[1]

Dr. Adams has a very different approach to healing. He adds laughter, humor, love, and compassion and friendship to the equation of health at Gesundheit Institute. Everyone works together, patients as well as practitioners as one happy family. Doctors and other healthcare individuals (from other alternative health care fields) teach the ways of wellness, helping each person to not only get well but to stay well. "Preventative medicine is most important," says, Dr. Adams. "There needs to be a trust, openness, and closeness for the patient to feel like a friend, not a spectator in his/her recovery but a willing participant."[1]

Dr. Patch Adams believes that house calls should be service oriented. The time spent with the patient nurtures the relationship.

People's homes tell so much about themselves. Patch states, "Relaxing in a person's home and enjoying his or her hospitality creates deeper bonds than can be forged in a doctor's office. The doctor becomes a person to the patient."[1] He takes the business out of medicine and puts love and caring in its place. Unfortunately, this advice isn't often heeded.

Endnotes

1. Patch Adams with Maureen Mylander, *Gesundheit!* (Healing Arts, 1998), 35.

CHAPTER 35

Organic Foods

One of the big businesses of the so-called health industries is that of organic foods. People are crying out for fresh, unadulterated, chemically free, and clean whole foods, free of all pesticides and industrial fertilizers. Fresh, raw whole foods are perfectly wonderful, and they are necessary for good health. It's the next best thing to farm-raised foods. The problem that makes it seem like big business with huge profits is that organic foods are higher in price than nonorganic or conventional foods. Another even bigger problem is involved with organic foods profits. Business has permeated the organic junk and processed food market. The word organic is becoming robbed of its integrity. It is becoming abused and misused, taken out of context. The worst of it is that some food manufactures have taken this as a magic word just to give the impression that these unhealthy processed products have suddenly become good for human consumption. Don't be fooled.

Let's start with the organic farming market. The best foods/produce one can buy in the markets are organic produce, if at all possible, the fresher the better. One must be very discerning in his/her shopping these days. The produce must be checked very carefully because it sometimes has been sitting in storage facilities and even comes from great distances, sitting too long between the picking and buying. It is best to buy locally. One must try and buy the freshest possible through examination, feel, smell, and touch. The local farmers markets are the better option as most are picked fresh that same day. It's best to go to a reputable farmer as some less honorable ones are into big business ventures and will hide the old produce under the good ones in the boxes or bushel baskets. Picking fresh is the best. It is best to examine each piece of produce before buying. It takes a little more time but is worth it.

Taste is the biggest reason for buying organic produce. I tell people to judge for themselves. People need to go to the market and pick up an organic apple and a conventionally grown apple. First of all, the organic one smells like an apple right off the tree and the other one has no smell at all. Then to really find out, they can buy both apples and take them home furthering their experimentation. Cut up each apple, taking a piece of the organic fruit, and savor each bite then eat the other. The conventional one has no taste and no flavor. It is *bland*. The tongue and the mouth just crave the fresh fruit's organic taste, and the other will leave you empty and hungry. That is where the nutritional aspect comes in. The body wants, desires, and needs nutrients. Conventional food lacks in that area, so a person will crave and continue to overeat until he/she gets the needed nutrients. Fresh whole foods fill the bill.

Organic products are free of pesticides, insecticides, and artificial fertilizers and are justly called clean produce. They meet specific growing standards or they cannot be called organic. The soils have to be a correct pH, no artificial chemicals will be allowed, and also no chemical sprays of any kind are used. Organic products that are bought in the store are higher in price but are good and healthy to eat. It's worth it for the health of the body.

Growing one's own produce is best, but not everyone has that luxury because of limited space and area. For optimal health, those who cannot grow their own organic foods should buy the very best raw, organic, clean, fresh whole foodstuffs and eat them in the proper food combinations. The body craves a raw organic diet consisting of fruits, vegetables, seeds, and nuts. When one feeds the body well, the body will respond favorably. This type of diet is an excellent alkaline diet unlike the standard American diet, which is very acidic. An acidic body is a poisoned, diseased body. An alkaline diet will continue to help the body to function and maintain optimal and abundant health free of diseases. These fresh whole foods are the necessary ingredient for staying out of doctors' offices and hospitals.

Many people do not want to pay the extra money for organic products. They would rather pay a cheaper price for cheap produce. Then they pay again for the supplements that they think are going to make them well. More money is shelled out as they continue in and out of the doctors' offices and hospitals, searching for cures for all of their disease symptoms. People are cheap and deceived. "You always get what you pay for," and "You are what you eat."

What bothers me is that the organic business has gone out of control, just as bad as the obesity diet industry has. It's all about money. Many stores now carry a line of some kind of organic packaged/canned foods and junk foods. Any processed/canned/bottled foods, organic or not, are unfit for the human body. Although many people will look at the label, and if it says organic, they look no further. They believe it's okay to buy and eat. After all, they conclude it's organic. That's the marketing behind it. The organic business has gotten so huge that they now have companies who will deliver your organic items to your business and home. They are delivering your groceries, luncheons, receptions, etc. Organics to Go and Organic. com are just a couple of names affixed to delivery trucks that travel throughout the San Diego area. As I have said before, the growing of all the produce must be in specific requirements, but what about all of the other businesses? What are the requirements for dead and processed foods? We do not get to look at the produce dumped on the doorstep like we can at the market. In my opinion, these businesses are organic in name only. Their products should still be avoided because they are fragmented, denatured, indigestible, and unfit for the human body. They only add to the accumulation of toxins within the body. People will still gain weight, become diseased, and age faster when they consume these junk products.

It's still considered junk food. They are still processed foods even if they use organic ingredients. No matter how noble and honorable the food manufacturer's efforts are, it will still be processed junk food. People need to be educated. Just because it says *organic* on the label doesn't mean it's healthy. After all, because it has a label, it is processed. God's food doesn't have labels.

It's confusing for people, especially children, because this junk food is organic and it should be good for eating, and it seems like the right thing to do. Whether or not it's a healthy food to eat depends on whether it adds nutrients to the body. Fresh whole foods are the only organic foods that fit that requirement—healthy and vitamin/mineral enriched, not synthetic. It's not a wise choice to eat what man made.

This organic food market started off in an innocent manner, to make available fresh wholesome foods. Food manufacturers then jumped on the bandwagon because they didn't want to be left out in the cold with less money in their pockets. How sad for those who just want their health. The world is coming to a fast crashing end. Technology is killing off humanity.

CHAPTER 36

Proper Food Combining

The human body wasn't created to eat complex meals and improper food combinations. Food combining is based on the theory that different food groups digest at different times and in different digestive modes. I appreciate how Hannah Allen puts it: "Hygienic food selection and principles of food combining are based on nutritional needs of humans and the limitations of our digestive systems."[1] The body's nourishment is received by how the digestive system digests and assimilates the food eaten. These correct food combinations eaten properly are the bases for digestion, assimilation of the nutrients, and elimination of the waste products by the body. Optimal digestion is utilized by eating the foods that have the same digestive times. The body dictates the principles and rules of food combining. If not eaten in proper combinations, the body will rebel.

Different foods are utilized in various manners by the chemistry of the body. There are acidic foods, such as proteins, that require an acidic medium to digest them. The enzyme pepsin starts the digestive process for the proteins. Starches and sugars begin their digestion in the mouth with the enzyme amylase. Even the smallest amount of acid destroys these enzymes. They require an alkaline medium for their digestion. Fats also require an alkaline digestive environment, and this digestion takes place in the small intestine. The important concept behind the principle of proper food combination is to eat starches and proteins at different meals, *never* together. If they are eaten together, the stomach will neutralize them and make the digestive process ineffective and incomplete and will retard the digestive process. These foods will be held up in the stomach, sometimes for hours.

This can lead to discomfort, indigestion, bloating, gassiness, stomachaches, heartburn, and abdominal distress as the stomach attempts to get rid of this mess. It may even reflux back into the esophagus, creating a weakness in the lower esophageal sphincter. A one-way valve into the stomach now becomes a swinging door for the stomach acid to ulcerate the esophagus and create cancers. The stomach needs to digest and empty quickly from these foods. In the meantime, this backup can cause the starches to decompose and ferment. The proteins will putrefy, producing gas, acid, and even alcohol that accompany the indigestion.

Eat fruits on an empty stomach only, never with starches or proteins although they can be eaten with lettuce or celery. Starches should be eaten with vegetables only for optimal digestions while proteins are to be eaten with vegetables only. This *is* the proper way to eliminate indigestion and disease. Never eat starches and proteins together because they will not digest. The digestive process is slowed and lengthened. When the stomach doesn't empty, this adds to the burden on the digestive system. If a protein and starch are consumed at the same meal, the enzymes are destroyed and the digestive juices that work parallel with these enzymes are neutralized. The food sits in the stomach at 98.6°F,[2] decomposing while waiting for the enzymes to generate and to be sent out of the stomach with more of the digestive juices; but the food, which is trying to escape, can't, so one feels the bloating, nausea, and indigestion. Sometimes vomiting may occur. Spoiled foods, not fresh, wholesome foods are spewed out and rejected.

It's best to keep the meals simple, eating foods without all the fanfare of condiments, spices, and improper foods so nothing will interfere with the digestive process. This simple way of eating decreases the cravings of the other unwholesome foods.

People are so afraid of being hungry. The raw food leaves the stomach and is digested quickly. Common statements are "I need food in my stomach" or "I can't just eat fruit. I'll starve." People are not used to having anything other than that stuffed-full feeling.

The body isn't burdened when the foods digest quickly. There are no toxic residues as the lymph and elimination systems keep the body clean and refreshed. Healing is maintained and the body has an overwhelming amount of energy.

Proper combining of foods ensures the eating and consuming only of foods that are of compatible digestive properties. Because of their similar digestive properties, these foods will digest and assimilate correctly for the wellbeing of the body.

The body is a self-healing mechanism, and nothing from the outside of the body will promote any healing; but taking away the causes of diseases, the body will continue to maintain good health. Using the principles of proper food combination and living the natural, hygienic lifestyle can and will help cleanse the body from disease and promote wellbeing.

There are definite ways to manipulate the foods one eats, what is eaten, when and how to eat to maximize digestion and minimize the time the food spends in the stomach. A person will learn to eat to live rather than live to eat. One will learn to sit down and enjoy a meal of wholesome foods, feeling refreshed and satisfied and alive and alert when the meal is done. Living foods *sustain* life. Most people, who eat the conventional American diet end up gorging themselves on lifeless, dead, processed, and cooked foods. They then feel stuffed, hungry, craving to eat continually, irritable, have indigestion, and experience heartburn. They feel dead and lifeless, just like the foods they just ate. Dead foods accelerate the aging process, take away health and generate disease.

It is wise to eat fewer foods. Eating less at each meal helps the digestive system to operate at its maximum peak. It offers the simplest load on the digestive system.[3]

Endnotes

1. Hannah Allen, "The Basis of the Food Combining System" (lesson 22, a course in Natural Health, Fit for Life Sciences Institute), 496.
2. Harvey Diamond, *Living without Pain* (VP Nutrition, 2005), 226–227.
3. Robert O. Young and Shelley Redford Young, *The pH Miracle* (Warner Books, 2002), 105.

CHAPTER 37

Nutrition: Nutrients, Vitamins, Minerals, Water

Are you a food lover? There are two categories or groups of food lovers: those who live to eat and those who eat to live. Those who live eating the standard American diet with all of the food additives will continue to experience the cravings and health challenges that this diet dictates.

Those who eat to live are those who experience health and have a desire to take care of their bodies. Natural hygiene is for those who want life, health, and happiness. They are those who desire to take care of themselves and eat just to live, thereby living in abundance. "We are what we eat" is the principle, and the food that they will consume is converted to human flesh to feed every cell of the body. Therefore, a certain number of nutrients are to be used for building cellular structures, replacing worn-out parts, and metabolizing and assimilating of these nutrients. Most foods are used as metabolic fuels for the energy of the body's cells so they perform their many activities. Nutrition needs to be a process of life. Nutrition refers to the process of which the body's cellular structure utilizes the elements of the foods consumed and the chemical energy processes by which these nutrients are assimilated throughout the entire organism at a cellular level. People do not nourish the body with what they consume; the body nourishes itself by the conditions that it is given.

By the way, it is important that a person maximizes the body's resources to promote the most efficient applications of the foods consumed. It becomes important in the way people eat; in what kind of conditions and environment (whether it is calm or stressful) they eat; whether the food is cooked or raw, whole, fresh; and the amount of food eaten along with the length of time it took to consume the meal. All of these factors have a deep-seated effect on nutrition as the nutrients in itself. The important factor is not just what one can eat but what and how our body appropriates at the cellular level, which will decide the state of the body's nutrition. Nutrients are a substance in food that the body uses to cultivate normal growth, repair, and maintenance.

Nutrients are considered more than vitamins although people think they're the same. There are six very important nutrients: carbohydrates, proteins (amino acids), fats, vitamins, minerals, and water. These are the absorbable components of foods and are extremely necessary for optimal health. Nutrients are necessary for energy, organ function and maintenance, food utilization, cell growth and repair.

There are two different categories of nutrients: micronutrients and macronutrients. Micronutrients, vitamins, and minerals do not provide energy by themselves. But the macronutrients, consisting of carbohydrates, fats, and proteins, do just that, provide the fuel for energy only when there are sufficient micronutrients to release them. So these two categories of nutrients work simultaneously and do not function independently.

Nutrients are worked through the digestive process that starts when the food is taken into the mouth, and then these raw foods are masticated, chewed, and mixed with the saliva. Amylase, an enzyme from the saliva, begins the digestion of the starches in the mouth. There are many different enzymes that work through the digestive process. The nutrients that have been consumed will be absorbed in the small intestine.

The liver has a remarkable ability to convert one type of molecule to another.[1] The organic chemicals found in these natural whole foods allow the body to use them and adjust to the variety of food intakes.

But there are many molecules that cannot make these conversions; these are the essential nutrients and must be provided only through the proper diet of raw whole foods for optimal health. Complex carbohydrates are produced from fresh produce. Glucose is the perfect food for the body for all of its cellular structures and functioning. It is the major fuel source and is readily used for all of the body's energy needs. Even a small drop in the amount of blood glucose will drastically reduce the function of the brain and can lead to the death of the neurons. The human body in all of its intelligence was created to carefully monitor and regulate the glucose levels. The human body thrives on a daily fresh whole plant produce diet. According to Elaine M. Marieb that if less than 50 grams per day are consumed, tissue proteins and fats are broken down for fuel energy.[1] Typically, the American diet varies between 200 to 300 grams of carbohydrates each day, but unfortunately, it consists of processed foods, sugars, refined flours, sodas, candies, etc.—all empty calories, energy only, but void of all nutrients. This just leads to deficiencies and disease.

Proteins are another extremely important nutrient. People use animal sources as proteins and these are pathological to the human organism, creating a heavy burden on the kidneys and liver. The people who consume an overload of protein end up with a protein poisoning.[2]

A high protein diet will eventually take its toll on the entire glandular system as the body is attempting to excrete and eliminate the overabundance of protein. In the process, it adds toxins to the body, and these will severely challenge the entire body. Arthritis symptoms seem to disappear when protein levels are decreased. The building blocks of protein consist of twenty-three amino acids of which eight are essential and the rest are less crucial and are called nonessential but are still needed by the body. The nonessential amino acids do not need to be present in the daily foods as long as there is a sufficient amount of essential ones in the diet. The essential ones are not produced within the body and must come from food. Most importantly, they must be of raw produce in order for the body to utilize them.

The body cannot use or assimilate protein in its original state. The proteins must first be digested and transformed into amino acids, and then the body can use these amino acids to form the protein that it needs. Mike Benton claims, "The ultimate value of a food protein lies in its amino acid composition. So it is the amino acids (Amino acid is the chemical building blocks used to create protein. The cells build protein by linking these amino acids in various combinations like tinker toys are used to build things), not the proteins, that are the essential nutrients. Amino acids are what the body uses to build on in the nourishing and repair of the body."[2]

Proteins, or amino acids rather, are important for the growth and the development of babies and newborn animals. The body uses them for the repair of tissues and replacement of worn-out parts.[2] Cell deterioration and waste removal occur because of the toxic lifestyle and diet that the standard American advocates. When a diet of fresh, raw whole fruits, vegetables, seeds, nuts, and fresh water is consumed, the tissue wastes are very minimal and the body's protein needs will be reduced. The optimal diet to have all of the body's sufficient protein met is the natural hygiene diet consisting of raw, fresh produce, seeds, nuts and sprouts. This can supply the body with the highest quality protein that is completely digestible and optimally assimilated.

It is best to eat the proteins raw because cooked proteins are coagulated, and when subjected to heat temperatures, enzyme resistant linkages are formed between the chains of amino acids, thus the body cannot break these down for use. When these aren't used, it goes through its chemical process as it tries to eliminate them, and it adds a toxic burden to the body. When wholesome, high quality proteins are consumed like in the natural hygiene diet, the body is left nourished, regenerated, and healed, not burdened with leftover toxic wastes. The natural hygiene diet provides the body with all the balance of vital nutrients that naturally occur in whole foods. According to Mike Benton, "For efficient protein use, an adequate amount of carbohydrates must be present."[2] Otherwise these proteins are converted to carbohydrate fuel for the body and the protein is not used for its original purpose. Fruits, vegetables, and nuts have a large amount of natural carbohydrates; therefore, the body can use all of the protein contained in these foods for its intended purpose, and there won't be any toxic byproducts through the unnecessary conversion of proteins. Many people do not realize the poisonous effects of their daily overuse of protein. It is no wonder that people have so many health challenges because of this factor.

These wholesome proteins are quite easily digested and assimilated. If eaten with the proper combinations of foods, it will make this process easier. Protein digestion is the most complicated of all gastric processes.[2]

Protein foods must be eaten with non-starchy vegetables, which also contain their own high quality amino acids. The standard American diet with its meat/bread sandwiches, hamburgers, and french fries, etc., requires different digestive methods and enzymes. When these are eaten together neither is completely digested nor can be used within the body for nutritional composition.

One who eats proteins on a natural hygiene diet is getting a good quality diet to meet all of the body's requirements. The whole raw fresh produce, seeds, nuts and sprouts contain all of the essential and nonessential amino acids. No one has to be concerned about how much protein to consume or calories to be counted. When eating a variety of fresh whole produce, the body is getting all of its needs met. The human body only requires 22–30 grams of protein a day. Plant protein is the highest quality protein because those who get their protein from animal sources suffer from diseases caused by the toxic overload within the body.

The body simply cannot digest an excessive amount of any protein. Nuts are a rich source of protein, but the human body can only digest and assimilate small amounts at a time. When one consumes large quantities, it will overload and burden the system, creating an acid accumulation, which throws the endocrine system out of balance. Animal proteins tend to cause more overeating than plant proteins do, and cooked animal proteins tend to be damaging to the body. It isn't any wonder that this society is in such a sad state of diseases, especially with cancer cases. Fruits, which are the body's natural food, contain the amino acids, which are completely ready for absorption without digestion.[3] This is the way to get the body's proteins. The body does not require the high amount that is claimed. One percent of the diet is all that's necessary.

T. C. Fry has stated in his Basic Health Library the conclusion of the research reported under the title "Mechanisms of Disease": "The conclusion *is* protein intake exceeding needs must be eliminated by the kidneys. The kidneys are stressed and gradually develop lesions and hardening. Eliminative capacity declines and disease (degeneration) becomes progressively more pronounced. This report shows that humans have poor capacity for eliminating proteins in excess of needs. Much kidney disease results on the high protein diet normal to most Americans."[3]

According to sources such as the American Society of Registered Technologist and Scripps Research Institute, among others, bone atrophy, another term for osteoporosis, is an epidemic at this time. The problem with this is that this disease begins in childhood. It used to be considered a disease for elderly women with the lack of estrogen as its primary cause. Now it seems to be a disease caused the intake of animal proteins, including milk drinkers; sugars; and processed food. Folks that have raw, plant-based raw diets seem to have less occurrences of osteoporosis.

The best way to prevent diseases of the bones, liver, and kidneys is to eat a diet based on principles of natural hygiene diet. The body stays healthier with raw foods, less food, and optimal foods for the human organism; and one will age slower and live longer with one's health at an optimal state.

Another major nutrient the body needs is lipids, also referred to as fats. Dietary fats do help the body to absorb fat-soluble vitamins. Lipids are very important for the functioning of the nervous system, for joint flexibility, and to help control inflammation. They also provide a protective cushion around the body's organs and nerves. It also adds an insulating layer of fat between the skin and the organs and is a source of energy that can be stored for future uses for the body.

There are saturated fats, which are found in animal proteins and coconuts, and unsaturated fats. The latter exist in avocados, raw nuts, and seeds. They are digested as fatty acids and are healthy for the body in small and limited daily amounts.[4]

Most people with a standard American diet consume more than 40 percent of their daily caloric intake by eating fats. The eating of animal proteins (saturated fats) and the trans fats from vegetable oils, processed foods, and fried foods is a contributing factor of obesity, heart disease, diabetes, and other debilitating diseases. Fat substitutes seem to be more prominent but are more damaging to the body than the real thing. Nutrients feed the body, help it to maintain homeostasis, allowing the body to regenerate and heal while also keeping the body functioning on an optimal level. Nutrients sustain the life of the body when they are received into the body through a natural raw food diet, which the biological needs of the body demands. The vitamins and minerals should be more than enough when supplied by the natural hygiene diet.

Vitamins are organic substances, which maintain the body's function, and more importantly, life itself.[5] These cannot be manufactured or chemically altered internally by the body but must be obtained from raw, fresh, natural whole foods. Many people believe that they get their vitamins from a bottle of supplements. These synthetic vitamins are very toxic to the body and do not metabolize or assimilate. The body treats these vitamins as poisonous drugs. Numerous people believe that the synthetic vitamins can replace foods, but they can't. They will never be healthy following this practice. Vitamins are essential for proper growth, vitality, function of the organ systems, and general wellbeing. Vitamins will govern and control the metabolism through the endocrine system. Through its intelligence, the body will maintain the proper balance if fed the foods that supply these components. Single deficiencies are rare. Most bodies are deficient because of improper diet and lifestyle. Therefore, the whole body suffers from this scarcity.

According to Earl Mindell, if one would eat the right foods in a well-balanced diet, a person would get all the vitamins that they need. He adds that very few people are able to arrange what he calls this mythical diet.[5] The reason it's called mythical diet is that much of humanity has adapted to the standard American diet and most are addicted to this way of life, including Earl himself, who takes many of his vitamins in supplement form. These only stimulate the body into so-called health, but it is a facade and a destructive lie. The truth of what he is saying is that yes, the standard American diet is extremely deficient and each person who succumbs to this is very malnourished because of the processed foods, sugars, white flours, additives, and cooked foods. Yes, the body thrives on vitamins, but only through the natural, raw whole foods, not pills. This cannot be repeated enough. As the Bible states in Romans 12:1–2, "I beseech you therefore, brethren, by the mercies of God, that you present your bodies a living sacrifice, holy, acceptable to God, which is your reasonable service. And do not be conformed to this world, but be transformed by the renewing of your mind that you may prove what is that good and acceptable and perfect will of God."[6]

God's will for humanity is to have good and perfect bodies that function properly and are maintained with appropriate foods as He created for us to eat. When this law/command is disobeyed, one will suffer the consequences in the most dramatic and tragic way.

True vitamins that are just a small portion of a group of organic substances already exist in relatively minute portions in natural, raw foods.[7] They are essential to the body's normal metabolism, and for whatever reason, they fall short. There are disease patterns that will start and continue until the health of the body is endangered. Degeneration starts, and if these patterns have not ceased and been corrected, the degeneration continues until there is destruction of the tissue and organs. This may occur over a short period or a lengthy portion of time (years) depending on the result of the deple-tion of nutrients and the damage created by this inadequate lifestyle. These vitamins need to come from natural sources, for any other way is inadequate. Popping pills is injurious to the body. It is similar to drugging.

The natural hygiene diet is a better way. All the vitamins the body needs come only from the raw natural foods: fresh fruits and organically-grown vegetables. Life scientists desire abundant health, which comes from obedience to nature's ways. Nature, not humanity, gives a guarantee of health. If at all possible, it's best to grow one's own produce to get a lifetime of disease-free health.

The healthy body requires fewer nutrients than an unhealthy one because the healthy body is much more efficient in the digestion, assimilation, and elimination of the nutrients and waste products.[8] This body is cleaner and purer than the sick body. The challenged body is void of health and requires a higher quantity of nutrients to get it well. That kind of body has higher needs and suffers from inadequate resources. The person who feasts daily on animal products; cooked foods with seasonings and condiments; and refined, processed and fermented foods will continue to have habitual addictions, such as for alcohol, tobacco, coffee, sodas, sugars, and drugs. The addictions and cravings are more prevalent in a body that is malnourished and desperately seeks to be healthy with the vitamins needed, not just for maintenance but for repair and regeneration. The sick body has much greater needs than the healthy one.

Vitamin intake is also lower for those who are emotionally stable and stress-resistant people. The person who exercises daily utilizes the vitamins in a more efficient way. The raw-food lifestyle also makes the digestive system more efficient in its processes, thus lowering its needs for large amounts of nutrients, as the needs of the conventional eaters are greater. The body in this nutritionally efficient state requires less sleep to restore the resources of nerve energy. On a natural hygiene diet, the vitamin intake is much greater, and yet the needs are decreased because of the effectiveness of the way the body assimilates them. This makes for a healthier body and for a long and prosperous life.

Each vitamin is either water- or fat-soluble. Fat-soluble vitamins will be absorbed into the body as fat and will be eliminated as fats through the feces. Water-soluble ones are absorbed in water and are urinated out through the urinary system. The fat-soluble vitamins are A, D, E, and K; the water-soluble ones are vitamin C and the B-complex vitamins.

Vitamins have their particular function in the workings of the body. Each one works together as a whole, one without the other will create a deficiency of sorts. Vitamins also work together with all of the other nutrients. They do not function alone, but together, working with the minerals, fats, proteins, carbohydrates, and water for the proper functioning of the body. Vitamins work together as coenzymes. When the needs of the body are great, the nutrients are supplied (raw foods) and the demands can be met. They are just a small part of the body's processes, which are used in unison. Dr. Alan M. Immerman's point is well taken and is very crucial: "The body acts on the vitamin, not the vitamin that acts on the body."[9] Vitamins are just a small part of the proficiency of the human body—the intricate human metabolic mechanism is of God's creation, which is wonderfully and fearfully made.

Mineral salts only in their organic form are usable by the human body. In their inorganic form, minerals exist naturally in the soil and in water, but in this inorganic form, they are useless and even dangerous to the human organism.[10] People need organic compounds for the body to function normally. Without it, life cannot go on. People and animals must eat plants to obtain their organic minerals.

According to Mike Benton, "Plants, when in their embryonic state, cannot use inorganic minerals in the soil but instead feed on the organic compounds contained within the seed."[10] Not until the roots and leaves are grown will the plant be considered as "mature," and then it can apply and use the inorganic minerals of the soil. Photosynthesis, with the presence of chlorophyll, is the manner by which the plant changes the inorganic matter into organic matter in the green leaves of the plant.

Critical changes occur in all minerals as they pass through the plant's structure. Chemists cannot isolate these processes in a lab as they try to analyze and duplicate these minerals for human consumption they destroy the plant. These synthetic substances are toxic and injurious to the body. The body can only use the organic minerals that are present in the natural diet of fresh varieties of fruits, vegetables, nuts, seeds, and sprouts in their whole unprocessed form. The person who adheres to this way of eating will always receive sufficient amounts of organic mineral compounds.

The purpose of minerals in the human diet is of vital importance to maintain human life. These salts enter into every cell tissue and fluid of the body. They are also the main element of the harder composition of the body, i.e., the bones, teeth, nails, hair, etc. The bones contain mostly calcium phosphate, which also is vitally important for maintaining the normal alkalinity of the blood. The mineral salts are also found in the body's secretions, saliva, tears, etc.; and if the body is deficient of these minerals, the secretions will also be lacking. They also help the body through its detoxifying and eliminating of its wastes purposes. When one consumes cooked and processed foods, which are lacking in minerals, acidosis is produced through the fermentation of the carbohydrates and putrefied proteins. The minerals help to restore the body's alkalinity.

According to *Human Anatomy and Physiology* author, Elaine Marieb, the human body does require moderate amounts of seven minerals: calcium, phosphorus, potassium, sulfur, sodium, chloride, and magnesium along with about a dozen trace minerals.[11]

Minerals are not used in isolation but along with vitamins and the other nutrients to make sure that the body functions smoothly. According to Marieb, there is a precise balance between the uptake and excretion states for it "is crucial for retaining needed amounts of minerals while preventing toxic overload."[11] For example, sodium, which is present in all natural foods and added in large amounts to processed and cooked foods, can cause high blood pressure if too much is consumed in refined states. Marieb claims that fats, sugars, and grains are void of all minerals while vegetables and legumes are the most mineral-rich sources of foods.[11]

The cells of the body have their balances because of their mineral exchange. Sodium is most abundant in the extracellular fluid while potassium is needed for maintaining intercellular pressure. Sodium and potassium are the main electrolytes in the blood. Both are needed for proper nerve and muscular functioning. All minerals work together yet separately, as well as other vitamins and nutrients. For example, calcium needs magnesium, vitamins D and K, phosphorus, and other trace minerals in order to be absorbed into the skeletal structure. Iron is essential for the hemoglobin to transport oxygen in the blood.

Minerals are the main workers to help the vitamins assimilate within the body. They work together as a team. The body can produce a few vitamins, but it cannot construct a single mineral. Vitamins cannot work properly without minerals, so the body needs both simultaneously to thrive and function.

Water is one of the essential nutrients of the body. Without it, there isn't any health, and death comes quickly. A body can live for three weeks without food, but a person can only live for three days without water. The human body is 70 percent water, and blood is 94 percent water. The human body is an enclosed sea of life. Water is essential for life and survival. It plays an important part of almost every body function from thinking to breathing. It's wise for the body to consume only pure, fresh, clean water. The body receives its nutrients of water from the fluids that are consumed and the raw foods that are eaten. The raw, fresh whole foods have high water content, which is healthy for the body. According to Austin L. Brooks, water is also regulated by the body's oxidation reactions. This process occurs with the combining of hydrogen in the foods that are eaten and with the oxygen that is breathed.[12]

The body uses water in some of the following ways:

- Water is required to carry nutrients through the bloodstream to all areas throughout the body.
- Water keeps the body temperature stable; it cools internally as well as externally.
- Water keeps the body hydrated, which also keeps the skin hydrated, soft, and supple.
- Water dilutes the cellular waste toxins produced during the metabolic processes and carries them away.
- Water is a part of every cell of the body, since the body consists of 70 percent water.
- Saliva is the first part of digestion, and a well-hydrated body keeps the mouth moist as to aid in foods downstream.
- Water dissolves the built-up minerals within the body, helping to eliminate heart disease and arthritis.

- Water is needed for the proper functioning of the glandular system, the endocrine systems, and the functioning processes of the pancreas.
- Water keeps the colon clean. The large intestine needs to be hydrated to keep the wastes moving through it.[13]

The large intestine is where the body's processes remove the fluids, and thus, feces are formed for removal through the sigmoid and rectal areas. Water is needed for a continuous removal of these wastes as not to become hardened, impacted, and constipated, creating mucoid plaque. Cooked foods, animal flesh, grains, and processed foods also lack the water content needed for proper elimination. It just continues its impacting process until the colon and the body itself is severely overloaded with accumulated toxins and waste products and then becomes severely distressed. Disease is the body's housecleaning system. Cancers are forming and yet the individual isn't paying attention. They are continuing to live this incorrect lifestyle and getting worse.

During the body's metabolic functioning, it loses four to six pints of water daily. Loss occurs through sweating, breathing, and urinating—all ensuring the necessary loss of toxins.[13]

The body's natural diet is sufficient for water intake. Raw fruits, for example, are 80–90 percent water. Vegetables have high water content but not as much. Nuts and seeds still have at least 5 percent water. Cooked foods do not contain the sufficient amount of water needed by the body. The body has to add more liquid to cooked food to make it more digestible. The problem with this is while one is eating, and if a person drinks enough liquid for the body to digest these cooked foods, the first stage digestive juices will be diluted, and this causes incomplete digestion.[13] This will result in the loss of energy. The food will putrefy in the colon, and the sugars will ferment in the stomach. On the other side, there isn't enough liquid consumed to assist the digestion of these cooked foods. The body will take the fluids from the blood supply, resulting in mild hydration. Therefore, in the body's created intelligence, it will protect the blood chemistry and pH level, thereby hindering the digestion. It is good to sip water throughout the day as thirst demands and stick with a raw produce diet, which produces the most optimal water in nature. Water may be consumed up to one-half hour before meals, but not during the meals and not until at least two to three hours after a meal depending whether it's a raw produce food meal or not. Some ill-combined meals may be a challenge because they will create excessive thirst, and raw foods do not.

Some people will add minerals or pH drops, hydrogen peroxide or chlorine dioxide to the distilled water to make it more alkaline because the distilling process and reverse osmosis processes make the water more neutral.[14] The water that the body needs shouldn't contain these poisons. Hallelujah Acres advocates purified drinking water using a steam distiller. Great, but then in this water a small amount of ionic trace mineral solution is added to lower the small loss of minerals from the body because of drinking low mineral water.[15] The claim is that this mineral loss is small, but over the years, this loss can be significant. They claim also that these trace minerals are easily absorbed by the body. Michael Donaldson states, "Foods as well as body fluids contain ionic minerals; the body cannot function without ionic minerals."[15] If the fresh produce contains these minerals, can't a person just get them fresh from the diet without having to add chemically processed synthetic minerals?

Unhealthy living practices can dehydrate the cellular structure of the body, which can create an excessive thirst. The body in its Supreme Creator's intelligence needs to clean and eliminate the excess sodium and toxins caused by cooked and processed foods, especially with the large amounts of sodium and seasonings in these foods. (The cooked foods needed sodium to make them palatable.) The water helps to hold toxic materials in suspension so that the cells and the tissues of the body will suffer less damage.

Edema is a condition in which the body takes on extra water to hold and keep the toxins in suspension within the body's soft tissues, especially in the legs and feet. A person who consumes a diet consisting of cooked and processed foods, especially with salts, seasonings, and other condiments, in most cases, will suffer with the effects of edema. The lymph system will run a bit sluggish and tend to back up. More and more toxins accumulate in the circulatory system and immune systems. This can prove dangerous to the body because, until all of this can be eliminated, it is all stored in the lower extremities. In the worst cases, the accumulation of toxins becomes excessive that it will be stored throughout the body. A few days of fasting helps the body to do its housecleaning. The body then can eliminate and rid itself of the waters, cleaning out the fluids and toxins from the cells and tissues.

Hospitals and doctors only add to the dilemma of the poisoned body by adding sodium chloride water in the IV to the so-called dehydrated person. Dehydration occurs because of lack of pure, fresh water intake from fresh, raw foods and pure distilled water. This IV procedure is a dangerous practice for the person to accept. Another problem is the prescribed diuretic water pills to end the edema situation. It does not get rid of the edema at all. The causes aren't addressed. Diuretics work by preventing aldosterone, therefore making the situation worse because it then causes further dehydration and more weakening of the adrenal glands.[16] The lower resistance of the body due to the toxic buildup weakens the whole body in its entirety. The adrenal glands weaken and exhaust their function. The body is out of balance.

On a cellular level, there needs to be a balance between the inner fluid within the cells and the fluid that surrounds the cells. This outer fluid is maintained by the minerals potassium and sodium. Potassium resides mostly inside the cell and sodium stays mostly in the fluid surrounding the cells. The fluid retention occurs when this balance between the sodium and potassium goes out of whack, and more fluid begins to accumulate either in the cells or in the area outside of the cells. This imbalance causes the puffiness and the bloating in the legs, feet, ankles, hands, and fingers. In extreme cases, the face tends to get puffy as well.

The body needs pure, fresh distilled water; a fresh, raw whole produce diet; and a fast to rid of these accumulated toxins and get the body to regenerate, heal, and maintain its God-given functions.

Endnotes

1. Elaine N. Marieb, *Human Anatomy and Physiology*, 5th ed. (Benjamin Cummings, 2001), 950.

2. Mike Benton, "Fit Proteins in the Diet," part II, lesson 8, course in Natural Health Fit for Life Sciences Institute, 210.

3. T. C. Fry, "Medical Research Finds America's Protein Intake Causes Disease," in vol. 1, bk. 2 of *Fit for Life – Basic Health Library*, 1.

4. Mike Benton, "Fats in the Diet" (lesson 11, a course in Natural Health, Fit for Life Sciences Institute), 278.

5. Earl Mindell and Hester Mundis, *Earl Mindell's Vitamin Bible* (Warner Books, 1991), 3–4.

6. The New King James Version, the Holy Bible, (Thomas Nelson, 1994).

7. Robert McCarter and Elizabeth McCarter, "A Statement on Vitamins," vol. 1, bk. 2 of *Fit for Life – Basic Health Library*, 5.

8. T. C. Fry, "Factors That Lower Vitamin Needs," in vol. 1, bk. 2 of *Fit for Life – Basic Health Library*, 14–15.

9. Alan Immerman with T. C. and Marti Fry, "The Metabolic Wizards of Life's Processes" (lesson 9, a course in Natural Health, Fit for Life Sciences Institute), 252.

10. Mike Benton, "Organic and Inorganic Minerals" (lesson 10, a course in Natural Health, Fit for Life Sciences Institute), 265.

11. Marieb, *Human Anatomy*, 954.

12. Austin L. Brooks, "Water Transports Nutrients to All the Body Needs" (lesson 14, a course in Natural Health, Fit for Life Sciences Institute), 334.

13. George Malkmus with Peter and Stowe Shockey, *The Hallelujah Diet* (Destiny Image, 2006), 183–184.

14. Robert O. Young and Shelley Redford Young, *The pH Miracle* (Warner Books, 2002), 94.

15. Michael Donaldson, "Clean, Pure Water," *Hallelujah Acres Diet and Lifestyle Magazine* 48 (January/February 2008): 13.

16. David G. Williams, "Fluid Retention: The Stress Connection," *Alternatives Magazine* 9, no. 2, 10.

CHAPTER 38

Enzymes

Enzymes are the living portions of foods, raw foods. They give life and are life. They are a gift from God to keep the body in optimal health. Enzymes are the life of the human organism and are derived from living foods, not the dead, processed foods of the standard American diet. Heat in any form will kill the life of these delicate enzymes, so all processed and cooked foods are void of any enzymes; thus, they are dead foods. Enzymes are the catalysts that help the foods to digest, assimilate, and are the life force to the body.

People think they can consume any kind of food as often as they desire, anytime they want, anyway they want, and then they wonder why they continue to get sick. This type of practice totally overloads the digestive system, constitutes overeating, which will fill the gut with all the particles of undigested foods, therefore, burdening the body with toxic waste products that are not eliminated. "More energy is used by the digestive system than any other system of the body," states Harvey Diamond.

Enzymes are very small protein chemicals that carry the necessary energy source that is needed for every chemical action that occurs within the body. There are numerous chemical activities that occur beyond the scope of vision, but if the body doesn't have all the necessary enzymes to accomplish these acts, the body would die.

Harvey Diamond very eagerly expresses the effects of enzymes on the body. "In all the building required, repairing and maintaining of any part of the body, inside or out, enzymes are involved. Without them, nothing will get done," Diamond says. The life of the body will cease to exist without them. The body would be under great stress if it had to produce all the enzymes to accomplish each and every task. Foods, raw, fresh foods, come into play to help out. These foods have the correct balance for the body.

There are three classes of enzymes: metabolic, digestive, and food enzymes. A metabolic enzyme, Harvey Diamond refers to as "the body's labor force, the constructive workers."[1] They keep the body functioning properly. The body needs enzymes for the eyes to blink, for swallowing saliva and foods, blood circulation, breathing, assimilation of foods, walking, talking, and the workings of the lymph system to keep the body clean. The lymph system helps to prevent disease, pain, and the destructive breakdown of the body.

According to Harvey Diamond, "Your body can produce a certain amount of metabolic enzymes and no more. You can and will run out of them."[1] When they are gone, there is death to the human organism. The functions of life will cease to exist. Anything that is cooked and processed uses up these enzymes at an accelerated rate. It's best to guard these enzymes so the body will have optimal health, slower aging processes, thus a longer, more productive, healthy life.

The second type of enzymes is food enzymes. Food, only in its whole, fresh, uncooked state keeps the body alive. In the beginning of the world, man ate only raw produce foods. After the flood upon the Earth, when God destroyed all of His creation (except Noah and his family) and there wasn't any vegetation left on the planet, man (Noah and his family) began to cook his foods, meats, and grains.[2] Thus, the age of death began to dramatically decrease in just a few generations because of his cooked food diet. Man is the only species on Earth who eats cooked foods, and man (along with his domesticated animals) is the only ones who suffer disease. The diseases of cancer, diabetes, obesity, osteoporosis, heart attacks, and premature death—all plagues modern mankind. The foods that people eat are supposed to keep the body healthy and alive. The cooking of these foods destroys the enzymes in them, *all* of them. The food will sit in the stomach because without enzymes, there isn't any way to digest it. The body will then be forced to use its metabolic enzymes in place of the destroyed food and digestive enzymes necessary to digest the foods. When this happens, people are destroying their health and shortening their lives. Harvey Diamond comments, "The reason this is so is that when you suddenly force the metabolic enzyme, mechanism to produce digestive enzymes, the work that the metabolic enzymes would have been doing to keep everything working efficiently and effectively is compromised and thwarted."[3] The body is kept from doing its job, which overburdens the systems. Un-eliminated toxins build up, back up, and allow the body to establish diseases. The raw foods that should be eaten, keep the body cleansed of waste toxins, thus free of disease. Diamond comments, "The very mechanism in the body designed to keep you healthy and energetic is kept from doing its job."[3]

The third types of enzymes are digestive enzymes, and these are the enzymes that are involved in the digestive process. There are different types of digestive enzymes and each has a special job to the breakdown of substances in water; building proteins, transferring organic substances, rearranging molecules and enzymes, and releasing enzymes in the presence of oxygen that change the color of foods.[4] They all have their enhancements and effects on the digestion of foods.

Virginia Verano, BSc, made a careful, but important, observation: "The human digestive tract is divided into three cavities: the mouth, the stomach, and the intestines. Each of these cavities possesses its own characteristic digestive juice, or juices, with which to do the digestive work of a particular cavity."[5] Each step of digestion, with its particular enzymes, prepares one stage to enter into the next. If they aren't prepared properly and efficiently, the food values are destroyed, thus the digestion is ineffective and no benefits to the human organism are received. "Without good digestion," claims Verano. "We rob ourselves of many important elements and permit decomposition and putrefaction."[5] Toxicity and diseases are becoming a part of the body as it attempts to do its housecleaning. Each enzyme is very specific in what it does, and with each food type, it will aid in its digestive process. It only acts on the one type and no other. The enzymes work at body temperature. If there is heat above that, they will be destroyed. The also work in an alkaline environment. If neutral, they are ineffective.

The enzyme of the mouth is amylase, which digests starches. If there is even a hint of acid, the digestion of the starches ceases. The gastric juice in the stomach is poured out in large quantities (1.5 to 2.5 liters) a day. Verano adds, "If no protein is eaten, the juice is almost neutral in reaction."[5] Stomach enzymes are pepsin and gastric lipase. Pepsin is for the proteins and gastric lipase is for the fats. The four to five enzymes of the intestinal secretions are considered to be alkaline in their reaction. Bile is an enzyme to split fats in the digestive process within the duodenum. These enzymes are there to aid in the digestive process of the foods for proper assimilation and elimination of its end waste products. Proper food combination is of the utmost importance in the digestion of salivary and gastric digestion.

Endnotes

1. Harvey Diamond, *Living without Pain* (VP Nutrition, 2005), 312.
2. Genesis 6:21 (NKJV).
3. Diamond, *Living without Pain*, 318–319.
4. Hannah Allen, "The Principles of Digestive Physiology Which Decree Correct Food Combining" (lesson 2, a course in Natural Health, Fit for Life Sciences Institute), 498.
5. Virginia Verano, "Basic Considerations in Food Combining" (lesson 22, a course in Natural Health, Fit for Life Sciences Institute), 513.

CHAPTER 39

Afterthought

By the way, before we actually leave this subject of chemicals in the destruction of our bodies, let's introduce one more avenue about the way chemicals enter our bodies—through our environment.

These can be in our city, air pollution, and other pollutants, and even our work environments. But probably the most chemically-infested area is our own home environment. The average American, claims Mike Benton, "spends 93 hours in his or her own home each week. About one-fifth of the population spends up to 150 hours weekly in their homes."[1]

I can hear you saying, "Now wait a minute. You've gone just too far." Let me explain. There are many surprising sources and these sources can and do disrupt the normal processes of our bodies as well as creating allergies and unknown diseases.

Fred Farmer, Hallelujah Acres Health minister, states, "According to the Consumer Product Safety Commission, 150 chemicals commonly found in homes have been linked to allergies, birth defects, cancer and psychological abnormalities."[2]

Let me name just a few of the culprits. Carpeting holds more pollutants, dust, toxins, and pesticides from the tracking in of the pets and the people walking into the home, also other toxins of which many cannot be vacuumed up. New carpets are the worst for they are treated with formaldehyde-type chemicals. Formaldehyde is a chemical that coats all new carpets, cloth-covered and foam-filled furniture, foam in mattress pads and pillows, and even new clothes. For this reason, it is wise to buy only machine washable clothes. Many children's clothes, especially pajamas, contain fire retardants that are very dangerous. When ignited, this stuff practically melts on the body rather than burns. Among other chemically-induced products are house paints, draperies, wood paneling, etc., but let's not stay focused on these alone.

What I'd like to focus on is the bath and beauty products and the household cleaners. The bar soaps, lotions, deodorants, and antiperspirants. These contain many different chemicals, some more toxic than others. The gauge should be not to use anything you wouldn't use on a newborn baby's skin. The skin contains many small surface capillaries, and through them chemicals can and will enter through the skin into the blood system. For example, I have known many people who have severe allergic reactions to underarm deodorants and antiperspirants including myself. Rashes, itching, sores, and hives are some common symptoms that are experienced. I now use what's called a crystal stick deodorant (see resources) and have had no more problems. It is a natural, chemical-free alternative.

In fact, once the diet is cleaned up and one is eating properly combined fresh whole foods, there isn't a problem with body odor. It's amazing how many people smell like the meals they eat. The foods are just trying to leave the body, and the skin, as well as the lungs, is the way for the body to do it.

The shampoos, conditioners, hairsprays and mousses, and other hair products are also filled with chemicals. We just wash the chemicals of these shampoos, conditioners right into our bodies. The warm water in the showers opens the pores of the skin, allowing these entrances into the body. It's best to buy organic products with the least amount of ingredients, especially harmful chemicals. Get in the habit of reading all labels.

Hairsprays are very dangerous to the lungs, eyes, and the skin. In fact, one of my husband's clients owns a beauty salon, and she is now developing macular degeneration and blindness because of the chemicals in the beauty products used in her salon. What's so sad is that she's not willing to give up her business until she's totally blind. In fact, Halleluiah Acres health minister, Aurdree Lee, states, "Speaking of beautifying the outside when it comes to cosmetics, women need to know that there are still a lot of chemicals in natural-sounding cosmetics. I've worked for a number of salons in Chicago and New Jersey, and I've seen it all. Even though a facial may be labeled as 'avocado facial' or a 'berry facial,' it still has a lot of chemicals in it. Ask to see the ingredients in it…if you wouldn't eat it, don't put it on your face."[3] It is best to change our diet and lifestyles first—inward beauty definitely shows outward. We can use coconut oil and avocados on our face and body, but we can eat them because they are good for us internally as well.

I have seen some women's vanities and dressers so cluttered and filled with these so-called beauty products and perfumes, and yet they don't look or smell beautiful because their bodies are a toxic dump. Many people look much older than their years because of the overwhelming load of toxic chemicals.

Nail polishes and nail salons have sprung up everywhere. The twenty nails of a woman's hands and feet are decorated and painted in all sorts of designs and will even include jewelry embedded into the nails. The toxicity of these products is outrageous. "It doesn't sink into the body through the nails," you may say. Somewhat correct, but when a woman does her cooking, eating finger foods, licking her fingers through a meal, etc., the toxins are going into her mouth or into the foods she's preparing, so beware! Formaldehyde, nitrocellulose dissolved in solvents, etc., is waiting to enter the body. Poisons are poisons. A little or a lot will still set up disease and kill the body. When I quit using nail polishes and polish removers (which I found out I was allergic to these poisons) and with a change of diet, I have long, hard nails instead of chipped, cracked, and peeling nails. I have to keep them trimmed every couple of weeks because they tend to grow too long.

Men are not to get off the hook. After all, the shaving creams, aftershaves, colognes, deodorants, hair tonics, etc., are also prone to create a chemical disaster. They are also just as diseased as their counterparts used by females.

Bar soaps, antibacterial and moisturizing bars are the one or the worst offenders of chemically-induced toxins. As with the shampoos, these gain their entrance into the human body through the skin's open pores in warm to hot showers. The antibacterial soaps do not get rid of any more bacteria than any others without these harmful ingredients, especially the ingredient triclosan. Many people have mild to severe allergic reactions to these soaps. The perfumes and scents added to the soaps are also without any health effects, as many brands are so nauseating in their aroma, which seems to linger on the body much of the day. That is the manufacture's agenda. Look for a homemade bar-soap recipe at the end of this chapter.

People will use moisturizing bar soaps (see resources) and lotions to rid their dry skin. In essence, they only add to the dryness by their diets, along with the soaps and lotions. Nutritionist, Hulda Clark, explained, "A part of every skin problem is due to the toxic elements found in the soaps themselves. For instance aluminum is commonly added as a 'skin moisturizer.' It does this by impregnating the skin and attracting water, giving the illusion of moist skin. In fact, you simply have *moist aluminum* stuck in your skin, which your immune system must remove."[4] The body lotions with the isopropyl alcohol tend to dry it out even more. The more one uses these products, the drier the skin becomes until it will crack and bleed. A more natural approach to the body splashes is rose water or even a 100 percent pure witch hazel (see resources). Witch hazel is a great aftershave because it closes the pores and soothes the irritated skin, allowing it to heal faster without itching and burning. Use it with a little vitamin C powder, and you have a wonderful skin conditioner. Witch hazel (only 100 percent) on a cosmetic pad can be very soothing and healing for hemorrhoids. Keep a few in an airtight container next to the commode for use as needed.

The biggest problem that is at bay right now is the hand sanitizers that are in every store, schools, hospitals, gyms, children's play areas, etc. It is the largest chemically-based poisonous attraction. Hand-washing is very important, but these are ineffective at maintaining one's health. If you won't eat it, do not put it on your skin. It is filled with ethyl alcohol, isopropyl alcohol, water, glycerin, carbomer, fragrance, aminomethyl propanol, propylene glycol, etc. "Alcohol-based hand sanitizers are poor at killing viruses," reported ABC News on February 5, 2013.[5] Hulda Clark wrote, "One hundred percent of cancer patients have the solvent isopropyl alcohol accumulated in their liver and in their cancerous tissues."[6] Many people may use these products and not develop cancer, but why take the chance? It's like playing Russian roulette with your body.

Children have ingested these products, and yet people will allow them in areas with children. These products are extremely flammable and poisonous. People need to teach their children to wash their hands often rather than using these concoctions. In fact, isopropyl alcohol is in many different drugs, household, beauty and food products. Mouthwashes contain much alcohol as well as many other ingredients, including triclosan, that are poisonous to the body. Like I said previously, sublingual is the fastest way into the body even if you don't swallow it. If ingesting a proper diet, the body will not have to experience bad breath or body odor of any kind.

Another problematic product is toothpaste. Not only do some toothpastes (please read labels) contain triclosan, a known carcinogenic, but glycerin as well. Glycerin is generally what makes up most of the product, as it may be the first ingredient on the label. It helps to make the toothpaste more fluid, but it also coats the teeth. It makes the teeth more sensitive, unable to be adequately cleaned, leaving them with an increased risk to cavities. The teeth will also be prone to a greater risk of plaque, dental and gum infections.

Earl Mindell advises, "There may be a connection between toothpaste (with its crystalline abrasives, foaming agents, and other additives) and bowel diseases such as ulcerative colitis, Crohn's disease, and irritable bowel syndrome."[7]

Be careful to buy toothpaste without fluoride (see resources), as fluoride is an extremely dangerous chemical. A study done in the year 2000 was uploaded on an online article: "About Fluoride—Truth Every Mother Should Know," stating that "Sodium fluoride is a hazardous industrial waste by-product of the nuclear and aluminum industries and is the primary ingredient in rat and cockroach poisons." In fact, T. C. Fry comments, "Fluorides in an organic form are toxic. The body defends against fluorides by at first hardening the teeth, then they become brittle and break down under ordinary eating."[9] All toxins are carcinogenic and do interfere with the normal body functioning. Yet it is allowed in our toothpastes, foods, drugs, and water systems. As I keep saying, the fastest way into the body's blood system is through the mouth, not just into the digestive tract. Sublingually, the blood vessels absorb these products instantly. I looked up sodium monofluorophosphate, the active drug first listed on a brand of toothpaste (are we brushing our teeth with drugs now?), and it's listed on the hazardous waste list. Many other chemicals in these toothpastes are toxic to the liver and kidneys. Sodium lauryl sulphate can make the teeth and gums extremely sensitive as well as creating mouth ulcers.

Many of us have never bothered to read labels on the products that are purchased for our use, especially toothpastes and personal care products. Little do we realize what these ingredients are/or what they actually do to the human body. Most people live with the concept that the manufactures of the brand name products would ensure and sell a completely safe product for everyone to use. We *need* to be more diligent in reading labels and finding out what these chemicals are and do to our bodies. When we knowingly buy and use these products then we are knowingly creating our diseases that destroy our body.

Well, now it's time to open our eyes to the truth. There are, according to Internet research, "close to 11,000 chemicals that have been developed over the last half century for potential use in personal care products (this includes skin care, hair care, and oral care) and cosmetics. The vast majority of these (around 9 out of 10) have never been subject to exhaustive tests (as a pharmaceutical product would require) to ensure that they are absolutely safe for use on the human body."[11] Fluorine can be found in food sources such as almonds, carrots, vegetable greens, and these are for the optimal health of the body, it does not need to be brought chemically into the body and destroy it.

People want their homes to smell nice, trying to mask the foulness of the lifestyles they live. The sprays and plug-in air fresheners have great amounts of toxins as they do not rid the odors but just cover them up and, at the same time, can destroy the lungs. Mike Benton states, "They may also coat the nasal passages with an oil film, irritate the eyes and airways, and deaden the sense of smell with a nerve chemical."[12] None of these air fresheners actually eliminates any odors; they simply contaminate the air. Open windows and a healthy lifestyle will mean most household odors will less likely occur. A nonsmoking household that follows a primarily raw food diet will not have most of the household odors that plague most Americans homes.

Household cleaners take a stand as being the most hazardous and dangerous toxins in the home. The kitchen, bathrooms, and laundry areas need to be cleaned up of these poisonous hazards to make the home a safe haven.

Most of the household cleaning should be mechanical, not chemical. Many women are terribly overworked, running a household and working a day job as well. But it is still no longer an excuse as there are natural cleaners (at least not as hazardous) that work just as well as the toxic-based chemical ones, and many are cheaper in cost.

Oven cleaner wouldn't be needed if eating a proper diet. If it does need cleaning, use baking soda as a scouring powder with Amway L.O.C. or Shaklee Basic H to cut through the grease. Pouring hot water slowly down the drain and then adding about ½ cup of washing soda can accomplish drain cleaning. Wait about one minute and flush again with more hot water and plunge as necessary to unclog and loosen the drain. There are too many people who burn themselves severely or fixate themselves trying to unclog a drain with the chemicals, which for me didn't work anyway.

Kitchens can be cleaned with 20 Mule Team Borax as a scouring powder with Amway L.O.C. (¼ cup L.O.C. or Basic H to 24 ounces distilled water into a spray bottle) or Shaklee Basic H. Windows can be cleaned with ⅛–¼ cup white vinegar to one quart of distilled water in a spray bottle. If needed a small amount of bleach can be used for sinks and grout, sparingly and when there's good ventilation only. Never mix bleach with any other cleaners. It will burn your lungs and possibly burn your eyes.

Mike Benton states, "During 1975 for instance, over 1,300 household soap detergents and 775 dishwasher product poisonings occurred."[12] Dishes can be washed by hand with the L.O.C. or Basic H, or use in the dishwasher the 20 Mule Team borax powder in the wash cycle. Works great. It was even approved by service men during the yearly maintenance checkup, he marveled at how clean the dishwasher was kept by this regimen.

Bathroom showers and tubs can be cleaned biweekly or once a month with LOC diluted with water sprayed on the walls and 20 Mule Team Borax on a scrub brush for the scouring. Rinse. It works as the best cleaner ever. If using regular chlorine bleach for mold, it must be extremely well-ventilated, being careful not to breathe in the fumes or you will burn your lungs.

For a good mildew cleaner, mix into a spray bottle the following ingredients: 1 teaspoon liquid castile soap, 1 teaspoon TSP (trisodium phosphate, found in hardware stores), 1 teaspoon 20 Mule Team Borax, 1 teaspoon vinegar, 1 liter hot water. This is for cleaning mildew and grease.

For cleaning my toilets, I scrub with a bowl brush and L.O.C., and for tough water deposits, I pour a can of Coke or Pepsi (any variety) and allow it to sit for a few hours (while I run errands or go to work). Swish and flush.

For the laundry there are various "natural" laundry detergents and soaps in the health food and grocery stores. Most people have different allergies that are due to the products their clothes are washed in. Shaklee and Amway do carry some also (see resources). Do not use fabric softeners as it makes the towels, for example, less absorbent. I do carefully use a product called De-Solv-it (see resources) for the salad dressing spills on my husband's shirts, it works great but use in a well-ventilated area (my laundry room is in the garage). Even though it is an orange-based cleaner, it still has fumes.

Ant and fly sprays can be replaced with a diluted solution of L.O.C. and water, (see above for kitchen cleaner). They drop dead and their trails are eliminated. You will continue to spray every so often, just as you would the old dangerous bug sprays, but only you are killing the ants, and not you. Spray plants infested with bugs in the garden area, let sit about five minutes, and rinse with the water from the hose.

My house has been free of harsh chemicals for a few years. I did have a lot of allergies because of these chemicals, plus the fact my lungs couldn't take the smells of the products. To keep the house clean needs to consist of only 20 Mule Team Borax, white distilled vinegar, regular chlorine bleach, Amway L.O.C. cleaner, Shaklee Basic H cleaner and their laundry cleaner. Most of the chemicals used by the general public are useless and would be better to be replaced by more natural, less caustic substances. I have replaced all of my toxic ones with natural ones. Many stores are now carrying different brands of chemical-free alternative cleaners.

We have an attached garage but have not parked in it for years. Even though the garage has a firewall, all of the vehicle's engine fluids, rubber fumes, etc., will permeate into the house. It's best to keep the environment free of pollutants. To those in the winter snow belt areas, it's still better to scrape windows (I do too in the San Diego winters) than to have your vehicle as part of your death from cancers. If you do have any chemicals that you do use, *do not* store them in the house. Please keep them in the garage.

Use an open window policy as much as possible to allow fresh air into your home. Use a room air cleaner or household air exchange filtration system to filter the home, especially for those folks who have airtight homes, particularly in the wintertime. Mike Benton states, "Stale air called 'human aerial excrete' is the primary source of pollution. Trapped in closed houses are the wastes of our breathing. These contain carbon dioxide, carbonic acid, and yet other waste products. They are deadly to man and beast alike in concentration such as they become in closed homes."[12]

It's important to keep our home environment safe and a clean place to live, free of toxic chemicals and other dangerous substances, which, by this practice, will achieve a higher level of health and wellness. There are so many more chemicals that I haven't even mentioned for lack of space. A wise person will learn about the chemicals in their environment. Research and learn and be well.

It is impossible to be well without living in a healthy lifestyle and environment. This is all a way of education to draw one out of the ignorance, which causes destruction. If you continue to use these toxic chemical products, their poisons will all accumulatively add to the destruction of your body. Follow the pathway to health or keep and suffer with your diseases. You are only given two choices. Choose wisely.

As an example of natural and safe cleaners, below is a recipe for homemade bar soap:

Homemade Bar Soap

Requirement:

A small (10" x 12") plastic dishpan or soap molds
A glass or enamel 2–4 quart saucepan
1 can of lye (sodium hydroxide)
16.9 ounces–40 ounces olive oil
10 ounces coconut oil (palm kernel and castor
    oil are also oils for lathering)
1.5–2.2 ounces of fragrance or essential oils
Plastic gloves or rubber gloves
3 cups water

(Note: This recipe can be cut in half for smaller amounts.)

Instructions:

1. Pour 3 cups of ice water into the 2–4 quart saucepan. (I use a bigger one as it gives more room for stirring and to prevent splashing.)
2. Slowly and carefully add the lye a little at a time, stirring with a wooden or plastic utensil (make sure you use plastic or rubber gloves.). Do not breathe the vapor over the container or keep children from the area. Above all, use *no metal*. The mixture will

get very hot. In olden days, a sassafras branch was used to stir, imparting a fragrance and insect deterrent for mosquitoes, lice, fleas, and ticks

3. Let cool at least one hour in a safe place.
4. Pour the oils into the dishpan then, very slowly and carefully, pour the lye solution into the dishpan. Mix thoroughly, at least 15 minutes until it looks like pudding.
5. Add the fragrance and essential oils if desired at this time and mix again. (Information on different oils: For moisturizing and conditioning, use olive oil, cocoa butter, soybean, sunflower, or canola oil. For lathering, use coconut, castor, or palm kernel oil.)
6. If using soap molds, pour into them at this time.
7. If making bars, let the dishpan sit until the next morning or until hard enough to cut into bars. Generally 24-36 hours. It will get harder after a few days. Package the bars.
8. Remove from molds and package after a few days.
9. The curing process takes about two weeks.

This recipe has been revised from Hulda Clark's book *The Cure for All Cancers*.

Endnotes

1. Mike Benton, "Chemicals in the Household Environment" (lesson 51 of Ecological Factors and Their Roles in Nutrition, Natural Health course, Fit for Life Sciences Institute), 1124.
2. Fred Farmer, "Household Cleaning Products and Your Children," *Back to the Garden Health News* 37 (March/April 2006): 17.
3. Audrey Lee, "How I Beat Cancer in 90 Days," *Hallelujah Acres Health News* 67 (Summer 2011): 7.
4. Hulda R. Clark, *The Cure for All Cancers* (New Century, 1993), 564.
5. ABC News, http://abcnews.go/Health/story?id=1003859
6. Clark, *The Cure*, 39.

7. Earl Mindell and Hester Mundis, *"Earl Mindell's Vitamin Bible,"* (Warner Books, 1991), 13.

8. A. True Ott, "The Truth about 'Fluoride' (or whatever every Mother Should Know)," August 2000 p. 1.

9. T. C. Fry, "Introducing Life Science Program For Perfect Health," (lesson 3 of the Foundation of Life Science, a course in Natural Health, Fit for Life Sciences Institute), 60. 2011

10. Ott, "The Truth about Fluoride," 6.

11. Go Natural and Organic, "Toxic Toothpaste Ingredients and Other Chemical Cocktails," http://www.gonando.com/toothpaste.html. 2011.

12. Benton, "Chemicals in the Household," 1127.

CHAPTER 40

In Conclusion

Everyone has his/her allotted time, the days and years of our lives upon this planet. But people are shortening their lifespan and dying prematurely because of disobedience to the laws of nature and God our Creator.

All the diseases that have plagued our society seem to be so different, affecting so many numerous areas of the body in unusual ways, but they all have a common denominator—an accumulation of chemicals and toxic poisons along with poor diet and poor lifestyle.

The chemicals that have been created in this age and in our society are of the environment and in the foods we consume. They are on the increase and are destroying humanity. The people who are supposed to protect its people are instead greedily part of those who are a part of the destruction. The more of these poisons that infiltrate the body, the sicker and more diseased it becomes. It's similar to the movie *Soylent Green*, trying to feed an overwhelming mass of humanity, but it's not food that we are eating. All of the chemicals overload the body's circuits with poison until the body ceases to function.

Inadvertently, the accumulation and abundance of chemicals and chemical reactions are due to the body's inability to digest improper foods, processed foods, and incorrect food combinations that are held up in the digestive tract. In the end, people must be held responsible for their own health, or it will definitely worsen. All people need to become aware of what they are putting into their mouths. The blind will continue to lead the blind and they will both fall into the same pit, the pit of disease and destruction.

People want convenience, but that includes the chemicals which lead to cancers. Raw foods, on the other hand, are the real ones. It requires more work, but it leads to rebuilding and rejuvenation of the body.

We must follow the laws of nature, the laws of God, for He made each human body in the most unique and perfect way, and gave us the tools (foods) to take care of that body. His creation consists of wonderful fruits, vegetables, seeds, nuts, and pure water. What God made, we can eat; what man made, we do not eat. If people could see beyond the scope of human vision, to see what our Divine Creator Himself sees, then we definitely would be more respectful of the one and only body given to us. The body and this life is a precious gift and needs to be appreciated and revered.

PART TWO

What Do I Do Now?

CHAPTER 41

Food-Combining Principles

1. Have fruit only in the morning from the time you get up until noon. Have a fruit smoothie for breakfast, and if you get hungry, have a piece of fruit midmorning for a snack. Nothing else but fruit should pass your lips, so your body and its cells may get cleaned out.
2. Do not eat fruit with any proteins or vegetables (except celery and lettuce as these help to absorb some of the sugar from the fruit).
3. Do not combine sweet fruits with acidic/citrus fruits.
4. Do not eat proteins and starches at the same meal; they will not digest.
5. Salads combine well with proteins *or* starches.
6. Eat your starches with vegetables or salads only.
7. Eat your proteins with vegetables or salads only.
8. If you must have milk or yogurt, have it alone not combined with anything else as a snack in midafternoon.
9. If you must eat cheese, have a small amount with vegetables or on top of a salad.
10. Melons: eat alone on an empty stomach or leave alone.
11. Sprouted grains with salads or greens.
12. Use fats very sparingly. Fats delay the digestion of other foods.

13. Rid your diet of any preservatives, additives, and chemicals of any kind, so the body can heal itself of disease.
14. Do not eat acidic foods (tomatoes, lemons) with starchy foods. It slows the digestive process.

Food Combining: Fruits

Sweet fruits will include:

Bananas	Persimmons	Thompson grapes (seedless)
All sweet grapes	Fresh figs	Dates
Prunes	Dried figs	Raisins
Muscat grapes	All dried fruit	Carob

All dried fruits must be organic, thus free of all preservatives.

These fruits may be eaten in combination with the sub-acid fruits, not acid fruits.

Sub-acidic fruits will include:

Sweet apples (Delicious)	Pears	Sweet peaches	Mangos
Sweet nectarines	Blueberries	Papayas	Apricots
Raspberries	Mulberries	Guava	Sweet cherries
Blackberries	Sweet plums	Huckleberries	Passion fruit
Most grapes	Papaya	Apricots	Raspberries
Mulberries	Guavas		

These fruits may be combined with the sweet or acidic fruits. Acidic fruits will include:

Oranges	Kumquats	Sour cherries
Grapefruit	Loquats	Sour apples
Pineapples	Carambolas	Sour grapes
Strawberries	Loganberries	Sour peaches
Pomegranates	Gooseberries	Sour nectarines
Lemons	Kiwi fruit	Sour plums
Limes		

Cranberries: not recommended they contain benzoic acid.

Tomatoes – an acidic fruit without the sugar content of other acid fruit. Used with vegetable salad or any green or non-starchy vegetable, but not a starchy meal, which will not digest well. May be used with nuts or cheese.

These fruits may combine with the sub-acidic fruits but not sweet fruits.

Melons may include:

Watermelon	Casaba	Honey Dew
Crenshaw	Cantaloupe	Persian

These do not digest well with any other foods. Eat them alone or with other only

Food Combining: Vegetable, Grains, Fats, Proteins

Starchy vegetables include:

Potatoes	Yams and sweet potatoes
Jerusalem artichokes	Parsnips
Beets	Winter squash

Mildly starchy vegetables include:

Mature corn	Carrots
Pumpkin	Sprouted grains

Non-starchy and green vegetables include:

Lettuce	Celery	Cabbage (young, sweet)
Cucumber	Cauliflower	Sweet peppers
Broccoli	Brussels sprouts	Kale
Collard greens	Dandelion greens	Turnip tops
Mustard greens	Okra	Turnips
Eggplant	Green beans	Zucchini

Yellow crookneck squash   Other summer squashes   Bok choy
Alfalfa sprouts

Grains and foods containing grains include:

Wild rice	Brown rice	Buckwheat
Groats	Millet	Oats
Wheat	Rye	Barley

Oils and fats include (use very sparingly):

Butter	Avocados	Coconut
Olive oil	Almonds	Pecans
Flax seed oil	Pumpkin seeds	Sunflower seeds

Starchy proteins include:

Peanuts	Lentils
Coconuts	Lima and other beans in a pod
Chestnuts	Mature green beans in a pod
Dry beans	Peas in a pod
Garbanzo beans (chick peas)	Dry peas

Nuts include:

Pecans	Almonds	Pignolas (pine nuts)
Filberts or hazelnuts	English walnuts	Indian nuts
Black walnuts	Macadamias	Beechnuts
Hickory nuts	Cashews	Pistachios

Seeds include:

Sunflower seeds	Sesame seeds
Flax seeds	Pumpkin and squash seeds

Other plant proteins include:

Soy beans (fresh, dry, or sprouted)	Sunflower seed sprouts

Low proteins include:

Avocados (may also be classified as a fat and as a neutral fruit and is best mixed with green vegetables or sub-acidic fruit)
Olives

Sprouts include (contain significant amounts of protein, especially in the early stages):

Soy sprouts	Alfalfa sprouts (may be used as a green vegetable)
Lentil sprouts	Mung bean sprouts
Sunflower seed sprouts	All seed, bean, and grain sprouts

Animal proteins (not recommended):

Milk	Eggs
Cheese (raw milk or unprocessed)	All flesh foods except fat

RECIPES, DIRECTIONS, AND RESOURCES

CHAPTER 42

Sample Meals

Sample Breakfasts

Sunday: strawberry, kiwi and orange smoothie
Saturday: berries of any kind, peaches, apricots
Monday: grapes, pears
Tuesday: watermelon, cantaloupe
Wednesday: fresh ripe pineapple, apple, and peach smoothie
Thursday: papaya, pear
Friday: 1 or 2 grapefruits, plums or nectarines
Saturday: banana, pear, mango and cherry smoothie
Sunday: grapefruit and 2 oranges
Monday: honeydew melon, cantaloupe
Tuesday: mango, pear and peach smoothie
Wednesday: pears, apples
Sunday: grape, banana and cherry smoothie
Monday: Granny Smith apples, grapes
Tuesday: mango, pear and blueberry smoothie
Wednesday: cantaloupe
Thursday: banana, papaya
Friday: strawberries, oranges
Saturday: grapefruit, mango

Sunday: kiwi, peach and pear smoothie
Monday: grapes, fresh berries
Tuesday: banana, pear, dates
Wednesday: oranges, papaya
Thursday: strawberry, kiwi and cherry smoothie
Thursday: fresh pineapple
Friday: plums, apricots, organic raisins
Friday: kiwi fruit, oranges
Saturday: honey dew melon, mango

Sample Lunches

Try to have a raw lunch if possible.
Prepare the night before if working.

Sunday: salad, avocado, tomatoes
Monday: salad, pecans, cucumbers
Tuesday: salad, tomatoes, Ezekiel 4:9 tortilla
Wednesday: finger food, bell peppers, cucumbers,
    cherry tomatoes, celery
Thursday: grapefruit, almonds
Friday: salad, sprouts (alfalfa or other choice),
    tomatoes, raw cauliflower
Saturday: salad, avocado, tomatoes, Ezekiel
    4:9 tortilla with guacamole dip
Sunday: homemade humus with assorted vegetables
Sunday: Waldorf salad with romaine lettuce
Monday: guacamole dip with celery stalks and romaine lettuce
Tuesday: marinated vegetable salad with Ezekiel 4:9 tortilla
Wednesday: salad, raw almond slices
Thursday: salad, English peas, raw broccoli, avocado
Monday: salad, raw zucchini, squash, tomatoes, raw cashews
Tuesday: marinated vegetable salad with Ezekiel 4:9 tortilla
Wednesday: finger foods, bell peppers, cherry or
    grape tomatoes, celery, cucumbers
Thursday: Waldorf salad with romaine lettuce

Friday: salad, tomatoes, Ezekiel 4:9 tortillas
Friday: salad, tomatoes, avocado, Ezekiel 4:9 tortilla
Saturday: salad with walnuts, flax oil, and lemon
Saturday: bowl of chopped assorted vegetables

Sample Dinners

This is your 15 percent cooked portion of
the day. Don't forget your enzymes.

Sunday: salad, mushroom stuffing
Monday: salad, steamed or baked potatoes,
    steamed vegetable of choice
Tuesday: salad, steamed vegetables, wild sage rice
Wednesday: salad, vegetarian vegetable chili
Thursday: salad, Ezekiel 4:9 English muffins
Friday: salad with vegan cheese or almond
    cheese, sliced raw almonds
Saturday: salad, leftover vegetarian chili
Sunday: salad, bowl of cut-up vegetables, raw vegan humus
Monday: salad, vegan corn bread, steamed vegetables
Tuesday: salad, raw vegan pizza
Wednesday: salad, vegetarian stir-fry
Thursday: salad, steamed vegetables or leftover stir-fry
Friday: salad, potato salad
Saturday: salad, steamed vegetables, dinner bread choice
Sunday: salad, eggplant parmesan
Monday: salad, steamed vegetables
Tuesday: salad, pasta salad
Wednesday: salad, quick raw tomato soup
Thursday: salad, salsa with vegetables, Ezekiel 4:9 tortilla
Friday: salad, Mexican black bean salad
Saturday: salad, steamed vegetables

CHAPTER 43

Recipes

Some of the recipes in this book do violate the ideal food-combining principles. But for those who are not fighting a serious illness, an occasional, less-than-perfect combination can be had without any ill effects. Spend the next few days eating more combinable meals.

Mother Nature has made some mis-combinations, foods that are a starch and a protein. These include lentils, black beans, navy beans, kidney beans, garbanzo beans (chickpeas), peas, as well as other beans that I didn't mention. The stomach treats them as one food. It simply digests the starch first, then the protein. So this is different from eating meat and potatoes. When eating beans, it is wise not to eat any starches with them; vegetables or huge tossed salads are a wiser choice, not interrupting the digestive process.

The desserts and sweet breads are unfortunately very mis-combined and/or can be acid forming. After one has been on a diet free of all chemicals, consisting of fresh whole foods, and the body has gotten into a more healthy alkaline state, one can and will bounce back easier from these so called "healthy desserts." Make sure the next day the meals eaten consist of at least 50 percent high water content foods to help cleanse the digestive system.

Please do eat fruits and vegetables that are in season rather than the eating canned and frozen produce. All canned products are void of their enzymes because they are cooked. Therefore, foods of little water content are not affected by freezing, for example, dried legumes, nuts, seeds, and dried fruits. But the produce that has high water content, when it is frozen, the cell wall bursts and the cell's life is destroyed. Oxidation occurs and the nutrients are lost. The idea of a healthy body is to impact it with the most optimal nutrients to enable healing and good health. So the freshest whole produce available is the only thing the body deserves. Go for flavor. With the exception of homegrown food, fresh organics are the most flavorful. If you don't, you'll be disappointed and will continue to overeat until your mouth is satisfied as well as the stomach. Keep your meals as simple as possible because your foods will be digested with more ease.

In place of honey or maple syrup in some of the recipes, you may substitute xylitol or stevia (not to be confused with Splenda, which is a dangerous poison).

Xylitol can be used for cooking and baking, but stevia is not to be cooked and is used in raw dishes only.

When cooking your foods, use stainless steel pots, pans, and cookware. Never use Teflon or any type of nonstick utensil because the chemicals from them will leach into your foods.

Smoothies

Fruit Smoothie

For each smooth use only 3–4 pieces of fruit per person.
See the food combining charts for the correct combinations
and suggestions to enhance the digestion and
cleansing properties of the body.

Place in a bottom of the blender the softer fruits first: pears, strawberries, oranges, mangoes, kiwi, peach slices. Then put the less juicy fruits on top: bananas, blueberries, cherries, grapes, papayas, apples.

You may add a few frozen cherries, frozen blueberries, frozen peaches or 3–4 ice cubes to make it more chilled, if too thick add a little distilled water to blend.

Blend on low to start then increase after about 10 seconds to high and pulse for 10–20 seconds until smooth.

Pour into glasses, sip slowly, allowing the fruit to mingle with the saliva. Do not *gulp* this down.

Banana-Berry Green Smoothie

(Recipe from Hallelujah Acres)

Green smoothies are a quick and easy way to get
loads of nutrition and to lose weight. Tasty combinations are virtually endless and can be customized to help
with everything from joint pain to low energy.

½ cup strawberries
1 small banana
1 handful of chopped kale or spinach
1 cup distilled water
1 tablespoon of B-Flax-D (Hallelujah Acres
    product: see resources)

Put all in a Tribest Personal Blender (or a regular blender) until a thick smoothie has formed. Experiment with ingredients for a different taste!

Tossed Salad, Suggested Ingredients

Lettuces (greens): romaine, red leaf (a delicate lettuce; don't over-buy), green leaf, spinach, Swiss chard, kale (small amounts as it can be bitter), Chinese cabbage, bok choy, Bibb lettuce, radicchio, red cabbage

Cucumbers: common, English/burpless, pickling cucumbers (large, firm), Persian (these are a small variety)

Sprouts: alfalfa sprouts, bean sprouts, broccoli sprouts, mixed bean sprouts

Mushrooms: white button, cremini, oyster, shiitake, portobello

Other vegetables suggestions: bell peppers, beets, broccoli, carrots, cauliflower, celery, radishes, corn, black olives, tomatoes, (cherry, grape, or other types of tomatoes), onions, (green, purple sweet, Spanish, leeks, or other onion types)

Beans and peas: black beans, garbanzo beans (chickpeas), green peas, other types of beans, there is a variety of different kinds.

Nuts and seeds: a small amount can be added to the salad as long as they are raw and unsalted.

Toss and use sparingly a dressing from the homemade dressing list.

I would not add any fruit to the salad because it will ferment in the stomach because the fruit does not combine well with anything except lettuce and celery.

Keep your salads simple as it aids in optimal digestion.

When buying your lettuces and vegetables, buy enough that you will eat in about four days to keep it at its freshest. When I get home from the store, I wash (I use a small amount of Shaklee's Basic H or Amway's L.O.C. in the water in the kitchen sink; see resources) my lettuces and spin dry. Also I wash the broccoli, cauliflower, and celery, so they are ready to eat and store them in Tupperware containers.

Blended Salads

Here is a wonderful idea from the folks at Hallelujah Acres to get all the nutrients from eating a raw tossed salad without all of the challenges of compromising a weakened digestive system. It may work wonders for those who are in need of extra healing from different digestive health predicaments. Some examples would be inflammatory bowel disease, constipation, gastric band surgery and gastric bypass, as well as dental and mouth surgeries.

Take the ingredients that you would use for your salad, including the homemade dressing or even some organic flaxseed oil and put them into a blender. Blend a few seconds until smooth. Serve immediately as it will start to oxidize. You want it to oxidize in your stomach, not on the counter. Sip it very slowly as you allow each sip to mingle with the saliva in your mouth. This gives you the fiber as well as the raw enzymes and nutrients so desperately needed by the body.

The raw fiber that travels through the digestive system is not the same as the juicing because that fiber has been removed in the juicer. Once the healing of the body has progressed from the blended raw foods then you will be able to go to your regular eating of the salads and meals.

Salads

Pasta Salad

Cook ahead one bag Mrs. Leeper's Organic Rice Vegetable Twists (cook according to manufacturer's directions). Stir into cooked pasta (16 oz. spiral or twist) 1 tablespoon extra-virgin olive oil before putting in the fridge to chill.

Place in fridge to chill until ready to serve. Thaw ahead 1½ cups frozen organic green peas. Place in the fridge until ready to serve. Prepare just before:

>   2–3 stalks of organic celery, diced
>   1 red bell pepper, diced
>   1 cup organic broccoli, chopped
>   1 cup organic cauliflower, chopped
>   1 can low sodium black olives, sliced
>   1 tablespoon Italian seasoning
>   1 teaspoon Redmond Real Salt sea salt
>   Italian basil dressing (see salad dressings recipes)

Place the pasta in a large bowl. Work the pasta apart with your hands as it will stick together. Add the peas and the rest of the vegetables that were prepared ahead of time. Add the Italian seasonings, sea salt, and the Italian basil dressing. Toss lightly to mix. Serve immediately or refrigerate until ready to serve.

Not Your Momma's Potato Salad

Cook ahead 4 medium organic red skin potatoes and 4 organic sweet potatoes, peeled and sliced in big chunks. I steam them just until cooked then allow them to cool a bit. Then I cut them into small bite-size pieces and put in the fridge in a covered bowl until ready to serve.

Thaw ahead:
1 cup of organic frozen peas.

Prepare just before:
1–2 stalks organic chopped celery
1/3 cup each red, green and yellow chopped bell peppers
½ cup organic cucumber chopped, (optional)
¼ cup organic carrot, grated dash of paprika
1 teaspoon Redmond Real Salt Sea salt dressing.

Use the Italian basil dressing, the grapeseed oil-based Vegenaise or the Hallelujah Acres ranch dressing. Place the potatoes in a large bowl. Add the peas and vegetables. Add the salad dressing of choice (keep it light or it will be overwhelming). Add the seasonings to taste. Serve immediately. These salads are the cooked portion of our evening meal served with a regular tossed salad or I have served it when entertaining guests.

Mexican Black Bean Salad

2 cups black beans, canned or soaked
    overnight and cooked fresh.
½ large red bell pepper, chopped
½ large oranges bell pepper, chopped
½ small onion, diced (optional)
1/3–½ bunch fresh cilantro, chopped fine
    through the food processor.
1 can low sodium black olives, sliced in half
1 cob of fresh corn (optional: can use canned corn)

1 medium jicama, chopped into small pieces
1½ cups of vine-ripened fresh tomatoes, chopped
juice of 1 lime
(If you like a kick to this, you may add jalapeno
        pepper or cayenne pepper)

Mix all of the ingredients together, toss with cilantro salad dressing. Serve on shredded romaine lettuce leaves. Serves 4–6.

Note: if you don't like a particular ingredient, leave it out and add one you do like.

Cilantro Salad Dressing

¼ cup fresh squeezed lemon juice
½ to 1 teaspoon ground cumin
1/3 cup extra virgin olive oil first cold pressed (Trader Joe's brand)
½ to 1 teaspoon Real Salt sea salt
1 teaspoon dry Italian basil or 6–8 leaves fresh basil
½ bunch (another ½ from the salad) fresh cilantro

Mix together all the ingredients in a blender until well-blended. Store in a glass jar and refrigerate to allow flavors to blend. To make the salad the night before: mix together all of the salad ingredients *except the tomatoes*. Toss with the dressing. The next day, just before serving, chop the tomatoes and mix into the prepared salad. Toss well. Serve on shredded lettuce leaves.

This salad is of all raw ingredients except the beans. It is great for the evening meal. We have a tossed salad in addition to this one.

Simply Coleslaw

½ medium head shredded green cabbage
½ cup shredded purple cabbage
1 small raw organic carrot (shredded)
grapeseed oil based Vegenaise (just enough to moisten)
Real Salt just to taste (optional)

Mix all the vegetables together in a large bowl and spoon just enough Vegenaise across the top of the salad then mix well to coat all of the salad. Serve immediately.

Waldorf Salad

2 large organic Granny Smith apples, peeled and cored.
2 stalks organic celery
¼–1/3 cup of chopped pecans and walnuts, mixed
¼ teaspoon cloves
¼ teaspoon nutmeg
Grapeseed Vegenaise, just enough to moisten.

Chop the Granny Smith apples and the celery into small pieces and place into a bowl. Add the nuts and the spices mix together with just enough of the Vegenaise to moisten. Serve on romaine lettuce leaves. This can be a wonderful lunch.

Sweet and Sour Marinated Vegetable Salad

juice of one lemon
juice of one lime
1 squirt stevia
1 ½ cups Trader Joe's Extra Virgin Cold Pressed Olive Oil
1 teaspoon Redmond Real Salt sea salt
½ cup xylitol

Blend all ingredients together in a blender for about 30 seconds until mixed.

Store in a glass bottle in the refrigerator. It can also be used as a salad dressing for regular tossed salads as well as for the marinated vegetable salad.

Then chop equal amounts of organic broccoli and cauliflower. Place in glass bowl along with some organic cherry or grape tomatoes. Pour sweet and sour dressing all over mix. Cover and refrigerate overnight. Serve with salad or over lettuce leaves as a lunch.

Salad Dressings

Dressings that will make your salads sing. These salad dressings do not have preservatives so they will store for about a week in the fridge; the lemon and oil ones a little bit longer. These are all fresh and homemade, a delight to the palate.

Russian Dressing

(Makes 1½ cups)

3 organic dates soaked for 20 minutes in distilled
    water (or squirt liquid stevia for sweetness)
1 cup chopped vine-ripened tomato
½ cup first cold-pressed organic extra virgin olive oil
½ cup fresh squeezed lemon juice
½ teaspoon Redmond Real Salt sea salt
1 teaspoon paprika
1 clove chopped garlic

Combine all ingredients in a blender and blend until smooth. Store in a glass bottle and refrigerate. This one tastes like the Big Boy Restaurant tomato-spice/French dressing. I add a scoop or so as needed of Sunrider's herbal Nuplus for thickening.

Italian Basil Dressing

(Makes 1 cup)

1½–2 cups first cold-pressed organic extra virgin olive oil **
½ cup fresh squeezed lemon juice
¼ teaspoon Redmond Real Salt sea salt
¼ cup chopped fresh Italian basil
squirt of liquid stevia (optional if you like a hint of sweetness)
Combine all ingredients in a blender and blend until smooth. Store in a glass bottle and refrigerate.

Green Goddess Dressing

(Makes 2 cups)

1 organic avocados, pitted and peeled
½ to ¾ cup distilled water
¼ teaspoon fresh squeezed lemon juice
1 teaspoon Redmond Real Salt sea salt

Combine all ingredients in a blender and blend until smooth. Store in a glass bottle and refrigerate.

French Dressing

(Makes 2 cups)

3 organic dates, soaked for 20 minutes in distilled water (or 1 squirt of liquid stevia for sweetness [optional])
1½ cups first cold-pressed organic extra virgin olive oil**
2/3 cups fresh squeezed lemon juice
½ teaspoon celery seeds
½ teaspoon paprika
¼–½ cup fresh chopped basil (try different varieties to see which you like best)
1 teaspoon Redmond Real Salt sea salt

Combine ingredients in a blender and blend until smooth. Store in a glass jar and refrigerate. The previous recipes are altered recipes from *Rawsome* by Brigitte Mars.

**I use Spectrum brand or Trader Joe's first cold-pressed extra virgin olive oil (the latter one is not organic though). These are the only two that do not harden during storage in the fridge.

Hallelujah Acres Café Signature Ranch Dressing

1 part distilled water
3 parts grapeseed oil-based Vegenaise

customizable herb blend (any combination of dill weed,
oregano, thyme, basil, marjoram: start with
¼ teaspoon and build from there)
dehydrated or fresh chopped parsley (for color)

Combine all ingredients in a bowl whisk thoroughly. Store in glass jar and refrigerator. This is a variation of an Hallelujah Acres website recipe.

These salad dressings do not have preservatives, so they will store for about a week in the fridge. The lemon and oil ones a little bit longer. These are all fresh and homemade, a delight to the palate.

Sweet and Sour Dressing

juice of one lemon
juice of one lime
1 squirt stevia
1½ cup Trader Joe's first cold-pressed extra virgin olive oil
1 teaspoon Redmond Real Salt sea salt
½ cup xylitol

Blend all ingredients together in a blender for about 30 seconds until mixed. Store in a glass bottle and refrigerate. It can also be used as a salad dressing for regular tossed salads as well as for the marinated vegetable salad

Cilantro Salad Dressing

¼ cup freshly squeezed lemon juice
½ to 1 teaspoon ground cumin
1/3 cup extra virgin olive oil first cold pressed (Trader Joe's brand)
½ to 1 teaspoon Real Salt sea salt
1 teaspoon dry Italian basil or 6–8 leaves fresh basil
½ bunch (the other ½ from the salad)
fresh cilantro leaves

Mix together all the ingredients in a blender until well blended. Store in a glass jar and refrigerate overnight to allow flavors to blend. Use for Mexican bean salad, or if you'd like, a Mexican tasting tossed salad. For use as a regular salad dressing, use 1 cup of oil instead of 1/3 cup.

Dips and Sauces

Raw Vegan Hummus

(A variation of a recipe from the Hallelujah Acres website)

16 oz. can garbanzo beans (drained and rinsed)
3 tablespoons almond butter
¼ cup lemon juice (freshly squeezed)
1 tablespoon extra virgin olive oil
1 medium garlic cloves (peeled)
1 teaspoon Redmond Real Salt sea salt
¼ teaspoon ground cumin
pinch of cayenne or white pepper
garnish with freshly chopped parsley leaves
    and shake of paprika (optional)

In a food processor with the S blade in place and running, drop the garlic into the chute and run until minced. With the machine still running, place the garbanzo beans into the chute. Then add the lemon juice, olive oil, almond butter, and seasonings.

Process until well mixed and creamy. Transfer to serving bowl and add garnishes. Cover and refrigerate until ready to serve.

Guacamole

In a bowl, mash with a fork one ripe (soft but not mushy) avocado. Add to that 1 vine-ripened tomato, chopped finely; 1 tablespoon onion, chopped finely; and ¼ to ½ teaspoon Redmond Real Salt sea salt. Mix well. This makes a very nice lunch. Instead of serving the chips and sour cream, which tends to only upset the stomach, serve this dip with crisp organic romaine lettuce and organic celery stalks, or other cut vegetables.

Yummy Pasta Sauce

6 organic sundried tomatoes soaked for 1 hour
6 large Roma tomatoes
6 fresh basil leaves
¼ cup chopped onion
¼ cup chopped mushrooms
½ tablespoon minced or chopped garlic clove
1 teaspoon fresh oregano or ½ teaspoon, dried
1 teaspoon sea salt
1 tablespoon extra virgin olive oil or unsalted organic butter

Sauté the onion, garlic, and mushrooms in the oil or butter until tender. Add the first four ingredients to the food processor. Pulse until chunky.

Add the mushroom mixture to the food processor and pulse 20–30 seconds. Serve on top of pasta or polenta.

There are so many variations to this sauce, cooked or all raw. Have fun and enjoy.

Tomato Salsa

(A Hallelujah Acres recipe)

4 cups chopped tomatoes
1 seeded jalapeno peppers
3 garlic cloves, finely minced
1 onion
½ cup cilantro leaves
½ cup fresh basil
2 limes, juiced
2 teaspoons sea salt (optional)
1 tablespoon ground cumin

1 tablespoon chili powder
1 red pepper, seeded
1 cup sundried tomatoes, soaked in warm
    purified water (for 1 hour)

Place garlic in food processor and chop into small pieces. Add jalapenos, cilantro, basil, lime juice, salt, cumin, and chili powder into the food processor and chop until very fine. Pour this mixture into the bowl with the chopped tomatoes.

Place red pepper in the processor, chop fine, and add to the tomato mixture. Place the onion in the processor, chop fine and add to the tomato mixture. Place the sundried tomatoes in the food processor and chop until smooth like tomato paste. Stir the sundried tomatoes with the salsa mixture.

This is better after the flavors have blended for a couple of hours. It has a shelf life of 7–10 days.

This recipe was evaluated, tested, and in some cases, altered by an evaluation team of friends and coworkers (since I am not a salsa fan). It came out an overwhelming success from the consensus of the team.

(According to many of the evaluators, this recipe offers a lot of flexibility. They claim it's even better made the day before or as leftovers.)

Marinara Sauce

(A revised Hallelujah Acres recipe)

12 sundried organic tomato halves
4–5 organic pitted dates
2–3 fresh vine-ripened tomatoes
¼ sweet red onion
¼ cup tomato soaked in water
1 clove garlic
¼ cup extra virgin olive oil
1 tablespoon fresh squeezed lemon juice
1 teaspoon Redmond Real Salt sea salt

2–3 white button mushrooms, cleaned,
    washed, and sliced (optional)
½ teaspoon oregano
1 teaspoon dried basil (or ½ cup fresh basil)
pinch of white pepper (optional)

Presoak sundried tomatoes and dates in distilled/purified water for at least 1 hour before using. Steam the chopped onion and garlic in a little purified water before putting in the blender with the tomatoes (unless you like them raw). Reserve ¼ cup of the soak water.

For smooth sauce, puree all ingredients together in blender except the herbs. Mix in the herbs and allow the sauce to sit for at least 1 hour before serving. For a chunky sauce, coarsely chop fresh tomatoes in the food processor then set aside in a bowl.

Process rest of the ingredients until it is as smooth as possible then mix into the bowl with the tomatoes. Mix in the mushroom slices into the sauce. Allow to sit for at least 1 hour before serving. For a thicker sauce, leave out the water for soaking.

You can substitute 3 cups of cherry tomatoes or 5–6 Roma tomatoes for the 2–3 fresh vine-ripened tomatoes. This is an amazingly great sauce.

Main Entrees

The cooked portions of the evening meal

Vegetarian Chili

1 tablespoon extra virgin olive oil
1 large chopped onion
2 bay leaves
1 teaspoon cumin
2 tablespoons dried oregano
2 jalapeno peppers, seeded and diced fine
    (optional if you like it spicy)
3 cloves of peeled and minced garlic

4 cups chopped small vine-ripened fresh tomatoes
    (approximately 16–20 small to medium tomatoes)
1 tablespoon Celtic or Redmond Real Salt Sea salt (or to taste)
2 diced celery stalks
2 diced red bell peppers
1 tablespoon chili powder (to taste)
⅛ teaspoon white pepper or cayenne pepper (to taste)
3 large fresh cobs of corn (cut off the cob)
1 15-ounce can garbanzo beans
1 15-ounce can black beans
1 15-ounce can kidney beans (I use ½ to ¾ cup each of fresh
    beans, soaked overnight and then cooked for 45 minutes.
    The fresher ingredients, the better the chili tastes.)

Start cooking the beans if using fresh and cut up all of the vegetables. Heat olive oil in a very large pot over medium heat. Stir in the onions and garlic until soft and onion is clear in color. Stir in the seasonings with the bay leaves and salt. Then stir in the celery, bell peppers, jalapeno (if using).

Cover, reduce heat to low, and simmer for 5 minutes. Add tomatoes and beans. Bring to a boil. Reduce heat to a low simmer for 30 minutes. Stir in the corn and simmer for another 15 minutes.

Serve with a huge tossed salad. The freshest ingredients make this a tantalizing meal and a tummy warmer on cold winter nights. It tastes even better as a leftover.

Vegetarian Stir-Fry

(A variation of a Hallelujah Acres recipe)

You can use one or all of the vegetables listed below in the order given. It's best to have all the vegetables prepared just beforehand and ready to go.

In a large wok, stainless steel frying pan, or stainless Dutch oven pan, heat ¼–½ cup distilled water with 1/3 teaspoon ground or grated fresh ginger. Add 1 small chopped onion. Stir for 5 minutes then add 1 cup each:

chopped organic broccoli
chopped organic cauliflower
sliced or grated organic carrots
snow pea pods
jicama (optional)

Steam for about 5 minutes. Cover then add 1/3 cup each of organic celery, sweet bell peppers, red, yellow, and green slivered almonds.

Stir and add 1 cup sliced mushrooms and 1 teaspoon sea salt to taste.

Cover and continue to steam for 3 more minutes or until the mushrooms are just slightly cooked. The vegetables should have a little bit of crispness to them. Serve with wild sage rice, which has been cooking ahead of time. (Start the rice at least 35 minutes before the stir-fry).

Wild Sage Rice

In a medium stainless steel pot with a tight-fitting lid, put in 2¼ cups distilled water, 1 tablespoon of rubbed sage (ground sage), and 1 cup wild brown rice. Let this come to a boil, stir, and cover (do not peek) for 45 minutes on very low heat. When done, fluff with fork and serve.

I sometimes stir in ¼ cup each chopped broccoli, celery, and mushrooms about 6–8 minutes before the rice is done, and at that time if it needs it, you may add a little more water. This is a wonderful side dish to compliment the meal. Serve with a large tossed salad.

Mushroom Stuffing

This is a great way to have Thanksgiving year-round (6–8 servings).

approximately 25 medium-sized white button mushrooms (may use a combination of different varieties), cleaned and washed, cut into quarters.
1 small chopped organic onion

3 stalks sliced organic celery
3 tablespoons organic unsalted butter
1 tablespoon ground sage
1 teaspoon Redmond Real Salt sea salt
½ cup distilled or purified water
8 slices Ezekiel 4:9 Sprouted Whole Grain Bread or Rice Bread
    Gluten Free cut into small cubes and placed in a large
    bowl. Set aside.

In a food processor, place part of the mushrooms and process until uniformly chopped. Place in a bowl. Set aside. Continue processing all of the mushrooms in the same manner.

In a large stainless steel frying pan, melt the butter and add the chopped onions and celery; sauté for 5 minutes until the onions are translucent. Add the processed mushrooms to the frying pan along with the sage and sea salt. Stir until mixed well. Cover and place on low heat for about 10 minutes and add the distilled water (if you like a moister stuffing add more water; drier, less). Heat 1 minute more. Pour the mushroom mixture over the bread cubes and mix until well combined. Serve with a large tossed salad.

Note: If you don't like mushrooms, add 3 or 4 extra celery stalks instead or zucchini in place of the mushrooms.

Eggplant Parmesan

(A revised Hallelujah Acres recipe)

1 peeled eggplant, sliced into ½» to 1" rounds
1 teaspoon extra virgin olive oil
1 jar organic marinara sauce (or homemade:
    see marinara sauce recipe)
1–2 minced garlic cloves
½ onion, cut into rings
non-casein, non-soy veggie cheese (try Vegan Rella) or use
    almond cheese mozzarella style (for transition cooking)
Distilled or purified water

Steam garlic and onion in a small amount of distilled water until tender. Set aside. Sauté eggplant in olive oil until lightly brown and tender on both sides.

Cover the bottom of a baking dish with a small amount of marinara sauce. Make sure that the pan is large enough to hold the eggplant without it overlapping.

Place eggplant in pan and top with more sauce to cover the eggplant. Place the onion and garlic on top of the eggplant then cover with the rest of the marinara sauce. Once covered with sauce, top with grated veggie cheese or almond cheese. Bake at 400–450ºF for 15–25 minutes (covered) or until the sauce bubbles.

Raw Vegan Pizza

The pizza dough yields enough dough for 2 large pizzas.

1 cup plus 2 tablespoons warm water (105ºF–110ºF)
1½ tablespoon olive oil
3 1/3 cup unbleached flour
½ teaspoon sea salt
1½ organic sugar
1 teaspoons dry yeast

This can be made in a bread maker by placing the ingredients into the bread machine pan in order listed or the old-fashioned way, mixing it by hand like your grandma used to, kneading it and letting it rise before cooking.

If using the bread machine, place the pan of ingredients into the machine and close the lid. Process on the pizza dough cycle (cycle takes 1 hour). When the cycle is finished, remove the dough and form into a ball. For each pizza, roll one ball of dough on lightly floured surface into a 14-inch circle, slightly less than ¼ inch thick. Sprinkle corn meal evenly over a large cookie sheet or pizza pan. (Do not use Teflon pans as they have chemicals to contaminate your food). Transfer dough to a cookie sheet. Place in warm oven (175ºF) for about 20–30 minutes until it has risen. Then take out of the oven and preheat oven to 450ºF.

Place the pans in hot oven for about 10–15 minutes until just slightly golden (alter your cooking time if the crust is too well cooked). Remove from oven and cover each with red pepper sauce. Sprinkle oregano and chopped vegetables generously. Place back in hot oven for 5 minutes just to slightly heat the vegetables. Serve immediately with a large tossed salad.

Red pepper sauce: Take 2–3 medium to large red peppers. Chop in a food processor until ground. Place in a blender until fine and smooth. Set aside.

Some vegetable suggestions: chopped bell peppers (use different ones to add color: orange, green, yellow, and red), sliced or chopped mushrooms, sliced black or green olives (low sodium only), chopped fresh basil leaves, chopped onions, and chopped spinach leaves.

You may get creative and add other vegetables that you like. The main thing about this pizza is that it is very digestible, easy on the stomach, and assimilates well. You won't go back to the comfort foods again because those will make you feel loaded down and miserable. You will definitely experience the difference.

Quick Raw Tomato Soup

(Approximately 2 vine-ripened fresh tomatoes per person)

¼ teaspoon fennel (I use fresh fennel caplets; see resources)
dash of Redmond Real Salt sea salt to taste
1 thinly sliced onion (optional)

Place these ingredients into a blender (I use a Vitamix Blender as it just heats the soup as it's blending).

Blend for at least 5 minutes. This soup can be served slightly heated or chilled.

While it's blending, chop the vegetables and place in a large bowl.

For a tomato Florentine, place chopped spinach leaves on the bottom with chopped tomatoes and red pepper.

Other vegetable suggestions: use chopped broccoli, cucumber, celery or shredded zucchini, chopped or sliced fresh avocado. Serve with a tossed salad and Ezekiel 4:9 Sprouted Grain Tortillas.

Dessert Breads

Zucchini Bread

(Makes 2 loaves)

5 egg whites, slightly beaten
2 cups xylitol and/or organic sugar
2 cups shredded zucchini
1 teaspoon Redmond Real Salt sea salt
1 teaspoon baking soda
1 teaspoon aluminum-free baking powder
1 cup extra virgin olive oil or organic coconut oil
2 teaspoons vanilla
3 cups unbleached flour
½ cup chopped walnuts
2 teaspoons cinnamon
½ teaspoon nutmeg
¼ teaspoon cloves
½ to ¾ organic raisins

Heat oven to 325ºF. Place parchment paper or grease (bottoms only) of two loaf pans 9" x 5" or 8" x 4". In large bowl, slightly beat egg whites, xylitol, zucchini, oil, and vanilla. Add remaining ingredients. Blend well by hand. Pour batter into prepared pans. Bake at 325º F for 50–60 minutes or until toothpick comes out clean. Cool for 10 minutes.

Hallelujah Acres Date Nut Bread

1 cup organic pitted whole dates, cut into pieces
1 cup organic raisins
1½ cups boiling distilled water
1 cup unbleached flour
1 cup whole wheat flour

1 teaspoon baking soda
1 teaspoon aluminum-free baking powder
2 slightly beaten egg whites
1 teaspoon vanilla
½ cup chopped pecans

Place cut dates and raisins in small bowl. Pour boiling water over them. Set aside to cool. Meanwhile, in a large bowl, stir together flour, baking soda and powder. Stir in pecans. Add vanilla to egg whites and blend.

Add dates and raisin mixture to the egg whites; stir until well blended. Mixture should be thick. Spread lightly into a 9" x 5" x 3" pan lined with parchment paper. Bake at 350ºF for 35–40 minutes or until it tests done. Cool in pan for 10 minutes. Remove from pan and cool on wire rack. Best wrap and store overnight before serving.

Banana Nut Bread

1/3 cup organic unsalted softened butter
½ cup Xylitol
3 organic egg whites
1¾ cups unbleached flour
1 teaspoon aluminum-free baking powder
½ teaspoon baking soda
½ teaspoon Redmond Real Salt sea salt
1 cup mashed organic ripe bananas
½ cup chopped walnuts

Mix together the butter and the xylitol, add egg whites and beat well. Stir together the dry ingredients; add to the creamed mixture alternating with the bananas, blending well after each addition. Stir in the nuts. Pour into a parchment paper-lined 9' x 5' x 3" loaf pan. Bake in moderate oven (350ºF), 50–60 minutes or until a toothpick poked in center it should come out clean. Test to determine if it's done. Remove from pan, cool on wire rack for 30 minutes. Wrap and store in the fridge.

Dinner Breads

Many people seem to have a hard time not eating their breads. Too much grain, especially in improper combinations, is hard on the digestive system. Breads are very addicting and can be acid forming. My suggestion is to have your breads only with a vegetable meal. We gave up eating any refined wheat and have been enjoying Ezekiel 4:9 Sprouted Whole Grain Bread products (see resources). They have a very special and unique method in their baking process. I had problems with gluten and the sprouting process seems to be much kinder on my body.

Suggestions:

Food for Life, The Original 100% Flourless Ezekiel 4:9
*New Mexico Style Sprouted Grain Tortillas
*Sprouted 100 percent Whole Grain Bread (sliced bread)
*Sprouted Grain English Muffins

The English muffins and the loaf of bread come in a variety of different flavors.

Vegan Corn Bread

(Revised recipe from *Totally Vegetarian* by Toni Fiore)

1 cup unbleached whole wheat flour (if you have allergies, use rice flour)
½ cup organic yellow cornmeal, fine or medium
½ cup white grits or Masarepa (fine white cornmeal) or yellow grits ground fine in a clean coffee grinder.
½ teaspoons aluminum-free baking powder
¼ cup extra virgin olive oil
1 tablespoons organic evaporated cane sugar
1 teaspoon Redmond Real Salt sea salt
1 cup plus 1 tablespoon warm purified or distilled water

Don't expect this corn bread to rise like regular corn bread made with eggs, but do expect the lovely, golden squares to be moist and very flavorful. For a variation, you may add one of the following: chopped scallions or chives, 1 tablespoon jalapeno pepper, or Italian seasoning.

Preheat the oven to 350°F. Line an 8" x 8" square baking pan, or a 9" pie dish with parchment paper. Mix the flour, cornmeal, grits, and baking powder in a bowl. In a separate bowl, whisk together 1 cup and 1 tablespoon warm water, the oil, sugar, and salt along with any combination of seasonings (like the chives, scallions, jalapeno or Italian seasoning). Add the liquid ingredients to the dry and mix by hand with a wooden spoon just until everything is blended. Be careful not to overmix as it will create a heavy, dense bread.

Pour the batter into the prepared pan and bake for about 30 minutes or until a knife inserted into the center of the corn bread comes out clean; over-baking will make it dry and crumbly. Serve warm or at room temperature.

Note: You may spread very lightly with organic virgin coconut oil (optional).

Desserts

Raw Chocolate Cake

This delicious chocolate cake is really tasty for a wannabe. It's rich and very easy to make, especially when you are craving a chocolate cake and don't want to blow your body out of whack. It's made from raw ingredients, of which the main ingredients of walnuts and dates are rich sources of vitamins and minerals. It's not on the combinable list, but an *occasional* splurge after your body is back into health, should be okay.

Fit your food processor with the S blade. Put in 1½ cup of raw walnuts and a dash of salt into the processor and process the mixture until finely ground. Add 10 pitted Medjool dates, 1/3 cup raw carob powder, and ½ teaspoon vanilla extract or 1 teaspoon raw vanilla powder (the vanilla is optional). Process until the ingredients are combined and are stuck together.

Add 2 teaspoons distilled water. Process briefly.

Transfer to a plate and form a 5-inch round cake with your hands or with a mold. Place in the fridge until ready to serve.

Sometimes people will like to add things to the cake like toppings because they are so used to having their "cake with its frosting" and this one doesn't have that, so don't be tempted. Old habits can be very hard to break. If you just have to, and only on your birthday, put raspberries or sliced strawberries on it just before serving.

Super Power Balls

This recipe was taken from the book *Rawsome* by Brigette Mars, but I perfected it to make it taste like Chunkie candies (for those who remember these delights).

> ½ cup raw sunflower seeds
> ½ cup chopped fine pecan halves
> ½ cup–¾ cup raw carob powder
> ½ cup each fresh ground almond butter and raw organic tahini
> ¾–1 cup organic pitted dates soaked in distilled water for 20 minutes then pureed in a food processor
> 1 teaspoon vanilla extract
> ½ teaspoon cinnamon
> ½ cup organic raisins
> 1 cup raw almonds ground fine for rolling the balls in (optional)
> ½ cup each organic unsweetened coconut and almonds ground together. Please be careful not to grind them too long as they will become oily and clump together; they just need to be powdery.

In a large bowl, combine the sunflower seeds, chopped pecans, carob powder, raisins, and the cinnamon. Mix and set aside.

Next, place the dates in the food processor and puree them then add the almond butter, the tahini, and the vanilla until mixed. Add the date mixture to the nut mixture and mix well with your hands until uniformly mixed. Shape into 1–1½ inch balls. Roll in the ground almonds (coconut) and place in a single layer with waxed paper between each layer in a freezer container.

These may be stored in the freezer or refrigerator.

I freeze them for at least 24 hours then leave them in the fridge, so they are chilled but soft enough to have great flavor.

Raw Apple Pie

This recipe is also an altered creation from *Rawsome* and is a winning delight for all of my guests and at parties.

Crust:
1 cup raw almonds
1 cup pecan halves
1½ cups organic pitted dates (soaked in
    distilled water for 20 minutes)

Filling:
¾ cup organic raisins (soaked in distilled water for
¾ cup organic/pitted dates (soaked in
    distilled water for 20 minutes)
5 large organic Gala or Fuji apples, peeled and chopped
1 organic banana, peeled and sliced 20 minutes)
1 teaspoon cinnamon
1 squirt liquid stevia added for extra sweetness (optional)
2 scoops of Sunrider Nuplus apple cinnamon flavor or
    plain (optional, I use it to make a firmer pie)

To make the crust: Combine the pecans and almonds in the food processor, pulse just until chopped, about 10 seconds or so, then add the ¾ cup dates and pulse until evenly ground and mixed. Place the mixture into a glass pie plate.

To make the filling: Place the dates, raisins, apples, cinnamon, and stevia in the food processor, run until the mixture is chopped and pureed. Add the banana and continue to puree until the mixture looks like applesauce. Add the Nuplus until it's mixed.

To finish: spoon the filling into the piecrust. Refrigerate for 1 day before serving for optimal texture and flavor.

Pooh Bear Ice Cream

This is an excellent dairy-less ice cream that everyone will love. It has pure, fresh ingredients and the one that Pooh Bear loves, honey.

> 4 cups chopped fresh strawberries (the more
>   you use, the fruitier the flavor)
> 1 1/4 cup raw cashews
> 2 cups distilled water
> ½ cup raw clover honey
> teaspoon nonalcoholic vanilla or 1/3 of
>   ground vanilla bean (optional)

Blend all of the above ingredients in the blender until very smooth. Pour into a Tupperware freezer bowl big enough to have stirring room. (This can be put into an ice cream maker.) For those who do not have an ice cream maker, place in the freezer for about 4 hours. Take it out and stir it (this procedure adds air so the ice cream will come out scoopable, not hard). Continue this regime every 2–3 hours throughout the day. Use a kitchen timer to remind yourself. The ice cream will start to become thicker as it freezes longer. When it becomes very frozen and thick, do one last stir and then place it back into the freezer and ignore it until the next day. Then enjoy.

Variations: use different fruits; peaches, blueberries, pitted cherries, etc.

Vanilla Ice Cream

(Makes about 1 quart; revised from a
Hallelujah Acres recipe)

2 vanilla beans (or 2 teaspoon nonalcoholic vanilla flavor)
2 cups organic raw cashews or cashew pieces

2 cups purified water
¾–1 cup pure maple syrup

Blend all of the above ingredients in the blender until very smooth. Pour into a Tupperware freezer bowl big enough to have stirring room. (This can be put into an ice cream maker.) For those who do not have an ice cream maker, place in the freezer for about 4 hours, take it out and stir it, (this procedure adds air so the ice cream will come out scoopable, not hard). Continue this regimen every 2–3 hours throughout the day. Use a kitchen timer to remind yourself. The ice cream will start to become thicker as it freezes longer. When it becomes very frozen and thick, do one last stir and then place it back into the freezer and ignore it until the next day. Then enjoy.

40-Carat Cookies

½ cup distilled water
½ cup organic raisins
½ raw honey
½ cup extra virgin olive oil
1 teaspoon cinnamon
2½ cups unbleached flour (or 1¼ each unbleached
 and whole wheat flour or use rice flour or
 gluten-free flour to avoid allergies)
1 teaspoon fresh squeezed lemon juice 1
 cup organic carrots, grated
½ teaspoon each: nutmeg, cloves, allspice
teaspoon vanilla
2 egg whites
1½ non-aluminum baking powder
½ teaspoon baking soda
½ teaspoon Redmond Real Salt sea salt

Preheat oven to 350ºF. Pour water over the raisins, soak for 20 minutes. Drain then set aside.

Beat honey, oil, egg whites, vanilla, and lemon juice. Stir in the carrots and raisins.

In a separate bowl, mix together the flour, baking powder, baking soda, sea salt, and seasonings. Combine with the honey-egg white mixture. Mix until well blended.

Drop by teaspoonful onto a parchment-paper-lined cookie sheets.

Bake at 350°for about 10–15 minutes until golden. Makes about 40 cookies. Store in a Tupperware container in the fridge.

(This recipe is revised one of an old recipe *The Richard Simmons Show* on TV.) Looking for other healthy cookie recipes, log onto the www.hacres.com/recipes website.

Resources

Hallelujah Acres
Website: www.hacres.com
Address: PO Box 2388, Shelby, NC 28151
Phone: USA. 800-915-9355
Canada. 866-478-2224
(BarleyMax, health tips, and recipes)

VP Nutrition
Website: www.vpnutrition.com
E-mail: info@vpnutrition.com
Phone: USA. 877-335-1509

Sunrider International
Phone: 310-222-6363 USA
(Nu Plus Herbal food, Sunnydew liquid stevia from recipes)

Self-Health Resources Chula Vista, CA 91911 USA
Phone: 800-837-1663
(Vitamin C powder to use with organic healthy lotions for sunscreen, non-aluminum baking powder, and fresh herbal caplets)

Redmond Minerals Inc.
Website: www.realsalt.com
Address: Redmond Real Salt, Redmond, UT 84652 USA
Phone: 800-367-7258

Burt's Bees
Website: www.burtsbees.com
Address: PO Box 13489, Durham, NC 27709 USA
(Natural personal care items)

Aloe Life International
Website: www.aloelife.com
Phone: 800-414-2563 USA
(Healthy body lotion)

Answers from Nature
Address: PO Box 139, Gardenia, CA 90248
Phone: 877-550-9600 USA
(Healing Springs Body Lotion)

Food for Life Baking Company
Website: www.foodforlife.com
Email: info@foodforlife.com
Address: PO Box 1434, Corona, CA 92878-1434
Phone: 800-797-5090 USA
(Ezekiel Sprouted Grain Bread Products)

Trader Joe's
Phone: 800-746-7857
Address: West Coast, PO Box 5049, Monrovia CA 91017
East Coast, 117 Fredrick St., Suite 700, Needham, MA 02494
(Cold pressed extra virgin olive oil)

Spectrum Organic Products LLC
Website: www.spectrumorganics.com
Address: Melville, NY 11747 USA
Phone: 800-343-7833
(Organic cold-pressed extra virgin olive oil)

Enzymedica
Website: www.enzymedica.com
Address: 752 Tamiami Trail, Port Charlotte, FL 33953
Phone: 800-918-1118 USA
(Digest enzymes taken with cooked meals)

Shaklee Corporation
Website: www.shaklee.com
Address: 4747 Willow Road, Pleasanton, CA 94588
Phone: 800-SHAKLEE USA
(Basic H Organic Cleaner and organic laundry soaps)

Amway Corporation
Phone: 800-253-6500 USA
(L.O.C. Organic Cleaner, laundry soaps)

Tupperware
Website: www.tupperware.com
Phone: 800-TUPWARE USA
(Storage containers)

DeBoles Consumer Relations
Websites::www.deboles.com; www.glutenfreechoices.com
Address: 4600 Sleepytime Drive, Boulder, CO 80301
Phone: 800-434-4246 USA
(Gluten-frees pastas and other healthy choice pastas)

Dr. Bronner's Magic Soaps Website: www.drbronner.com
Address: PO Box 28, Escondido, CA 92033
Phone: 760-743-2211 USA
(Pure organic Castile bar and liquid bath soaps)

World Finer Foods Inc.
Website: www.worldfiner.com
Address: Bloomfield, NJ 07003 USA
(Mrs. Leeper's Organic Vegetable Twists; gluten/ wheat free)

Orange-Sol Household Products Inc.
Website: www.orangesol.com
Address: Gilbert, AZ 85233 USA
Phone: 800-877-7771

Go Natural and Organic: Look up safe products
Website: www.safealternative.com

StarWest Botanicals, Inc.
Website: www.starwest-bonticals.com
Address: Rancho Cordova, CA 95742 USA
(Rose water and 100 percent pure Witch Hazel extract)

Website for Alternative Chemical-Free Household Cleaners:
http://www.marksdailyapple.com/natural-cleaners/

Fluoride Free Samples
Clearly Natural Toothpaste (all-natural, fluoride free)
Website: www.clearlynaturalsoaps.com

Tom's of Maine
Website: www.tomsofmaine.com Facebook, Twitter, or watch on
YouTube
(Natural chemical-free and fluoride-free toothpastes; also children's
fluoride-free toothpastes)

JĀSÖN Natural Products: Pure, Natural, and Organic
Website: www.jason-natural.com
Phone: 877-527-6601
(Natural chemical-free and fluoride-free toothpastes)

Which Toothpaste Is the Best?
Free unbiased reviews and top picks toothpaste reviews.
Website: consumersearch.com/toothpaste

Guide of Less Toxic Alternative Cleaners
http://lesstoxicguide.ca/index.asp?household

Books

Toxic Free by Debra Lynn
Dadd Publisher, Penguin Group

The Pantry Cleaner by Mysti Reutlinger
ISBN 9781456546854

Chemical Free Kids by Allan Magaziner, Linda Bovie, and Anthony Zolezzi
Publisher; Twin Streams Kensington ISBN 07582-0369-1

Chemical Free Kids by Dr. Sarah Lantz, PhD
Publisher: Joshua

The Safe Shopper's Bible: A Consumer's Guide to Nontoxic Household Products, Cosmetics and Foods, by David Steinman

ABC News, http://abcnews.go.comHealth/story?id=1993859.

Adams, Patch, with Mylander, Maureen. Gesundheit! Rochester, VT: Healing Arts, 1998.

Alcoholics Anonymous. Alcoholics Anonymous, 3rd ed. Alcoholics Anonymous World Services, 1976.

Allen, Hannah. "Fasting Does Not Make the Body Disease Proof," Lesson 48, Fasting, Natural Health course, Fit for Life Sciences Institute.

———. "How to Break a Fast." Natural Health course, Fit for Life Sciences Institute.

———. "The Basis of the Food Combining System." Lesson 22, Human Physiology, Anatomy, and Our Dietary Nature, Natural Health course, Fit For Life Sciences Institute.

———. "The Organic Gardening: Avoid Commercially Produced Foods—Why?" Ecological Factors and Their Role in Nutrition, Natural Health course, Fit for Life Sciences Institute.

———. "The Principles of Digestive Physiology Which Decree Correct Food Combining." Lesson 22 of Human Physiology, Anatomy, and Our Dietary Nature, Fit for Life Sciences Institute.

———. "Protein Supplements." Lesson 85 of Getting to Know Other Dietary Schools, Natural Health course, Fit for Life Sciences Institute.

———. "Why We Should Reduce Our Meat Intake." Lesson 32 of Foods Not Suited to the Human Diet, Natural Health course, Fit for Life Sciences Institute.

———. "Overeating, Fasting Fanaticism, and Diet Fanaticism," Lesson 44 of Natural Health course, Fit for Life Sciences Institute.

Anatomical Chart Company. Anatomy and Pathology. 4th ed. Stokie, IL: Lippincott Williams & Wilkins, 2005.

Anderson, Kristina. "Gastoesophageal Reflux Disease." Radiologic Technology 18, no. 4 (January/February, 2010): 251–266.

Appleton, Nancy. "Don't Let Stress in Your Life Become Distress." Hallelujah Acres Diet and Lifestyle 49 (March/April 2008): 18.

Bazell, Robert. Her-2: The Making of Herceptin, a Revolutionary Treatment for Breast Cancer. New York: Random, 1998

Benton, Mike. "Proteins in the Diet," Lesson 8 of The Nutritional Basis of Life, Natural Health course, Fit for Life Sciences Institute.

———. "Fats in Our Diet." Lesson 11, Natural Health course, Fit for Life Sciences Institute.

———. "Organic and Inorganic Minerals." Lesson 10, Natural Health course, Fit for Life Sciences Institute.

———. "Dangers of a High Protein Diet." Lesson 85 of Getting to Know the Other Dietary Schools, Natural Health course, Fit for Life Sciences Institute.

———. "Fermented and Putrefied Foods in the Diet, Studies on Other Junk Foods." Lesson 37 of What's Wrong with Junk Food? Natural Health course, Fit for Life Sciences.

———. "Herbs." Lesson 42 of Harmful Practices to Avoid, Natural Health course, Fit for Life Sciences Institute.

———. "The Harmfulness of Beverages in the Diet." Lesson 34 of Foods Not Suited to the Human Diet, Natural Health course, Fit for Life Sciences Institute.

———. "Symptoms during Dietary Transition." Lesson 21 of Human Physiology, Anatomy, and Our Dietary Nature, Natural Health course, Fit for Life Sciences Institute.

———. "Sociological Benefits and Economic Ramifications of the Avoidance of Junk Foods," Lesson 38 of What's Wrong with Junk Food? Natural Health, Fit for Life Sciences Institute.

———. "Proteins in the Diet." Lesson 8 of The Nutritional Basis of Life, Natural Health course, Fit for Life Sciences Institute.

———. "Stress Management, the Life Science Approach." Lesson 64 of Natural Hygiene: A Better Way of Living, Natural Hygiene course, Fit for Life Sciences Institute.

———. "This Is A Lite Diet." In Junk Foods, Vol. 1, bk. 2 of Fit for Life – The Basic Health Library, 28.

———. "Why Condiments Should Not Be Used in the Diet." Lesson 29 of Foods Not Suited for Life, Natural Health course, Fit for Life Sciences Institute.

————. "Chemicals in the Household Environment." Lesson 51 of Ecological Factors and Their Role in Nutrition, Natural Health course, Fit for Life Sciences Institute.

Berry, Matthew E. "Adrenal Gland Disorders." Radiologic Technology 81, no. 1 (September/October 2009).

Blau, Danniella, and Alisa Scherban. "The Facts on Sugar Substitutes." ScrippsWellness.com. 2010, 1–3.

Blaylock, Russell. "Vaccines, What You Should Know." Hallelujah Acres Health News 59 (January/February 2010): 6–7.

————. Excitotoxins—The Taste That Kills. Albuquerque, NM: Health Press NA, 1997.

Brooks, Austin L. "Pure Water Is Essential to Proper Body Functioning." Lesson 14 of Non-Dietary Factors in Nutrition, Natural Health course, Fit for Life Sciences Institute.

Brooks, Austin. "Water Transports Nutrients to All the Body Cells." Lesson 14 of Non-Dietary Factors In Nutrition, Natural Health course, Fit for Life Sciences Institute.

Calabro, Rose Lee. Living in the Raw. Summertown, TN: Book Publishing Company, 1998.

Campbell, Colin T., and Thomas M. Campbell II. The China Study. Dallas, TX: Benbella Books, 2006.

Challen, Jack. "Medicalizing Life." Let's Live (September 2002): 22.

Charla, Tom. "Diary of a Dad." Living Without, April/May 2009, 10–12.

Cheraskin, E., and Marshall Ringsdorf Jr. New Hope for Incurable Diseases. New York: Exposition Press, 1971.

Chesnut, Dan E. Lying with Authority. Oklahoma City, OK: Restoration Health, 2008.

Church, Elizabeth. "Imaging Diabetes." Radiologic Technology 80, no. 4 (March/April 2009): 340–357.

Cinque, Ralph C. "Nutrition: A Hygienic Perspective." In Vol.1, bk. 2 of Fit for Life – The Basic Health Library, 4.

————. "Devising a Lifestyle That Includes Vigorous Exercise." Lesson 97 of Exercise and Its Role in Healthful Living, Natural Health course, Fit for Life Sciences Institute.

————. "Exercise: A Hygiene Perspective."

———. "Protein." Lesson 8 of Proteins in the Diet, Natural Health course, Fit for Life Sciences Institute.

Clark, Hulda Regehr. The Cure for All Cancers. Chula Vista, CA: New Century, 1993.

Colon-Kidney-Detoxification, (Internet Research Paper), detoxification.htm. Copy. 2/8/2010.

Contreras, Francisco. "Foods That Fight Cancer" Hallelujah Acres Health News 54 (March/April 2009): 7

Cousins, Norman. Anatomy of an Illness as Perceived by the Patient. New York: W.W. Norton, 1979.

Diamond, Harvey. Living without Pain. Osprey, FL: VP Nutrition, 2005.

Divine, Jeanette. "Adrenaline and Stress…Book Review." Hallelujah Acres Diet and Lifestyle 49, (March/April 2008): 13–14.

Donaldson, Michael, and Olin Idol. "ADD/ADHD: Are There Alternatives to Drugging Our Children." Back to the Garden Health News 33 (July/August 2005): 9, 24, 26.

Donaldson, Michael. "Why Eating Right Is Not Enough." Hallelujah Acres Health News 59 (January/February 2010): 10.

———. "Fresh Juice or Powder." 11.

———. "Johnny, Get Moving." 12–13.

———. "Cholesterol and Health Blitzing the Confusion, Back to the Garden Health News 32 (Summer 2005): 8.

———. "Clean Pure Water." Hallelujah Acres Diet and Lifestyle 48 (January/February 2008): 12–13.

———. "The Fine Line of Immunization…Johnny and His 88 Vaccines." Hallelujah Acres Health News 56 (July/August 2009): 26–27.

———. "Fish Oil Risk vs. Benefits." Hallelujah Acres Diet and Lifestyle Health Tip. MyHDiet.com, Archive 2005.

———. "The Heart Attack Helper." Back to the Garden Health News 37 (March/April 2006): 15.

———. "Help! Autism Stole Johnny!" Hallelujah Acres Health News 55 (June/July 2009): 10.

———. "Is Johnny Getting Old Before He Grows Up?" Hallelujah Acres Health News 57 (September/October 2009): 12–13.

———. "Lupus: Disarming the Robber of Vitality, Hallelujah Acres Diet and Lifestyle 48 (January/February 2008): 22.

———. "The State of Diabetes." Back to the Garden Health News 45 (July/August 2007): 18.

———. "Will Johnny Get Cancer…Hot Dogs Can Put Children at a 9.5 Times the Risk." Hallelujah Acres Health News 54 (March/April 2009): 6.

———. "Why Are We So Sick?" Back to the Garden Health News 34 (September/October 2005): 8.

———. "Why Is Johnny Fat?" Hallelujah Acres Health News 53 (January/February 2009): 5.

Dye, Michael. Protein and Propaganda, God's Way to Ultimate Health. Shelby, NC: Hallelujah Acres, 1995.

Farmer, Fred. "Household Cleaning Products and Your Children." Back to the Garden Health News 37, (March/April 2006): 17.

Farndon, John. Human Body. San Diego, CA: Miles Kelley, 2006, 39.

Ferrigno, Lou, and Douglas Kent Hall. The Incredible Lou Ferrigno. New York: Simon and Schuster, 1982.

Fielder, John L. "Relax with Music." INHS Hygienic Review, February 2004.

Flore, Toni. Totally Vegetarian. Philadelphia: Da Capo, 2008.

Flynn, Margaret. "Restructuring the Way We Produce Our Foods." Lesson 99 of Taking Charge of Our Destiny, Natural Health course, Fit for Life Sciences Institute.

Frahm, David and Anne Frahm. Reclaim Your Health. New York: Jeremy P. Tarcher/Putnam, 1995.

Frost, Robert. "The Road Less Traveled." (1920).

Fry, Marti. "Carbohydrates: The Fuel for the Human Body." Lesson 7 of the Nutritional Basis of Life, Natural Health course, Fit for Life Sciences Institute.

Fry, T. C. "Factors That Interfere with Vitamin Utilization." In Vol. 1, bk. 2 of Fit for Life – The Basic Health Library, 14–15.

———. "All Life Conditions and Activities Affect Nutrition." Lesson 5 of The Foundations of Life, Natural Health course, Fit for Life Sciences Institute.

————. "Debunking the Myths about Onion and Garlic." In Junk Foods, Vol. 1 of Fit for Life Sciences – The Basic Health Library, 18–19.

————. The Advisor, p. 16-17, 31.

————. "Factors That Lower Vitamin Needs." In Vol. 1, bk. 2 of Fit for Life – Basic Health Library, 14–15.

————. "Healthful Living Produces Health." Lesson 3 of The Foundations of Life, Natural Health course, Fit for Life Sciences Institute.

————. "Medical Research Finds America's Protein Intake Causes Disease." In Vol. 1, bk. 2 of Fit for Life – The Basic Health Library, 3.

————. "The Nature and Purpose of Disease." Lesson 2 of The Foundations of Life, Natural Health course, Fit for Life Sciences Institute.

————. "Introducing Life Science Program for Perfect Health." Lesson 3, Natural Health course, Fit for Life Sciences Institute.

Furlow, Bryant. "Preventing Drug-Resistant Infections in Health Care." Radiologic Technology 80, no. 3 (January/February 2009).

————. "Pain Management Imaging." Radiologic Technology 80, no. 5 (May/June 2009).

Go Natural and Organic. "Toxic Toothpaste Ingredients and Other Chemical Cocktails!" GoNandO.com. http://www.gonando.com/toothpaste.html.

Goldberg, Paul. "What Is Natural Hygiene?" INHS Hygienic Review.

————. "What is Inflammatory Bowel Disease?" The Goldberg Clinic. Access Date(?), URL.

Gordon, James S. "Foods and Supplements That Boost Mood." Bottom Line Personal 30, no. 8 (April 15, 2009): 9–10.

Gordon, James. "Food Sensitivities Can Cause Depression." Bottom Line Personal 30, no. 8 (April 15, 2009): 10.

Gower, Mary Ann. "Hallelujah Diet Too Late." Hallelujah Acres Health News 54 (March/April 2009): 4.

Graff, Jackie. "How I Got Fat Eating No Fat." Back to the Garden Health News 36 (January/February 2006): 23–24.

Gross, Robert. "Hay Fever and Asthma." Lesson 71 of Common Illnesses and Diseases and How Hygienic Living Can Help, Natural Health course, Fit for Life Sciences Institute.

Hazard, Susan. "Allergies, Hay Fever, and Other Chronic Illnesses." Lesson 71 of Common Illnesses and Diseases and How Hygienic Living Can Help, Natural Health course, Fit for Life Sciences Institute.

———. "Sugar and Carbohydrate Metabolism Disease." Lesson 73, Natural Health course, Fit for Life Sciences Institute.

———. "Garlic." In Junk Foods. Vol. 1, bk. 2 of Fit for Life – The Basic Health Library, 21.

———. "Onions as Medicine." 19–20.

———. "The Dangers of Drug Medication: Over-the-Counter and Prescription Drugs." Lesson 40 of Harmful Practices to Avoid, Natural Health course, Fit for Life Sciences Institute.

———. "Natural Approach to Overcoming Addictions." Lesson 69, Natural Health course, Fit for Life Sciences Institute.

Home Medical Dictionary, Ottenheimer Publishers Inc, Copy. 1998.

Hoseus, Suzy. "She Once Came Close to Ending Her Life, Now She Embraces It." Back to the Garden Health News 43 (March/April 2007) 8–10.

Howard, Pierce J. The Owner's Manual to the Brain. 3rd ed. Austin, TX: Bard Press, 2006.

Howenstine, James. "Natural Healthcare Is Your Responsibility." Hallelujah Acres Health News 59 (January/February 2010): 18.

Idol, Olin. "Rebuilding a Cancerous Body." Hallelujah Acres Health News 54 (March/April 2009): 15.

———. "Vitamin D—The Neglected Anti-Cancer Nutrient?" 15.

———. "Arthritis." Back to the Garden Health News 47 (November/December 2007): 20.

———. "Breast Cancer: Prevent It Rather Than Treat It." Hallelujah Acres Diet and Lifestyle 49 (March/April 2008): 20–21.

———. "The Cause of Most Cancers Revealed." Hallelujah Acres Diet and Lifestyle Health Tip. MyHDiet.com, May 5, 2009.

————. "Conventional Cancer Therapies and the Hallelujah Diet…The Role of Nutrition in the Process of Healing." 17.

————. "How Inflammation Promotes Cancer…Stopping Free Radical Damage." 17.

————. "Cancer Questions and Answers." 19.

————. "Food And Behavior: A Natural Connection (a book review)." Hallelujah Acres Diet And Lifestyle 50 (May/June 2008): 22–23.

Stitt, Barbara Reed Food & Behavior; A Natural Connection, Publisher: Natural Press 2004d

————. "Toxicity Refined Sugar: How Sweet Is It?" Hallelujah Acres Health News 55 (May/June 2009): 24.

————. "The Solution to the SAD State of America's Declining Health." Back to the Garden Health News 40 (September/October 2006): 16.

————. "What's Hot! Stevia Popularity Is Skyrocketing." Hallelujah Acres Health News 55 (June/ July 2009): 29.

Immerman, Alan, T. C. Fry, and Marti Fry. "Vitamins, The Metabolic Wizards of Life's Processes." The Nutritional Bases of Life, Part II, Natural Health course, Fit for Life Sciences Institute, 252.

Immerman, Alan, and Alec Burton. "Introduction to Fasting." Lesson 45 of Fasting, Natural Health course, Fit For Life Sciences Institute.

Juicing For Health, Vegetable Juicing, Internet Research Paper. health.htm/. Copy. Feb. 8, 2010.

King James Version of The Bible, Thomas Nelson Inc Publisher, Copy 1994

Kirchmeier, Leslie. "Cancer: As Long As There's Breath, There's Hope." Back to the Garden Health News 54 (March/April 2009): 1–2.

Kling, Joyce M. "Prenatal Cares for Better Infant and Maternal Health and Less Painful Child Birth." Lesson 55, Healthy Infants and Children, Natural Health course, Fit for Life Sciences Institute.

Lee, Audrey. "How I Beat Cancer in 90 Days." Hallelujah Acres Health News 67 (Summer 2011): 7.

Lee, John R., with Virginia Hopkins. What Your Doctor May Not Tell You About Menopause. New York: Warner Books, 1996.

Living Without, Winter 2002.

Luzajic, Lorette C. "Spilling the Beans, the Trouble with Soy." Hallelujah Acres Health News 56 (July/August 2009): 12.

Malkmus, Ann. "Killing Cancer From Within…Alkaline and Oxygen Levels Working Together." Hallelujah Acres Health News 54 (March/April 2009): 8

Malkmus, George, Peter Shockey, and Stowe Shockey. The Hallelujah Diet. PA: Destiny Image, 2006.

Malkmus, George. "Why Not All Raw?" Rev. Malkmus's Health Tip. MyHDiet.com, Aug. 16, 2005, URL.

———. "Alcohol Does the Body Bad." Rev. Malkmus's Health Tip. MyHDiet.com, July 29, 2008.

———. "Are You Living to Eat or Eating to Live?" Hallelujah Acres Health News 58 (November/December 2009): 6–7.

———. "Caffeine Does the Body Bad." Rev. Malkmus's Health Tip. MyHDiet.com, July 8, 2008.

—.——— "Caffeine—A Dangerous Drug." Hallelujah Acres Internet Research Paper, Issue 170, Archives 2001.

———. "Diabetes—A Natural Approach." Rev. Malkmus's Health Tip. MyHDiet.com, May 20, 2011.

———. "Does Everyone Who Adopts The Hallelujah Acres Get Well?" Rev. Malkmus's Health Tip. MyHDiet.com, November 10, 2009.

———. "Fruits, Veggies Don't Stop Cancer's Return (Summary)." Rev. Malkmus's Health Tip. MyHDiet.com, August 14, 2007

———. "Grain Does the Body Bad, Part 2." Rev. Malkmus's Health Tip. MyHDiet.com, June 17, 2008.

———. "NBC's Tim Russert Dies of Heart Attack at 58—Why?"

———. "The Hallelujah Diet—America's Best Weight Loss Program." January 5, 2010.

————. "Let's Start the New Year Right—Make 2010 the Start of a New Life." Hallelujah Acres Health News 59 (January/February 2010): 4–5.

————. God's Way to Ultimate Health: A Common Sense Guide to Eliminating Sickness through Nutrition. Shelby, NC: Hallelujah Acres, 1995.

————. "Milk Does the Body Bad." Rev. Malkmus's Health Tip. MyHDiet.com, May 6, 2008.

————. "The Origin of Sickness." Rev. Malkmus's Health Tip. MyHDiet.com, April 27, 2009.

————. "Rev. George Malkmus Experiences a Stroke—How Could This Happen?" Hallelujah Acres Diet and Lifestyle 49 (March/April 2008): 10–12.

————. "Sugar Does the Body Bad, Part I." Rev. Malkmus's Health Tip. MyHDiet.com, May 27, 2008.

————. "Sugar Does the Body Bad, Part II." Rev. Malkmus's Health Tip. MyHDiet.com, June 3, 2008.

————. "Thank God for Allowing Me to Have Cancer." Hallelujah Acres Health News 54 (March/ April 2009): 5.

————. "Toxicity: Refined Sugar: How Sweet Is It?" Hallelujah Acres Health News 55 (June/July 2009): 24.

————. "Stress-Related Aging." Hallelujah Acres Health News 57 (September/October 2009): 16.

————. "Vaccinations: Blessings or Curses." Back to the Garden Health News 34 (September/October 2005): 11, 14, 26.

————. "Why Most Cancer Treatments Fail." Rev. Malkmus's Health Tip. MyHDiet.com, September 23, 2008.

————. "The World's Most Affordable Health Care." Hallelujah Acres Health News 56 (July/August 2008): 8

Malkmus, Paul and Ann Malkmus. "You Are What You Eat, Counteracting the Threat of Cancer." Back to the Garden Health News 54 (March/April 2009): 3.

————. "Yes, You Can Afford to Be Healthy." Hallelujah Acres Health News 56 (July/August 2008): 8.

Manich, Clint. "The Incredible Shrinking Man." Hallelujah Acres Health News 53, 1–2.

Marchione, Marilynn. "Fat Kids Found to Have Arteries of 45-Year-Olds." Nov. 11, 2008.

Marieb, Elaine N. Human Anatomy and Physiology, 5th ed. San Francisco: Benjamin Cummings, 2000.

Mars, Brigitte. Rawsome. North Bergen, NJ: Basic Health, 2004.

Mattarella, Anne. "Medical Imaging's Role in Bariatric Surgery." Radiologic Technology 82, no. 4, (March/April 2011): 347–362.

McCarter, Robert and Elizabeth McCarter. "A Statement on Vitamins." In Vol. 1, bk. 2 of Fit for Life – The Basic Health Library, 5.

———. "Fallacy of Vitamin Supplementation."

———. "Food Supplements." Lesson 39 of Harmful Practices to Avoid, Natural Health course, Fit for Life Sciences Institute.

———. "Methods for Inducing a Lifestyle Change." Lesson 91 of Teaching Health-Building Practices, Natural Health course, Fit for Life Sciences Institute.

McLemore, Jodell L. "Inflammatory Bowel Disease." Radiologic Technology 78, no. 4 (March/April 2007): 291–294.

McMillian, Beverly. The Illustrated Atlas of the Human Body. Argosy, 2008.

———. Damage to Blood Vessels, p. 138-139.

———. Diabetes, p. 122.

———. Eating Disorders, p. 192-193.

McMillian, Beverly. The Illustrated Atlas of the Human Body. Sidney: Weldon Owens, 2008.

Mindell, Earl and Mundis, Hester. Earl Mindell's Vitamin Bible. New York: Warner Books, 1991.

Mindell, Earl. Earl Mindell's Herb Bible. New York: Simon & Schuster, 1992.

Moritz, Andreas. "Tony Snow—Was It Cancer or Chemotherapy That Killed Him." Hallelujah Acres Diet and Lifestyle Health Tip. MyHDiet.com, Sept. 30, 2008.

Mosby's Medical, Nursing & Allied Health Dictionary, 3rd Edition, The C.V. Mosby Company, Copy. 1990.

Natural Organic Lifestyle. "Benefits of Juicing." Natural Organic Lifestyle. Accessed Feb. 8, 2010. www.naturalorganiclifestyle. com/benefits-of-juicing.html.

Nelson, Dennis. "Air, Sunshine, and Light: Essential to Health." Lesson 13 of Non-Dietary Factors in Nutrition, Natural Health course, Fit for Life Sciences Institute.

Odle, Teresa. "Name Your Poison." ASRT Scanner 41, no. 6 (August/September 2009): 44.

Olive, Diane. Think Before You Eat. Glendale, CA: Griffin, 1994.

Ott, A. True. "The Truth about 'Fluoride' (or What Every Mother Should Know)." August 2000, p 1, 6.

Oxford Dictionary of Current English—4th Edition, Oxford University Press, New York, NY, Copy. 2006. Webster's Dictionary, Book Essentials Publications, Larchmont, NY, Copy. 1990.

Padgett, Chris. "Silent Attack: Depression the Other Type Of 'SAD'." Hallelujah Acres Diet and Lifestyle 50 (May/June 2008): 14–15.

Pick, Marcelle. "Splenda—Is It Unsafe? Or Truly the Perfect Artificial Sweetener?" Woman to Woman, 2005.

Plous, F.K. 20 Year-Study Links Disease To Sugar, Detroit Free Press (article, printed Sunday Nov. 12, 1972.

Quillin, Patrick, with Noreen Quillin. Beating Cancer with Nutrition. Carlsbad, CA: Nutrition Times Press, 2005.

Reynolds, April. "Obesity and Medical Imaging Challenges." Radiologic Technology 82, no. 3 (January/February 2011): 219–237.

Root, Leon, and Betty Kelly Sargent. Beautiful Bones without Hormones. New York: Gotham Books, 2004.

Salmon, Beth. "When ADHD Kids Grow Up." Let's Live, (Dear Editor: Question and Answers For The Editor and Chief) Oct 1999, p. 12, 14.

Scott, Anne M. "Thyroid Cancer in Adults." Radiologic Technology 80, no. 3 (January/February 2009).

Servan-Schreiber, David. "The Anti-Cancer Diet from a Doctor Who Survived Cancer." Bottom Line Personal 30, no. 3 (February 1, 2009): 1–3.

Shelton, Herbert. "Living vs. Dieting." In Vol. 1, bk. 3 of Fit for Life – Basic Health Library, 7.

———. "The Necessity of Proper Food Combining." In Fit for Life – Basic Health Library. Vol. 1, bk. 1, 8–9.

———. "Allergy." Lesson 71 of Common Illness and Diseases and How Hygienic Living Can Help, Natural Health course, Fit for Life Sciences Institute.

———. "Carbohydrates." Lesson 7 of The Nutritional Basis of Life, Natural Health course, Fit for Life Sciences Institute.

———. "The Fountain of Life," Lesson 14 of Non-Dietary Factors in Natural Health, Natural Health course, Fit for Life Sciences Institute.

———. "The Minerals of Life," Lesson 10, The Nutritional Basis of Life, Nutritional Health course, Fit for Life Sciences Institute.

———. "Natural Hygiene: What Is It?" INHS Hygienic Review. Accessed date? URL?

———. "Nine Rules for Proper Food Combining," http://chetday.comfcprins.htm/.

———. "Water—The Fountain of Life." INHS Hygienic Review (February 2004).

———. Health for Millions, 1968.

———."What Is Health? The Healthy Body Laughs At Viruses, Health for Millions," 1968.

Smith, Andrew F. Encyclopedia of Junk Food and Fast Food. Westport, CT: Greenwood Press, 2006.

Smith, Tammie. "Evidence Shows Food Allergies Are Increasing." Richmond-Times Dispatch, March 19, 2009. Access Date(?). URL.

Sprague, Ken, and Bill Reynolds. The Gold's Gym Book of Bodybuilding. Chicago: Contemporary Books, 1983.

Sunrider. Simply the Best! Product Information. Sunrider International, 1990–2000.

The Artificially Sweetened Times, Winter 2005.

Tilden, John H. "The Importance of Pure Water." Lesson 3 of the Foundations of Life, Natural Health course, Fit for Life Sciences Institute.

Vertrano, Virginia. "Basic Considerations in Food Combining." Lesson 22 of Human Physiology, Anatomy, and Our Dietary Nature, Natural Health course, Fit for Life Sciences Institute.

Weisburger, John. "Diet and Cancer…The Power of Fruits and Vegetables." Hallelujah Acres Health News 54 (March/April 2009): 1.

Wheeler, Marti. "The Enormous Value of Resting and Fasting in Disease." In Basic Health Library, bk. 3, 7.

Williams, David G. "A Sweet Solution to Brittle Bones." Alternatives Newsletter 10, no. 3 (September 2003): 18.

———. "Excitotoxins Don't Excite Me." Alternatives Newsletter 10, no. 4 (October 2003): 31–32.

———. "Fluid Retention: The Stress Connection." Alternatives Newsletter 9, no. 2 (August 2001): 10.

———. "When It Comes to Instinct: Trust, Not Verify." Alternatives Newsletter 9, no. 14 (August 2002) 106–107.

Winston, Kenneth Caine, and Brian Paul Kaufman. "The Prayer Prescription, Special Report Booklet." Prevention (2002).

Winter, Ruth. A Consumer's Dictionary of Food Additives. New York: Crown Publishers, 1984.

Yagoda, Janet Shagam. "Unlocking the Secrets of Parkinson's Disease." Radiologic Technology 79, no. 3 (January/February 2008): 231.

Young, Robert O., and Shelley Redford. The pH Miracle. New York: Warner Books, 2002.

Contributors

All of these people have contributed funds to help with the editing and other costs of this book and I want to thank each and every one of you by placing your name on this page. And a big thanks to all of those who want to remain anonymous.

John DiMercurio, Jill Miglia, Zhi James Zhang and Jin Ma, Mary Goucher, Les Sherman, Amy Wu, Maria Medeircos, Marina Cerqueira, Lenna Omarson, Roberta Orndorff, Doris Walsh, Alfonzo and Penny LeAleala with their family, Anila Jonnala, Keith and Shae Hanna, Patricia Sherbo, Anna Song Peterson, Susan Calcaterra, Gene and Jeanny Snowden, Barbara Harris, Mark Heuslein,

Mike and Nancy Covher, Bill and Eva Schneider, Judy Goldman, Debbie Harris, Trish Hilderman, David Webb, Darlene Bilbrey, Susan Mayes, Helen Roberts, Dave Johnson, Victor Mireles, Gene and Lynelle Glasser, James Usselman, Bert Byington, John II, and Nicole DiMercurio, Carol Holler, Caroline Edminster,

Anthony Gomez, Frank Nagy, Ruben De La Mora, Eric Ricketts, Jeffrey Tan, Daniel, Chavez, Eva Toledo, Mark Koholt, Vern Eaton, Jerry Jerome,

Richard and Marja-Liisa Rachubka, Dusty and Jean Holycross, Jason, Tanya, Emily and Michael Vezza, Forest and Kay Lewis, Donna Sass, Angela Allen, Bryan Cavero, Mo Khan, JoAnn Pastori,

Kristie Tiso, Gino and Lori Ruscitto, Justin Piatt, David Moncayo, Jorge Puga, Brady K Huang, Joe Juszczyk,

Raymond Juszczyk, Steven Juszczyk, Denzel and Betty Morris, Lisa Marra, Shannon Karwowski, Ken and Mindy Mazur, Bart and Reva Greim, Laura Reinia, Cheryl Marshek, Debbie Lombardi, Dennis and Darlene Welch, Nick and Laura Vaiasuso, Marty and Alice Nyari, Daniel and Gabriela Betancourt

About the Author

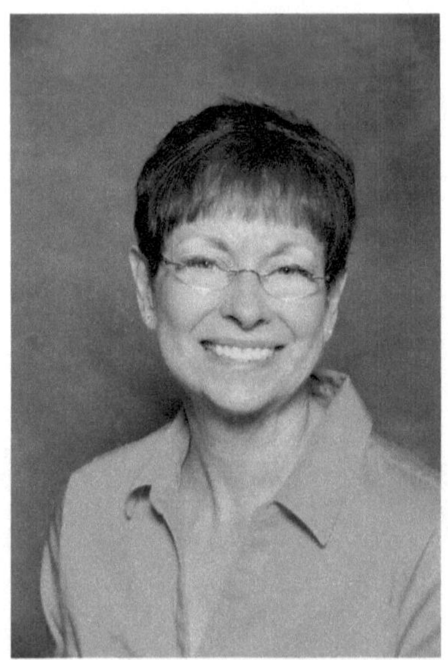

Marie DiMercurio RT(R)MHSc lives and works as a (registered) radiologic technologist in a small community in Southern California. She's passionate about the study and health of the human body. With that in mind, she returned to school and continued her education, graduating with a master's degree with honors from the Fit for Life Sciences Institute and the College of Natural Health. As a life scientist and health educator, she wants to share her gift with everyone.

www.ingramcontent.com/pod-product-compliance
Lightning Source LLC
Chambersburg PA
CBHW051431250726
48655CB00001B/12